Second Edition

ETHICAL
and
LEGAL ISSUES

For Imaging Professionals

Second Edition

ETHICAL and LEGAL ISSUES

For Imaging Professionals

DOREEN M. TOWSLEY-COOK, MAE, RT(R), FAERS
Former Radiologic Sciences Program Director
Allen Memorial Hospital
Waterloo, Iowa
Private Educational Consultant
Creative Enterprises Unlimited
Cedar Falls, Iowa

TERESE A. YOUNG, JD, RT(R) (retired), CNMT (Emeritus)
Health Educator
Solo Law Practitioner
Polk City, Iowa

Illustrated

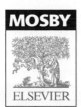

MOSBY

ELSEVIER

11830 Westline Industrial Drive
St. Louis, Missouri 63146

Ethical and Legal Issues for Imaging Professionals

ISBN-13: 978-0-323-04599-5
ISBN-10: 0-323-04599-5

Previous edition copyrighted 1999

ISBN-13: 978-0-323-04599-5
ISBN-10: 0-323-04599-5

Acquisitions Editor: Mindy Hutchinson
Developmental Editors: Christina Pryor, Alaina Webster
Publishing Services Manager: Patricia Tannian
Design Direction: Margaret Reid

Printed in the United States of America

Last digit is the print number: 9 8 7

REVIEWERS

Gina M. Augustine, MLS, RT(R)
Director
School of Radiography and Specialty Programs
Jameson Healthsystem
New Castle, Pennsylvania

Joseph R. Bittengle, MEd, RT(R) (ARRT)
Assistant Professor
Division of Radiologic Imaging Sciences
University of Arkansas of Medical Sciences
Little Rock, Arkansas

Gary M. Carlton, BS, RTR
Clinical Instructor
Bonsecours School of Medical Imaging
Richmond, Virginia

Ellen Colbeck-Taylor, BA, RT(R)
Radiography Program Director
Richland Community College
Decatur, Illinois

Andrea J. Cornuelle, MS, RT(R)
Associate Professor
Radiologic Technology Program
Northern Kentucky University
Highland Heights, Kentucky

Janice D. Dolk, RT(R), RDMS, MA
Consultant to Sonography Projects
Performance Improvement Coordinator
Adjunct Faculty
Community College of Baltimore County
Owings Mills, Maryland

Charles Francis, MEd, RT(R)(QM)
Department Chairperson
Associate Professor
Radiographic Science
Idaho State University
Pocatello, Idaho

Rose K. Goeden, RHIA
Instructor
HIM Program
Dakota State University
Madison, South Dakota

Sergeo Guilbaud, BS, RT(R), LRT, AERTSNY, ASRT
Vice-President of AERTSNY
Chairman of Hospital Affairs Committee of AERTSNY
Long Island College Hospital
Brooklyn, New York

Martina Harris, BS, RT(R)
Clinical Coordinator
Medical Radiography Program
Cooper University Hospital
Camden, New Jersey

Nancy Hawking, EdD, MEd, BS, RT(R)
Director of Imaging Sciences
University of Arkansas-Fort Smith
Fort Smith, Arkansas

Kathleen O. Kienstra, MAT, RT(R)(T)
Program Chair
Radiation Therapy Program
Barnes-Jewish College of Nursing and Allied Health
St. Louis, Missouri

Alice Pyles, MSRS
Radiology Program Director
Mississippi Delta Community College
Moorhead, Mississippi

Jean R. Robinson, RT(R), BA
Program Director
Assistant Professor
Radiologic Technology Department
Roan State Community College
Oak Ridge, Tennessee

Jeannean Hall Rollins, MRC, BSRT, (R)(CV)
Associate Professor
Radiologic Sciences
Arkansas State University
Jonesboro, Arkansas

Francine J. Todd, MEd, RT(R), ARRT
Bowling Green State University-Firelands College
Huron, Ohio

Lynette Kay Watts, MSRS, RT(R)
ARRT, Texas State Lisence
Assistant Professor
Midwestern State University
Wichita Falls, Texas

In memory of my husband, Donald Young, MD, whose dedication to the field of radiology helped to keep me focused through the trials and tribulations of this book

TERESE YOUNG

To the captain of the AT EASE III, Jerry Cook, my husband, whose humor and patience kept me and the boat afloat when I traded my time on the water to be an author

DOREEN TOWSLEY-COOK

PREFACE

Education's purpose is to replace an empty mind with an open one.

MALCOLM S. FORBES

WHY STUDY ETHICS AND LAW?

Many people believe that ethics—including biomedical ethics—is just using good common sense and that medical legal issues are topics to occupy attorneys. Therefore a value system and appropriate behavior should be inherent factors in an imaging professional. Problem solving should just be an exercise in being practical and simply determining the best answer. Unfortunately, this is not true. Ethical and legal problem solving begins with an awareness of ethical and legal issues in the imaging sciences. The sum of ethical and legal knowledge, common sense, personal values, professional values, practical wisdom, and learned skills will enable imaging professionals to tackle and solve the problems they will face.

ORGANIZATION

This text provides a good balance of ethical and legal knowledge. It familiarizes the student and the imaging professional with ethical and legal terminology, definitions, methods, and models. Each chapter is divided into two sections: ethical issues and legal issues. Although the discussions of ethics and law were difficult to separate, they do require individual and specific attention. The study of ethics provides the necessary foundation for technologists to apply professional standards and exercise personal integrity in responding correctly to the ethical challenges they will encounter. The investigation of legal issues that have an impact on technologists provides a basic understanding of applicable law and equips them with knowledge to allow them to become their own risk managers. After the reader becomes familiar with each topic, problem-solving skills in the imaging environment—which frequently presents ethical and legal dilemmas—will be enhanced.

Many questions are raised throughout the text materials. Some of these, particularly those involving ethical dilemmas, have no completely right or wrong answer, and the student or imaging professional may consider the authors biased. It will be the reader's choice to agree, disagree, question, and pursue solutions appropriate for his or her own conscience. This is the stuff of ethics.

The second edition of this text reflects new technology and imaging environments that provide many new ethical and legal dilemmas for the imaging professional in the 21st century. Health law is changing rapidly to keep pace with these new challenges in imaging. The legal policies discussed reflect the state of the law at the time of publication. In addition, as is stated many times within the text, the applicable law depends on the particular jurisdiction. Consultation with local counsel is recommended when specific legal issues arise.

DISTINCTIVE FEATURES

- Balanced coverage of ethical and legal issues provides a basic foundation of ethical and legal knowledge and gives readers the ability to tackle and solve the problems they will face daily in the clinical setting.

- Case studies present real world scenarios, allowing students to practice problem-solving and decision-making skills.
- Coverage of relevant current events places ethical and legal issues in a realistic light and enhances the descriptions and explanations of ethical and legal issues.
- Bulleted, key point summaries make it easy to locate information and to study one area at a time, assimilating details in a logical sequence.
- The standardized heading scheme and chapter outlines make chapters easy to navigate.
- Margin definitions and a glossary are easily accessible resources for the student.

NEW TO THIS EDITION

- Discussion of limited radiographers, health care literacy, HIPAA, employee rights, whistleblowing, and relevant new technologies such as digital imaging, PET, and genetic testing is included.
- Relevant and revised case studies have been added to update existing content and to illustrate new discussions in ethical and legal fields.
- More content on the history of ethics has been added.
- Updated legal terminology refreshes the content.

PEDAGOGICAL FEATURES

- Imaging Scenarios spark classroom discussion or can be used for written assignments. They encourage students to apply what they are learning and to develop critical-thinking and problem-solving skills.
- Review Questions allow the students to test their retention of the information presented in the chapter.
- Critical Thinking Questions and Activities ask students to examine their personal responses to various situations. Students may be asked to expand on their knowledge of policies and procedures through various activities.
- Professional Profiles present a brief glimpse into how ethics and law will affect readers' daily lives as professional imaging technologists.
- Learning Objectives and Chapter Outlines focus students on the most important content.

ANCILLARIES

Evolve Learning Resources is an interactive learning environment designed to work in coordination with *Ethical and Legal Issues for Imaging Professionals*, second edition. Instructors may use Evolve to provide an Internet-based course component that reinforces and expands the concepts presented in class. Evolve may be used to publish the class syllabus, outlines, and lecture notes; set up "virtual office hours" and e-mail communication; share important dates and information through the online class calendar; and encourage student participation through chat rooms and discussion boards. Evolve allows instructors to post examinations and manage their grade books online. The Evolve site for *Ethical and Legal Issues for Imaging Professionals* includes the following:

- An image collection of approximately all figures, tables, and boxes
- A test bank of approximately 200 questions in Exam View with page references and correct answer rationales
- PowerPoint presentations to accompany each chapter in the book

- An instructor's manual
- Weblinks

For more information, please visit http://evolve.elsevier.com/Towsley-Cook/ethical/ or contact an Elsevier sales representative.

ACKNOWLEDGMENTS

Ms. Young would like to thank Cindy Vest from the University of Iowa Hospitals, Dr. Carter S. Young, Medical Director of the Department of Radiology at Methodist Medical Center in Peoria, Illinois, and Dr. Donald C. Young, former Director of Breast Imaging at the University of Iowa Hospitals, for their assistance throughout this project.

Ms. Towsley-Cook expresses her thanks to all of her past students, who provided her with an environment that continually facilitated her "critical thinking," and to the many imaging patients who reminded her of the importance of empathy and practical wisdom.

The goal of this book is to assist in the education of the imaging professional by raising ethical and legal awareness. We hope that this awareness will allow the imaging professional to implement critical thinking and problem-solving skills to make appropriate choices in the challenging imaging environment of today and an ever-evolving tomorrow.

Terese A. Young
Doreen Towsley-Cook

Anyone who thinks he knows all the answers isn't up to date on the questions.

FRANK LAWRENCE

CONTENTS

Second Edition

ETHICAL
and
LEGAL ISSUES

For Imaging Professionals

1 ETHICAL AND LEGAL FOUNDATIONS

We don't receive wisdom; we must discover it for ourselves after a journey that no one can take for us or spare us.

MARCEL PROUST

Chapter Outline

Ethical Issues
History
Values
Professionalism
Ethical Schools of Thought
Ethical Models
Patients' Rights

Legal Issues
The Law
The Lawsuit
Risk Management
Quality Assurance

Learning Objectives

After completing this chapter, the reader will be able to perform the following:

- Define ethics.
- Explore the history of ethics.
- Identify three types of values that have an impact on the imaging professional's ethical decision making.
- Define professionalism.
- List and explain ethical schools of thought and models.
- Explore the schools of thought and models to choose guidelines acceptable to the reader's individual style.
- List the questions involved in the problem-solving framework.

- Define law and describe the three foundations on which it is established.
- List the three basic divisions of law and the subdivisions that most frequently have an impact on the imaging professional.
- Identify the three phases of a lawsuit, and define the imaging professional's role in each.
- Define risk management and the imaging professional's role.
- Define quality assurance and its implications in the hospital.
- Identify additional information needed to minimize risks effectively.

Key Terms

common law
consequentialism
critical thinking
deontology
ethics
judicial decisions
law, the

legislation
professionalism
quality assurance
risk management
statutory law
values
virtue ethics

Professional Profile

Legal and ethical issues surround me daily in my professional career as I carry out my responsibilities as a picture archiving and communication system (PACS) coordinator and radiologic technologist. As I maintain the PACS system, which requires great emphasis on computer security and information (according to standards set by Health Level Seven [HL7] and the Health Insurance Portability and Accountability Act [HIPAA]), and perform radiographic procedures, I must constantly observe a level of ethical behavior and be cognizant of my legal responsibilities toward maintenance of information, care of my patients, and protection of their rights. Legal and ethical concerns influence the way I and every other technologist perform procedures, the way we interact with patients, and even the way we dress.

When performing any radiographic procedure, I try to maintain focus on the code of ethics set forth by the American Society of Radiologic Technologists (ASRT) and the provisions of the American Registry of Radiologic Technologists (ARRT). As a registered radiologic technologist, I must carry a sense of morality and ethical traits. My choice to become a radiographer was driven by a desire to have technical involvement in the care and treatment of sick and injured people. The care I give in the radiology suite and elsewhere implies my sense of responsibility and accountability.

Professional ethics must be adhered to in the radiology department and in all other locations in health care. Allied health professionals must practice decorum both in the workplace and in the community. Radiologic technologists share a commitment to the patient and the physician to perform procedures as well as possible, whether that be securing the proper view, handing off the proper contrast pharmaceutical, or ensuring the use of the correct technique. We must be conscious of patients' rights while maintaining a civil and caring demeanor. We should treat all persons with the utmost respect and put our personal beliefs aside to work with others as a united team.

Radiographers provide health care services while maintaining the patient's dignity and meeting specific needs. We are patient advocates in maintaining high-quality care, which includes ensuring patients' rights to privacy and confidentiality. We act together with other members of the health care team to make professional decisions and enhance personal accountability. Professional conduct and a conscious awareness of our and our patients' ethical and legal rights are key to success in delivering health care in the 21st century.

Charles V. Carpeaux, RT(R), PACS Coordinator
Oakwood Southshore Medical Center, Trenton, Michigan

ETHICAL ISSUES

Imaging and radiation science professionals face a variety of ethical challenges within medical imaging services. Because of their differing diagnostic applications, individual modalities present specific ethical dilemmas. Imaging professionals should consider these dilemmas to be challenges and opportunities for growth. When faced with such challenges, imaging professionals and radiation science practitioners must apply professional standards and exercise personal integrity to respond correctly to the situation. A firm grounding in ethics may help imaging professionals, radiation therapy specialists, and other health care professionals respond positively to the dilemmas they encounter in the workplace.

ETHICS
Ethics is the system or code of conduct and morals advocated by a particular individual or group.

Ethics may be defined as the system or code of conduct and morals advocated by a particular individual or group. It is also the study of acceptable conduct and moral judgment.[1] Ethics is a system of understanding determinations and motivations based

BOX 1-1	THE SEVEN PRINCIPLES OF BIOMEDICAL ETHICS

Autonomy: respect for the patient as a person
Beneficence: performance of good acts
Confidentiality: duty to protect the privacy of the patient
Justice: moral rightness
Nonmaleficence: avoidance of evil
Role fidelity: faithfulness and loyalty
Veracity: obligation to tell the truth and not to lie

on individual conceptions of right and wrong. It is not determined by strict rules or rigid guidelines, and although it is relatively stable, it can change over time.

The preceding description of ethics is broad and general. For the imaging professional, biomedical ethics may be defined as the branch of ethics dealing with dilemmas faced by medical professionals, patients, and their families and friends. Biomedical ethics may also be described as guidelines for proper activities and attitudes toward patients and peers. In this case, biomedical ethics suggests a standard of conduct that is expected of members of the profession. These standards are based on the seven principles of biomedical ethics. They are displayed in Box 1-1 and are discussed later in the text.

High ethical standards must be the foundation of professional practice to ensure the recognition of the imaging technologist as a competent health care professional: "The development of a code of ethics is one of the identifying steps in the sequence of the transformation of a semiprofession into a profession."[2] Professional codes of ethics help ensure a high standard of practice. A well-designed code lists the principles and rules defining ethically sound practice. It encourages those within the profession to consider the implications of their actions and educates those outside the profession about the sort of care they may expect. A good code of ethics also serves a regulatory function by specifying a standard of conduct by which all members of a profession must abide. Although many certifying bodies in the imaging and radiation sciences have developed codes of ethics (see Appendix A), unification remains a challenge. The American Society of Radiologic Technologists (ASRT) Code of Ethics considers various aspects of the imaging professional's role in health care. These areas include conduct, respect, diversity, technical applications, decision making, aid in diagnosis, radiation protection, ethical conduct, confidentiality, and education.

No code of ethics provides the answers to the dilemmas faced by the imaging professional, nor is a code of ethics merely a set system of conduct. Ethics is also a personal study and investigation. Thus the purpose of a code of ethics is to present a framework for a systematic examination of beliefs that may lead the technologist to an understanding of personal and professional morality and responsibility.

The creation of an ethical framework requires critical thinking. **Critical thinking** has been defined as "purposeful, self-regulatory judgment which results in interpretation, analysis, evaluation, and inference."[3] It is an ethical problem-solving tool that allows the imaging professional to perform the following tasks:

- Adequately interpret and analyze ethical theories and models
- Evaluate the application of those theories and models to a given situation
- Plan an appropriate course of action

Critical thinking allows the professional to process personal experience and knowledge and incorporate them into daily decisions. Through critical thinking the professional

CRITICAL THINKING
Critical thinking is purposeful, self-regulatory judgment resulting in interpretation, analysis, evaluation, and inference.

BOX 1-2	**ATTRIBUTES OF CRITICAL THINKERS**

Able to cut through pretense and fads
Confident and energetic
Courageous
Decisive
Flexible yet systematic
Honest
Imaginative
Intellectually curious and skeptical
Objective
Open to new ideas and respectful of others' views
Persistent
Responsible
Willing to take risks and consider novel ideas

internalizes and personalizes ethical concepts. Attributes of critical thinkers are listed in Box 1-2.

HISTORY

Ethics was born of necessity when humans first realized that they required certain behaviors to get along as a group.[4] As time passed, certain individuals were credited with providing bricks in the foundation of ethics (Figure 1-1).

Ethics has continued to evolve with societal changes. This evolutionary process will be evident to the imaging professional as new technology is developed. Each new technology will provide new ethical dilemmas for the patient and the professional.

VALUES

VALUES
Values are qualities or standards desirable or worthy of esteem in themselves; they are expressed in behaviors, language, and standards of conduct.

Values determine both personal and professional ethics; therefore ethical questions generally involve conflicts between values. A **value** is a quality or standard that is desirable or worthy of esteem in itself. Values are expressed in behaviors, language, and the standards of conduct the imaging professional endorses or tries to maintain.[5] A person's daily experiences influence and guide the expression of values. For example, a professional who attempts to maintain honesty with co-workers and patients has honesty as a personal value.

Values clarification developed by Louis Rath enables the individual to discover, analyze, and prioritize what he or she has.[6] Rath explains that an individual should make choices only after careful consideration of the alternatives. The person should take pride in these choices and be willing to defend them. An example of this might be an imaging professional who has, after careful consideration of personal values, made the choice to become a radiation therapy professional. The individual takes great pride in this decision and is willing to discuss and defend this choice. The imaging professional has based this decision on a desire to enhance the quality of life for patients who may be dealing with life-threatening illnesses.

Values clarification enables the imaging professional to organize values into a personally meaningful system. The individual's set of beliefs about truth and reality is defined by this system. Thus the imaging professional who values honesty may believe that others are honest with him or her because of this personal value.

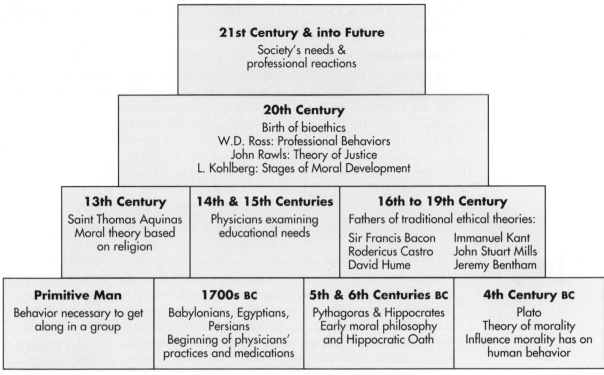

FIGURE 1-1 Historical foundations of ethics.

Imaging professionals prioritize their values, creating a hierarchy. For example, an imaging professional who values honesty may also value privacy to a greater or lesser degree. Depending on the way each of these values ranks within the personal hierarchy, the professional may take several different courses of action when faced with a dilemma in which both privacy and honesty are involved. This hierarchy may change over time as a result of life experiences and individual reassessment.[7]

Values guide and motivate the decisions and choices of imaging professionals, often without their realizing it.[8] Because the motivations and actions of others may be based on different hierarchies and different value systems, awareness of individual values improves communication.

Imaging professionals should use self-analysis to determine their own values before they begin ethical problem solving, which is discussed later in this chapter. Understanding the values of others and recognizing their importance are important steps in ethical decision making. Imaging professionals must recognize that others' values are as valid as their own.[9] The three basic groups of values are personal values, cultural values, and professional values.

Personal Values

Personal values are the beliefs and attitudes held by an individual that provide a foundation for behavior and the way the individual experiences life.[9] For example, an imaging professional may personally value timeliness and organization. These values influence the way the imaging professional makes decisions and judgments. Religious convictions, family, political beliefs, education, life experiences, and culture influence the imaging professional's personal values. Each person's values differ.[10]

Cultural Values

Values specific to a people or culture are known as cultural values. They may also guide the imaging professional's decision making because they influence opinions about health care. The value of individual choice may be important to an imaging professional from the United States. An imaging professional from an Asian culture may place more emphasis on the value of elderly people than would some professionals from other cultures.[9] Multiculturalism and diversity integrated into the imaging curriculum facilitate discussions of cultural values and their importance to high-quality imaging services (see also Chapter 9). The imaging professional must acknowledge the impact of culture on decision-making processes. Figure 1-2 presents continua of cultural values.

IMAGING SCENARIO

The director of radiology services receives a memo from the institution's chief executive officer (CEO) concerning a patient complaint. He begins the investigation by listening to all the parties involved and remains objective while visualizing the overall situation. With this approach, he realizes that the complaint has arisen from a difference in cultural values. These cultural differences caused confusion and emotional discomfort to the patient and involved issues of being touched, privacy, and communication.

The female patient, who speaks little English, was scheduled for a mammogram, which a male technologist was to perform. Because English is not her primary language and she was uncomfortable being undressed with a man touching her, the patient became upset and left without her examination. On questioning, the mammographer reports that he tried his best to explain the procedure to the patient and that he was pleasant and considerate. Each person involved in the situation sees the problem from a different perspective.

The significance of this situation for the patient is the emotional trauma involved and the lack of completion of the examination. The mammographer failed to complete the procedure. The director of radiology services has been advised by the CEO that mammography is heavily marketed and that these types of situations should not happen and are not to happen in the future. How best can the situation be resolved while including recognition of all the parties' values?

The director first interviews persons from varying cultural backgrounds to make himself more knowledgeable. He then provides a brainstorming session for radiology personnel and asks them to compile a list of possible solutions. One solution is to initiate focus groups that include community members from a variety of cultural backgrounds. The patient is invited and participates in a focus group to work out solutions to situations such as the one she experienced. After the many solutions and alternatives are evaluated, several are implemented at different levels, including educational activities within the department and the development of a department procedure and policy to promote recognition of all patients' cultural values in future situations.

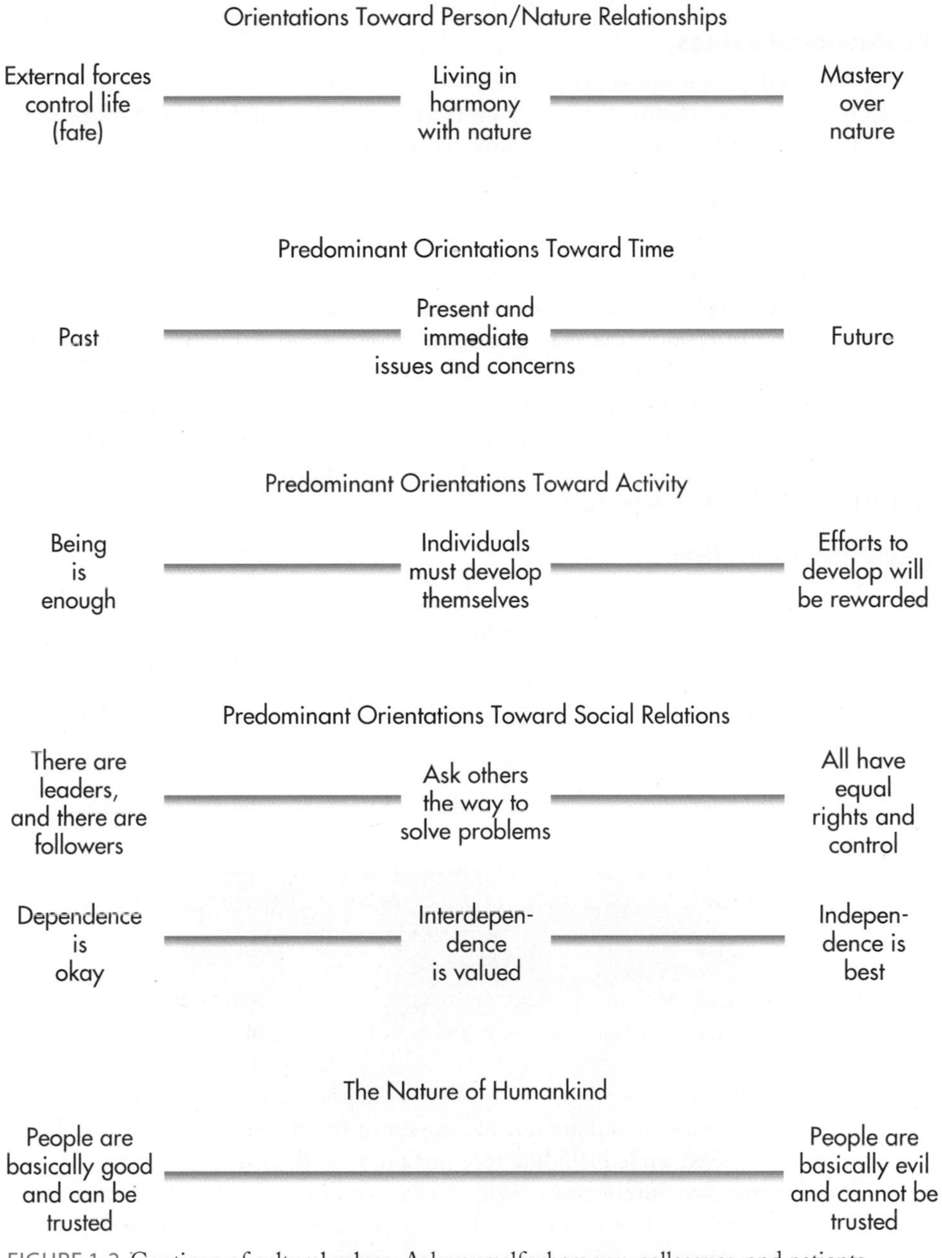

Orientations Toward Person/Nature Relationships

External forces control life (fate)	Living in harmony with nature	Mastery over nature

Predominant Orientations Toward Time

Past	Present and immediate issues and concerns	Future

Predominant Orientations Toward Activity

Being is enough	Individuals must develop themselves	Efforts to develop will be rewarded

Predominant Orientations Toward Social Relations

There are leaders, and there are followers	Ask others the way to solve problems	All have equal rights and control

Dependence is okay	Interdependence is valued	Independence is best

The Nature of Humankind

People are basically good and can be trusted	People are basically evil and cannot be trusted

FIGURE 1-2 Continua of cultural values. Ask yourself where you, colleagues, and patients fit on each continuum.
From Creasia J, Parker B: *Conceptual foundations of professional nursing practice,* ed 2, St. Louis, 1996, Mosby.

Professional Values

Professional values are the general attributes prized by a professional group.[9] Imaging technologists may learn about their profession's values, standards, and motivations through codes of ethics, formal instruction, and role modeling.

Values in Practice

Values may conflict with one another, with the imaging professional's duties, and with patients' rights. Personal, professional, and cultural values may provide conflicting guidelines.[8] The computed tomography (CT) specialist's value of providing good care for the patient during the examination may conflict with the value of honoring the patient's right to choose, especially if the patient is hesitant to have the examination. The radiation therapy technologist's value of carefully giving safe therapeutic doses of radiation may conflict with the patient's value of relief from suffering. In each of these situations, imaging professionals must identify the values involved in the decision-making process and determine the most important ones.

PROFESSIONALISM

PROFESSIONALISM
Professionalism is an awareness of the conduct, aims, and qualities defining a given profession, familiarity with professional codes of ethics, and understanding of ethical schools of thought, patient-professional interaction models, and patient rights.

The imaging professional works in a challenging and changing environment. To respond appropriately to the many biomedical ethical dilemmas they will face, imaging professionals must be able to apply the basic concepts of **professionalism**—an awareness of the conduct, aims, and qualities defining a given profession (Figure 1-3).[11] Familiarity with professional codes of ethics and understanding of ethical schools of thought, patient-professional interaction models, and patients' rights prepares imaging professionals to address future ethical dilemmas. When difficult situations arise, they

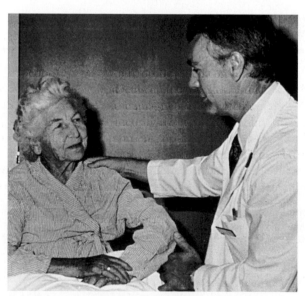

FIGURE 1-3 Professionalism and an awareness of personal standards of ethics are essential for imaging technologists.
From Ehrlich RA, Daly J: *Patient care in radiography*, ed 6, St. Louis, 2004, Elsevier.

have already thought through the various courses of action and can respond in keeping with their personal standards of ethics.

ETHICAL SCHOOLS OF THOUGHT

Ethics may be divided into three broad schools of thought:
1. Consequentialism
2. Deontology
3. Virtue ethics

Consequentialism, deontology, and virtue ethics are ways of establishing a value hierarchy in ethical decisions. Each school of thought offers different guidelines for ethical problem solving. No one school is better than the others; imaging professionals must choose the one that best serves individual, professional, and institutional goals.

Consequentialism

Consequentialism, or teleology, bases decisions on the consequences or outcomes of a given act. It evaluates the good of an activity by assessing whether immediate harm is balanced with future benefit. For example, a patient undergoing radiation therapy for cancer may experience some discomfort now, but the palliation or cure of the cancer is the desired beneficial consequence of the therapy. Consequentialism advocates providing the greatest good for the greatest number.

Within a teleologic framework, an imaging technologist assisting in triage for trauma patients would assign services to the most critically injured patient last to serve a greater number of less seriously injured patients. Are decisions based on final outcomes appropriate? Is this a reasonable philosophy for health care providers? In what way would an imaging director using consequentialist ethics determine ways to cut staffing in a department?

CONSEQUENTIALISM
Consequentialism is an ethical school of thought in which decisions are based on the consequences or outcomes of a given act; the good of an activity is evaluated based on whether immediate harm is balanced with future benefits.

Deontology

Deontology bases decision making on individual motives and morals rather than consequences. It is therefore the opposite of teleology. Deontology examines the significance of actions themselves. For example, members of certain religious groups refuse blood transfusions because they believe the act is morally wrong. Although they may be concerned about the consequences of this refusal, they are making the choice based on their religious beliefs regarding blood transfusions. Personal rules of right and wrong derived from individual actions, duties, relationships of all kinds, and society are used for reasoning and problem solving in the deontologic school of thought.

Drawing from the previous example, would the imaging technologist find deontology any more useful in decision making regarding triage for victims of a radioactive spill? Can absolute rights and wrongs in triage be determined? In what way would an imaging director using deontologic ethics determine ways to reduce staff? Should the moral significance of each individual be considered in department restructuring?

DEONTOLOGY
Deontology is an ethical school of thought that bases decision making on individual motives and morals rather than consequences and examines the significance of actions themselves. Deontologic problem solving uses personal rules of right and wrong derived from individual actions, relationships of all kinds, and society.

Virtue Ethics

Virtue ethics is a relatively new school of thought. It focuses on the use of practical wisdom and moral character for emotional and intellectual problem solving. Virtue ethics incorporates elements of teleology and deontology to provide a more holistic approach

VIRTUE ETHICS
Virtue ethics is a new ethical school of thought that focuses on the use of practical wisdom for emotional and intellectual problem solving. It incorporates elements of teleology and deontology to provide a more holistic approach to solving ethical dilemmas.

to solving ethical dilemmas. Careful analysis and consideration of consequences, rules established by society, and short-term effects play significant roles in decision making in virtue ethics.

Virtue ethics lends itself to many situations in which imaging professionals may become involved. For instance, an imaging technologist assisting in triage needs to recognize the significance of each individual and the way triage decisions affect the family and friends of injured persons. However, the technologist also works under time constraints and must understand that victims suffer from varying degrees of trauma. A department manager should understand the way staffing decisions will change lives and directly affect the quality and type of imaging services available through the department but must also be aware of the cost and resources necessary to provide high-quality imaging services.

ETHICAL MODELS

Models for ethical decision making in health care broadly describe different types of interactions with patients. They provide frameworks for understanding expectations and responsibilities (Table 1-1). Individual health care professionals must choose the model or models they feel are appropriate. Some models may work in certain situations and not in others (Figure 1-4). All the models may be applied to any of the ethical schools of thought presented in the previous section. Each imaging professional will discover or develop the ethical problem-solving method that works best for him or her.

Engineering Model

The engineering model identifies the health care provider as a scientist concerned with facts and defines the patient as a condition or procedure, not a person. A health care professional using the engineering model tends to view the patient as a collection of body systems rather than as a whole. Under this model a diagnostic imaging technologist considers the patient a gastrointestinal or skull series, not an anxious human patient. A vascular imaging professional using the engineering model believes that primary importance should be placed on the circulatory system, not on the patient's emotional or psychologic needs.

Paternal or Priestly Model

The paternal or priestly model casts the caregiver in the omniscient, paternalistic role of making decisions *for* patients rather than *with* patients. The magnetic resonance technologist who powerfully urges a feeble 90-year-old man onto the table when the patient

TABLE 1-1 **ETHICAL MODELS**

Model	Precept
Engineering	Provider views patient as condition or procedure
Paternal/priestly	Provider thinks he or she knows what is best for patients
Collegial	Mutual cooperation between provider and patient
Contractual	Business relationship in which both provider and patient have obligations, rights, and responsibilities
Covenantal	Agreement between provider and patient grounded in traditional values

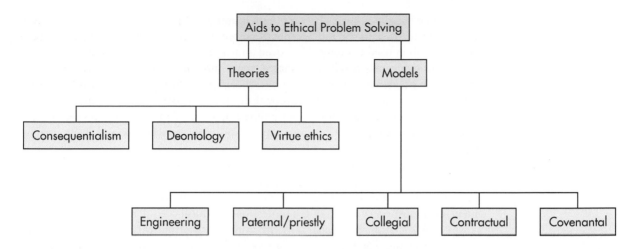

FIGURE 1-4 Aids to ethical problem solving.

explains that he cannot make the move is exhibiting paternalism. So is the imaging professional who dismisses the needs of patients who want to know more about procedures by telling them not to worry, that everything will be fine. Those who subscribe to the priestly model generally believe they know best and tend to discount the patient's feelings.

Collegial Model

The collegial model describes a more cooperative method of providing health care for the patient. It involves sharing, trust, and the pursuit of common goals. An imaging professional who takes time to get to know the patient and works with the patient to reach a mutual understanding is working within the collegial model. This model may be helpful in addressing patients' emotional needs and engaging their cooperation. However, it requires that the health care professional have enough time to spend with the patient.

Contractual Model

The contractual model defines health care as a business relationship between the provider and patient. A contractual arrangement serves as the guideline for decision making and provision of services. That is, the patient and provider are seen as parties to a contract in which both sides have obligations, rights, and responsibilities. This model is exemplified in the informed consent process. The imaging professional who explains an invasive procedure to a patient is involved in the contractual process.

Covenantal Model

The covenantal model recognizes that many areas of health care are not always covered by a terse, businesslike contract. Instead, care is based on an agreement between the patient and health care provider, an agreement often grounded in traditional values and goals. These include trust in the professional's integrity and confidence that the professional has the patient's best interests in mind. Many imaging procedures require the patient to trust in the radiographer's competence and professionalism. Therefore the model often used combines the covenantal and contractual models to build a business relationship and implement shared goals and values. The ability to trust often depends on previous experience with health care procedures. A patient experiencing a difficult pregnancy may trust the sonographer's skills based on values inherent in the covenantal model. Similarly, a person injured in an accident may ask to be taken to a specific hospital because of previous satisfaction with services received in its imaging department.

PATIENTS' RIGHTS

Patients' rights are among the most important issues involved in biomedical ethics, influencing almost every aspect of the professional's ethical considerations. The American Hospital Association has recognized the importance of patients' rights and has published a brochure, *The Patient Care Partnership* (see Appendix A), to help patients understand expectations, rights, and responsibilities.

Patients' awareness of their rights and needs and of the availability of various imaging techniques provides both opportunities and complications for the imaging professional. However, the patient's knowledge and participation facilitate high-quality imaging. The patient's role should include active participation in health care based on accurate information.

Dowd Problem-Solving Model

The Dowd Model was developed to aid in ethical problem solving for imaging professionals. The six steps of this model, listed in Box 1-3, are specific and valuable tools that will enhance imaging case study analysis (Box 1-4).[12] The Dowd Model first requires assessment of the problem. Thorough data gathering and awareness of all sides of the situation are integral to this step. Next, isolating the issues calls for recognition of what values, principles, and ethical dilemmas exist. This is followed by analysis of the data to provide an objective framework for review of all the issues involved. After assessing the problem, isolating the issues, and analyzing the data, the imaging professional must develop a plan of action and institute the plan. The final step, analysis of the outcome, shows whether the problem was handled in a satisfactory fashion or whether another approach should be considered.

BOX 1-3	DOWD MODEL

Assessment of the problem
Isolation of the issues
Analysis of the data
Development of a plan of action
Institution of the plan
Analysis of the outcome

IMAGING SCENARIO

An imaging student is preparing to complete a final competency on a patient requiring a cervical spine (c-spine) exam. It is the deadline date for this competency. The student has been procrastinating with this competency and feels uncertain of his preparedness.

The patient arrives from the emergency room (ER) in more serious condition than was expected. He is on a backboard with a cervical collar. An ER nurse, who is monitoring his vital signs, explains that he has lost sensation in his lower limbs. The ER physicians want the c-spine images STAT.

Much to the student's dismay, the radiographer explains that the student will not be able to demonstrate competency on this patient. The situation requires expediency, and the staff technologist believes the student is not capable of performing a good-quality exam quickly. Unless another c-spine patient arrives before the student's afternoon class, the student will fail the competency.

Discussion questions
Using the case study analysis described in Box 1-4, consider the following questions:
• How did this problem occur?
• How many sides are there to this problem?
• What are the values of the parties involved?
• Whose values are the most important?
• What is the significance of the values of each of the parties?
• How can the problem be resolved?

IMAGING SCENARIO

An imaging program at a local college has several students inquiring about the new radiologist assistant program. The program has only three vacancies. The competition for these positions has become fierce with each applicant believing he or she is more than qualified. The selection committee is considering the fairest and most ethical way to make the choices. They agree to use the Dowd Model to determine the selections.

Discussion questions
• How will each step of the Dowd Model lend itself to the selection process?
• How would each step of the Dowd Model lend itself to the applicants' pursuit of the RA student position?

| BOX 1-4 | **CASE STUDY ANALYSIS** |

The health care professional considering an ethical problem may ask four questions to provide a framework for case study analysis[9]:

1. What is the context in which the ethical problem has occurred?
2. What is the significance of the values involved in the problem?
3. What is the meaning of the problem for all the parties involved?
4. What should be done to remedy the problem?

What Is the Context in Which the Ethical Problem Has Occurred?

With contextual information, the health care professional may discover the way the problem arose, learn the various sides to the problem, and begin to understand the values of the parties. Determining the context of the problem requires the gathering of facts and information about values relevant to the conflict. The professional must listen to all aspects of the story to create a complete picture.

What Is the Significance of the Values Involved in the Problem?

The resolution of most conflicts requires compromise on the parts of those involved. The goal of the imaging professional involved in an ethical conflict should be to help individuals prioritize their values to preserve those most important to the issue. The professional must understand which values may be subordinated by the parties at the cost of the least harm. To do this, the professional must determine the significance of all values involved.

What Is the Meaning of the Problem for All the Parties Involved?

Ethical problems have a history and context that render them significant or insignificant to the parties involved. The imaging professional needs to discover some of that context to determine the significance of the problem for all the involved parties. In answering this question the professional may discover the roots of recurring value conflicts and be able to aid in the formation of a policy to avoid future difficulties.

What Should Be Done to Remedy the Problem?

Using information gathered and processed, the professional should be able to offer a variety of ways to resolve the conflict. The involved parties may wish to explore several options before coming to a decision. Imaging professionals should keep in mind that although some options might be ethically permissible, they may not support the values of those involved. Other options (such as assisted suicide or abortion) might be ethically permissible for one party but not for another.[7]

LEGAL ISSUES

Imaging technologists face many legal issues in addition to the ethical dilemmas they encounter. Although they cannot be expected to have a thorough understanding of all legal issues, they should have a basic knowledge of the law and its branches (Table 1-2), the legal system, the legal issues they are most likely to encounter, the legal facilities of the institution, and institutional regulations regarding the patient care they provide. An understanding of other legal matters that influence the professional life of the technologist (e.g., student rights, diversity issues, employee-management relations, whistleblowing) is also important. These matters are discussed thoroughly in later chapters. Imaging

TABLE 1-2 **BRANCHES OF THE LAW**

Branch	Area of Responsibility	Penalties for Violation
Administrative	Deals with licensing and regulation	Can include suspension and revocation of license
Criminal	Addresses wrongs against the state	Can include fines, restitution, community service, and incarceration
Civil	Addresses wrongs committed by one party harming another	Can include monetary damages to compensate for loss and to punish

technologists should begin their exploration of legal implications for their practices with a broad overview of the law and some of its components, especially the lawsuit and the function of risk management. Specific legal issues faced by technologists and their facilities that influence patient care are discussed more thoroughly in Chapters 2, 4, and 5. Methods to decrease the risk of litigation are also provided in these chapters.

THE LAW

The law is a body of rules of action or conduct prescribed by controlling authority and having binding legal force.[13] The basis for the controlling authority of the law in the United States includes common law from England but has been molded by statutes and judicial decisions (case law) since the birth of the United States (Figure 1-5).

Common law, which forms the basis for the current law in 49 of the 50 states, includes all the statutory and case law background of England and the American colonies before the American Revolution.[14] This common law encompasses principles and rules that derive their authority solely from ancient usages and customs or the judgments and decrees of courts supporting those usages and customs.[13] Louisiana is the only state in which English common law does not form the basis for current law. Louisiana's law is based on Roman law and derived from the Napoleonic Code, which was established in France after the French Revolution.

Legislation, as provided for in the U.S. Constitution, includes all the laws or statutes put into place by the elected officials in federal, state, county, and city governments. Judicial decisions may interpret the statutes and therefore further refine their application. Judicial decisions may reinforce common law principles or change them to match the changes in society.

Common Law

The following example regarding the origins of the tort of negligence may help to illustrate the common law basis of our current law system. The tort of negligence originated in the liability of those who professed to be competent in certain "public" callings. In England and the colonies, a carrier, an innkeeper, a blacksmith, or a surgeon was regarded as holding himself out to the public as one in whom people should have confidence. This act of holding themselves out as knowledgeable in their field created an

THE LAW
The law is a body of rules of action or conduct prescribed by controlling authority and having binding legal force.[14] Its basis is in common law from England, but it has been molded by statutes and judicial decisions since the birth of the United States.

COMMON LAW
Common law encompasses principles and rules based on ancient usages and customs.

LEGISLATION
Legislation is all the laws and statutes put into place by elected officials in federal, state, county, and city governments.

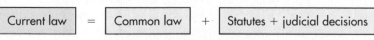

FIGURE 1-5 Sources of current law.

obligation to give proper service. If such service was not delivered through their personal fault, they might be held liable for any damage or injury caused.

The imposition of a duty of care based on the special position of professionals and the possibility of liability if that duty was not performed correctly was based on custom. Ancient judicial decisions imposed liability based on this custom. Thus common law regarding negligence was established through custom and judicial decisions supporting that custom.

The current law regarding negligence, which is discussed thoroughly in Chapter 2, originated from the same custom. Under current law, negligence can be found only if a duty is owed, that duty is breached, and demonstrable harm has resulted from the breach.

Statutes and Judicial Decisions

STATUTORY LAW
Statutory law includes all laws enacted by federal, state, county, and city governments.

Continuing the example of negligence may help to illustrate the role **statutory law** and judicial decisions play in current law. Negligence can be found only if a duty exists. This duty can be imposed in several ways. A statute may create such a duty. In Iowa, for example, a statute lists the risks that a physician must disclose to obtain informed consent from a patient. The statute has established a duty to disclose those risks before the procedure is performed. Judicial decisions that interpret the statutes may further refine the details surrounding physician disclosure.

In a state that has no statute defining a physician's duty to disclose risks, or has a statute that is not specific, the obligation of disclosure still exists but has a different basis. Previous judicial decisions (or precedents) in a state's courts form the basis for the duty of physicians in that state. The reasoning on which those decisions are based may well be common law principles that have been adapted to meet the changes in society. For example, some states have adopted, through **judicial decisions**, the standard that a physician must disclose to a patient information that a reasonable medical practitioner similarly situated would disclose. This is called the *physician-based standard*.[15] Other states have adopted the reasonable patient standard, which means that the physician must disclose information that a reasonable patient needs to make an informed decision.[16]

JUDICIAL DECISIONS
Judicial decisions are previous cases that either interpret statutes or adopt and adapt common law principles.

Simplistically, current law is a product of common law, statutory law, and judicial decisions. As is evident from these examples, however, current law can vary depending on the jurisdiction. In addition, although courts often look to decisions from other jurisdictions for guidance, they are not bound to follow those decisions. Moreover, the law can change as society changes. Therefore imaging professionals need to know the current law in their jurisdictions.

Administrative law, criminal law, and civil law are components of the legal system that have an impact on the medical imaging sciences. Administrative law determines the licensing and regulation of the practice of imaging professionals and regulates some employer-employee relations. Criminal law seeks to redress wrongs against the state. Civil law attempts to compensate for wrongs committed by one party resulting in harm to another party (see Table 1-2). The same set of circumstances may be the basis of a civil, criminal, and administrative case.

Each branch of law has separate and distinct penalties. For example, the imaging scenario on p. 17 resulted in all of the following: an administrative action involving the technologist's license to practice; a criminal charge of battery possibly involving incarceration; and a civil lawsuit alleging medical malpractice, which may require the insurance company of the hospital, the technologist, or both to pay monetary damages.

IMAGING SCENARIO

An elderly patient comes to the imaging department for lumbar spine films. The patient attempts to be cooperative but because of pain is unable to lie flat on the imaging table and refuses the examination. The imaging technologist assures the patient that she will be able to lie flat and assists her to lie down against her will.

The patient complains to her son, an attorney, about her treatment, and he contacts protective services to investigate. As a result of the investigation, criminal battery charges are pending against the technologist. In addition, the patient files a civil lawsuit against the technologist and the hospital. The suit alleges medical malpractice based on the hiring of the technologist, the negligence of the technologist, and the failure to train and supervise the technologist properly. Protective services has brought the investigation and charges to the attention of the regulatory division of the state public health department, and they are investigating the incident.

Lawsuits involving the medical imaging sciences are generally brought under tort law, a subdivision of civil law. A tort action is filed to recover damages for personal injury or property damage occurring from negligent conduct or intentional misconduct.[17] The types of torts that imaging professionals might encounter include assault, battery, false imprisonment, defamation, negligence, lack of informed consent, and breach of patient confidentiality. The tort most often involving imaging professionals is negligence. Subsequent chapters explain torts in detail. Imaging professionals must have a basic understanding of the elements of torts, strategies to protect themselves and the facilities in which they work from lawsuits, and the role of risk management in minimizing the number and effect of lawsuits.

The imaging professional is exposed constantly to situations that can become the subject of litigation without warning. As providers of medical imaging services, they can be required to participate in litigation. To be prepared, the imaging professional must have a basic understanding of the mechanics of a lawsuit.

THE LAWSUIT

A lawsuit is generally composed of a pleading phase, discovery phase, and trial. During the pleading phase a complaint is lodged and an answer given. During the discovery phase the attorneys seek the facts of the case by questioning the involved parties. During the trial the case is presented to a judge or jury for a decision (Table 1-3).

Statutes of limitation set forth the time period after the cause of the complaint in which lawsuits can be brought against a physician or other health professional. These time limits vary by jurisdiction. In addition, attorneys are required to make a reasonable inquiry into the facts of the claim before filing lawsuits. Settlement negotiations can and usually do occur before a lawsuit is filed and generally continue throughout the lawsuit. Many lawsuits are settled before trial.

Pleading Phase

A lawsuit is begun when a plaintiff files a complaint (also called a claim or a petition, depending on the court in which it is brought) against a defendant with the court. In a medical negligence lawsuit, this complaint may allege that the defendant has failed to provide treatment, has provided inadequate treatment, or has committed misconduct. The lawsuit

TABLE 1-3 **PHASES OF A LAWSUIT**

Phase	Action
Pleading	Complaint lodged
	Answer given
Discovery	Facts sought in several ways:
	Written questions: requests for information, including interrogatories, requests for admissions, requests for production of documents, e-mail, audio and video information
	Oral questions (deposition)
Trial	Presentation of facts to judge or jury
Decision	
Postdecision appeal process	Decision may be reversed or reviewed

alleges that the plaintiff has been injured as a result of the action or inaction of the defendant. Lawsuits may have many defendants, including physicians and individual care providers. In addition, the health care facility may be sued for the actions or lack of action of any of its employees and students. Notice of the filing of the lawsuit must be given to the defendant by very specific methods dictated by the particular court in which the lawsuit has been filed. The defendant must file a written answer to the allegations in the complaint within specific time frames set by the court in which the lawsuit has been filed.

Discovery Phase

The lawsuit then proceeds to the discovery phase. The purpose of discovery is to ascertain the truth concerning the incident. During the discovery phase, questions may be asked of any of the parties (including employees and students of a party) either in writing (interrogatories, requests for admission, and requests for production of documents) or orally (depositions). Parties are under oath regardless of whether questions are oral or written. These interrogatory answers, admissions, and statements from depositions will be used at trial if testimony contradicts or does not agree with these earlier statements. Because discovery is such an important part of any lawsuit, it must always be conducted with the supervision of the defense attorney.

The Trial

After the discovery phase is complete, the lawsuit advances to trial. The lawsuit may be dismissed or settled at any time before or during the trial. Dismissal or settlement generally occurs if the discovery phase reveals facts that make the success of one party or the other unlikely at trial. Settlement negotiations often involve attorneys for the plaintiff, defendant, and defendant's insurance company, as well as the parties themselves, which may include a representative for the hospital and the physicians who are themselves involved. These negotiations can be through correspondence, telephone calls, and informal or formal meetings. Negotiators, mediators, and arbitrators (generally highly experienced attorneys or retired judges) are often used to bring objectivity to the negotiations and encourage the parties to settle the lawsuit. If a lawsuit proceeds to trial, any potentially relevant witness may be called. A student or staff medical imaging professional may be a party or a witness in a medical negligence case.

RISK MANAGEMENT

Litigation may arise from patient care in which the technologist is involved. Therefore the imaging professional must understand the importance of minimizing risk by thoroughly documenting information, ensuring that informed consent has been obtained, maintaining patient confidentiality, practicing radiation protection, and maintaining a safe environment for patients and employees.

Risk management is the system for identifying, analyzing, and evaluating risks and selecting the most advantageous method for treating them.[18] The goal of risk management is to maintain high-quality patient care and conserve the facility's financial resources. An effective risk management program has three primary goals:

1. Elimination of the causes of loss experienced by the hospital and its patients, employees, and visitors
2. Reduction in the operational and financial effects of unavoidable losses
3. Coverage of inevitable losses at the lowest cost

Risk management seeks to maintain high-quality patient care and the safety and security of the facility's patients, employees, visitors, and property. The risk manager must also be concerned with public and patient relations, since dissatisfied patients are more likely to sue for medical errors.[18]

QUALITY ASSURANCE

Hospital quality assurance programs are directly concerned with assessing and improving patient care. **Quality assurance** focuses more narrowly on patient care than does risk management. It is broader than risk management, however, in that it considers a wide range of quality concerns and uses hospital committees to oversee the quality of various hospital functions. These committees carry out functions mandated by standards of the Joint Commission on Accreditation of Healthcare Organizations (JCAHO) and in

IMAGING SCENARIO

A patient arrives at the imaging department for an intravenous pyelogram (IVP). The imaging technologist assigned to IVPs that day proceeds to take the patient's history. During the course of the history the patient responds to a question regarding food allergies by saying that she is allergic to seafood. This allergy may indicate an allergy to the iodinated contrast material used to perform an IVP. The discovery of this allergy leads the technologist to consult the radiologist, who determines that the iodinated contrast should not be used.

Discussion

The discovery of this seafood allergy and the taking of appropriate action by the technologist have prevented what could have been a situation likely to involve litigation. The technologist discovered this allergy because of a consistent, systematic, and thorough approach to documentation of the patient history. The advantage of the consistent, systematic, and thorough approach is that the technologist follows the same procedure with every patient, eliminating the risk of overlooking an important item of patient history.

some states by standards required by statute or regulation. Functions performed by these committees range from overseeing the quality and necessity of surgery to determining which doctors may practice in the hospital and what procedures they may perform.[18] Quality assurance and risk management are important and closely related functions in providing high-quality care. We discuss both throughout the text, but for purposes of this text we discuss risk management as including quality assurance (Box 1-5).

Health care facilities generally employ a risk manager or a team of risk managers to maintain efficiency and quality of care. Each student or staff imaging professional, however, must take responsibility as a risk manager and be aware that risk is always present.

Policies and procedures are formulated in facilities and individual departments to minimize risk exposure (Box 1-6). Examples of important procedures include taking

---

BOX 1-5   **QUALITY IN HEALTH CARE   WHERE ARE WE NOW?**

Improving patient safety and quality has been a top priority for hospitals. Health-related organizations, including the Institute of Medicine, have worked hard to develop a way to improve hospital quality. An Institute of Medicine report published in 2003 targeted 20 areas that needed quality improvement. As a result of this report and input from many physician organizations, the Patient Safety and Quality Improvement Act of 2005 was signed into law. Physicians believe this law to be a major win for patient safety. Its purpose is to make it easier for physicians to report medical errors in the hopes that others might learn from the mistakes. The new law will encourage physicians and others to report errors, with the intent of helping individuals in similar situations avoid the same mistakes, according to Dennis O'Leary, MD, president of the Joint Commission on Accreditation of Healthcare Organizations. Under this new law physicians and those they work with can report errors and near-misses and this information will be entered in a nonidentifiable way into central databases. Health and Human Services can access these databases to produce recommendations on how quality can be improved on a national level. Reports on errors and near-misses stay confidential and cannot be used in any criminal, civil, or administrative actions. Information from sources outside the patient safety system, including medical records, is still open to legal discovery.

Compiled from Priority Areas for National Action: Transforming Health Care Quality, *Institute of Medicine Report*, 2003; and Patient Safety Gets Boost from Law Easing Fear of Reporting, *AMA News*, Aug. 15, 2005.

BOX 1-6   **COMMON RISK MANAGEMENT GUIDELINES**

Follow facility and departmental policies and procedures.
Take a thorough, consistent, and systematic approach to informed consent and documentation.
Strictly respect patient confidentiality.
Practice consistent radiation protection.
Be aware of safety issues.
Report hazardous conditions.

IMAGING SCENARIO

A young woman in her sixth month of pregnancy arrives in the imaging trauma center after being involved in a head-on collision. Fortunately, her seat belt and airbag kept her from contact with the windshield, but they caused severe bruising. She is having chest pain and has not felt the baby move since the accident. She is frantic with fear. As she lies in the imaging suite, she overhears someone talking from the adjoining room. She hears partial sentences with such phrases as crushing injuries, fetal death, oxygen deprivation, and internal injuries. The imaging professional caring for her rushes to close the door, but not before the young woman becomes hysterical. She demands an explanation from the radiographer. The imaging professional is at a loss for words, angry to be placed in this situation by his peers and becoming very concerned about the patient's welfare.

The woman goes into premature labor, and the baby spends months in the NICCU. The mother also spends weeks in the hospital. A medical malpractice lawsuit charging negligence and breach of confidentiality is later filed.

Discussion questions
- How did unethical behavior turn into a lawsuit?
- How would problem-solving models aid the resolution of this scenario?
- What legal issues may arise during this lawsuit?
- What standards of care were violated?

a thorough, consistent, and systematic approach to informed consent and documentation (see imaging scenario on p. 19), strictly respecting patient confidentiality, consistently practicing radiation protection, being aware of safety issues, and immediately reporting hazardous conditions. These procedures limit the litigation risks inherent in the imaging professions.

SUMMARY

- Ethics or codes of behavior evolved from the need of humans to get along as a group. Several people through history provided foundational structure for the ethics we recognize today. Ethics for imaging professionals will continue to evolve as technology evolves. Imaging professionals must deal with these ethical dilemmas.
- Imaging professionals rely on personal ethics derived from their value systems, values clarification, and professional ethics as defined in codes of ethics to make decisions. These decisions involve appropriate activities and attitudes concerning patients and other health care professionals. The personal, cultural, and professional values of imaging professionals also affect the ethical decision-making process. These values may conflict with one another and with those of patients and other health care providers during ethical dilemmas.
- Ethical theories and models serve as tools in problem solving. The three schools of ethical thought are teleology, deontology, and virtue ethics. Imaging

professionals also use ethical models to guide interaction with patients. Common models include the engineering, paternal or priestly, collegial, contractual, and covenantal models.

- Case study analysis is aided by a decision-making framework in which the imaging professional asks questions about the context of an ethical problem and ascertains the significance to the other parties of the conflict and the values involved to determine a satisfactory outcome and avoid future ethical dilemmas.
- Legal matters may affect imaging professionals. Law has been established through common law, case law, and statutes, all of which have binding legal force. Law may also be divided into administrative, criminal, and civil law. Lawsuits involving the imaging professional are generally brought under tort law, a subdivision of civil law.
- Imaging professionals are exposed constantly to situations that may result in liability for themselves, the facilities in which they work, and the physicians with whom they work. These lawsuits usually allege that harm has occurred because of negligent conduct or intentional misconduct by a health care provider. Imaging professionals may be involved in a civil lawsuit as a witness or defendant. Both roles require participation in the pleading, discovery, and trial phases of the lawsuit.
- Litigation may be reduced through risk management and quality assurance, which seek to improve patient care and minimize litigation risks through standardized procedures and guidelines. In addition to the established risk management team, each imaging professional must be a risk manager.

REFERENCES

1. *Webster's new world dictionary of the American language*, ed 2, New York, 1982, Simon & Schuster.
2. Warner SB: Code of ethics: professional & legal implications, *Radiol Technol* 52(5):485, 1981.
3. American Philosophical Association: *The Delphi Report: research findings and recommendations prepared for the committee of pre-college philosophy*, ERIC Document Reproduction Service No. ED 315-423, Newark, Del, 1990.
4. MacIntyre A: *A short history of ethics*, New York, 1966, Macmillan.
5. Omery A: Values, moral reasoning, and ethics, *Nurs Clin North Am* 24(2):488, 1989.
6. Rath L, Simon S, Merrill H: *Values and teaching*, Columbus, Ohio, 1966, Merrill.
7. Rokeach M: *Beliefs, attitudes, and values*, San Francisco, 1968, Jossey-Bass.
8. Fry ST: *Ethics in nursing practice: a guide to ethical decision making*, Geneva, Switzerland, 1994, International Council of Nurses.
9. Creasia J, Parker B: *Conceptual foundations of professional nursing practice*, ed 2, St Louis, 1996, Mosby.
10. Burnard P, Chapman CM: *Professional and ethical issues in nursing*, New York, 1988, Wiley.
11. Anderson KN: *Mosby's medical, nursing, and allied health dictionary*, ed 5, St Louis, 1997, Mosby.
12. Dowd SB: *Ethical decision making* (Computer Program), Edwardsville, Kan, 1994, Educational Software Concepts.
13. *Black's law dictionary*, ed 6, St Paul, Minn, 1990, West.
14. *People v Rehman*, 253 C.A. 2d 119, 61 Cal. Rptr. 65, 85 (1967).
15. *Smith v Weaver*, 407 N.W. 2d 174 (Neb. 1987).
16. *Korman v Mallin*, 858 P. 2d 1145 (Alaska 1993).
17. Schwartz V, Kelly K, Partlett D: *Prosser, Wade, and Schwartz: cases, and materials on torts*, ed 10, Westbury, NY, 2000, Foundation Press.
18. Furrow BR, Greaney TL, Johnson SH, et al: *Health law: cases, materials and problems*, St Paul, Minn, 2004, West.

1 Ethics is defined as:_____.
2 **True or False**   Ethics was born of necessity.
3 Biomedical ethics includes which of the following?
   a. Exact rules
   b. Feelings and beliefs of the imaging professional
   c. Legal issues and judicial decisions
   d. Guidelines from the American Medical Association
   e. All of the above
4 Consequentialism is another name for which of the following?
   a. Virtue ethics
   b. A contract
   c. Exact rules
   d. Teleology
5 Deontology emphasizes which of the following?
   a. Significance of the motives
   b. Good of the majority
   c. Emotional problem solving
   d. Practical reasoning
6 The imaging professional may encounter biomedical ethical problems because of which of the following?
   a. Value conflicts
   b. Patients' awareness or lack of awareness of rights
   c. Differing hierarchies of values
   d. All of the above
7 Describe two major functions of a code of ethics.
8 The ethical model that treats the relationship between the health care provider and patient as a business agreement is the _____ model.
9 The _____ model treats the provider as an omniscient or fatherlike figure.
10 The _____ model is based on traditional values and goals.
11 Three types of values are _____, _____, and _____.
12 What four questions may help the imaging specialist solve ethical problems?
   a. _____
   b. _____
   c. _____
   d. _____
13 The _____ problem-solving method was developed specifically for imaging professionals.
14 **True or False**   The patient has the right to refuse treatment.
15 **True or False**   Patients have the right to know the immediate and long-term effects of their treatment choices.
16 The origin of the current law is which of the following?
   a. Common law
   b. Statutes
   c. Judicial decisions
   d. All of the above

17 An incident between a patient and an imaging technologist could involve which of the following?
   a. Administrative law
   b. Criminal law
   c. Civil law
   d. All of the above

18 Lawsuits involving the medical imaging sciences generally are brought under which kind of law?
   a. Criminal law
   b. Administrative law
   c. Civil law, tort division
   d. Common law

19 Risk management strives to do which of the following?
   a. Eliminate the causes of loss in the facility
   b. Lessen the effects of unavoidable losses
   c. Cover inevitable costs at the lowest price
   d. All of the above

20 Common law is which of the following?
   a. The law of common sense
   b. The laws of the particular jurisdiction
   c. Based on ancient usages and customs
   d. The law of the common persons in England

21 Risk management is performed by which of the following?
   a. A risk manager
   b. A risk management team
   c. The imaging technologist
   d. All of the above

22 Quality assurance uses which of the following?
   a. Report cards for employees
   b. Hospital committees to oversee quality issues
   c. Hall monitors to watch for mistakes
   d. Inspection teams to check cleaning of the facility

23 Risk management tools include which of the following?
   a. Knowing and following policies and procedures
   b. Respecting patient confidentiality
   c. Practicing radiation protection
   d. All of the above

24 **True or False**   Professionalism promotes the good of the individual and depends on high ethical standards.

25 **True or False**   Patients share in the responsibility for their health care.

26 **True or False**   Because health care facilities have legal counsel, imaging professionals do not need to know anything about the law.

27 **True or False**   Current law has been established through common law, statutes, and judicial decisions.

28 **True or False**   Lawsuits involving imaging professionals are most frequently brought under criminal law.

29 **True or False** A tort action alleges harm caused by the negligent or intentional act of another.

30 **True or False** An imaging professional never has to worry about answering questions or testifying in a lawsuit.

31 **True or False** An imaging professional's role in a lawsuit may include being a witness or a defendant.

32 **True or False** Written answers to interrogatories are not important; the only information that is important is that presented at trial.

33 **True or False** Risk management is performed by the risk management department, and the imaging professional does not have to be concerned with it.

34 **True or False** The imaging professional should understand the elements of torts.

35 **True or False** Since all states have the same laws, the imaging professional does not need to know anything about the law in any particular state.

36 **True or False** When faced with interrogatories, the imaging professional should go ahead and just answer them.

37 **True or False** Tort actions can be brought only if a patient is harmed by the intentional act of an imaging professional.

38 **True or False** An imaging professional's involvement in the discovery phase of a trial has no influence on whether the case proceeds to trial.

39 **True or False** An incident involving an imaging professional can be cause only for a case filed in civil court.

40 **True or False** Administrative law involves the administration of justice in a criminal case.

CRITICAL THINKING *Questions & Activities*

1 Why is ethics important to the development of professional status for imaging professionals?

2 If you had to pick an ethical theory with which you felt most comfortable to aid in problem solving in imaging, which one would you choose and why?

3 To what extent should imaging professionals' religious beliefs, cultural views, values, and understanding of professional codes of ethics influence their decision making? In what way do ethical models give structure to problem-solving techniques? Give an example and justify your decision.

4 Describe the way the roles of the imaging professional and patient interact when a biomedical ethical problem develops in one of the imaging modalities. Do the roles ever conflict? Explain your reasoning.

5 Do you believe that ethics is a necessary academic course for imaging professionals, or that ethics is just common sense? Defend your answer.

6 Does imaging practice provide unique ethical dilemmas? Discuss them.

7 What is your possible involvement in each of the three phases of a lawsuit?

8 If a case proceeds to trial, in what way would your involvement in the discovery phase influence the trial?

9 Describe ways in which each imaging professional can be a risk manager.

Continued

CRITICAL THINKING *Questions & Activities —cont'd*

10 What strategies do you need to learn from the next three chapters to protect yourself, your facility, and the primary care physician from liability?

11 Discuss an ethical dilemma you have personally experienced.

12 Analyze your current problem-solving skills for strengths and weaknesses.

13 Interview imaging professionals who have been in practice for 10 years or more and ask about ethical dilemmas they have observed and experienced.

14 Keep an ethical diary (individually or as a class). Include situations, questions, and personal thoughts.

15 Prepare a table listing the three schools of thought for ethical problem solving, citing the precepts of each and how it is similar to and different from the others.

16 Assign teams to role play an ethical problem-solving situation in one of the imaging modalities. The ethical problem should be the same for each team, but the model and theory should vary. After the team assignments are completed, discuss application of models and theories. Cite the positive and negative aspects of each.

17 Videotape a procedure for further team development. Evaluate images, adequacy of protection, and appropriateness of positioning, and discuss patient care.

2 PRINCIPLES OF BENEFICENCE AND NONMALEFICENCE

A person may cause evil to others not only by his actions, but by
his inaction, and in either case he is justly accountable to them
for the injury.

JOHN STUART MILL

Chapter Outline

Ethical Issues
Proportionality
Beneficence
Nonmaleficence
Differences Between Beneficence and
    Nonmaleficence
Medical Indications Involving Principles of
    Beneficence and Nonmaleficence
Justice

Contractual Agreements
Surrogate Obligations
Imaging Professional's Role
Patient's Role
Legal Issues
Standard of Care
Negligence
Methods to Decrease Risk

Learning Objectives

After completing this chapter, the reader will be able to perform the following:

- Distinguish between beneficence and
  nonmaleficence.
- Identify the four conditions used to assess the
  proportionality of good and evil in an action.
- Demonstrate an ability to make appropriate
  decisions by applying the principles of beneficence
  and nonmaleficence.
- Identify medical indicators involved in imaging.
- State the imaging professional's role in doing good
  and avoiding evil.
- Provide patients with the knowledge necessary to
  ensure their participation in decision making.

- Identify and define the legal concept of standard
  of care.
- List the many sources of standards of care.
- Define negligence, medical negligence, and
  res ipsa loquitur.
- Identify methods to decrease risk, including
  documentation, technical detail issues, radiation
  protection, and safety.
- Identify and justify which information is appropriate and inappropriate for documentation.

Key Terms

beneficence
medical negligence
negligence
nonmaleficence

principle of double effect
reasonable care
res ipsa loquitur
standard of care

Professional Profile

The ethical and legal issues that face radiographers take on new dimensions as technologic advances are made. Issues of patient confidentiality have become a greater concern in my practice as a radiographer and educator because of changing methods of communication. Today radiographers have access to more personal information that has the potential to do harm, and we must be cautious in how and when we communicate about our patients' health and personal status. Just because I have access to patients' medical records, that does not mean I have permission to read their private information. As a patient myself, I view the confidentiality statement as a contract ensuring that my information is private and confidential. It is my responsibility to provide the same level of assurance to patients. The use of electronic transmission of confidential information requires me to be mindful of the profession's code of ethics and my moral and legal obligation to protect each patient's and student's right to privacy.

Students and patients make assumptions about the ethical standards that guide my practice. Because I bring earned credentials to my job, they believe I will treat them fairly, ethically, and within the standards of practice. This is a level of expectation I wish not to disappoint.

Advancements in radiographic equipment have created an environment in which it may seem that the technology can select and administer the radiation and that, as long as the images are of diagnostic quality, the amount of radiation exposure to patients is incidental. Students and radiographers must be more diligent than ever in selecting radiation exposure techniques to maintain the "as low as reasonably achievable" (ALARA) principle. Radiographic imaging is a major contributor to patients' radiation exposure, and the use of medical imaging for diagnosis and treatment continues to increase.

When computed radiography was introduced into our radiology department, we were not knowledgeable about this technology and how it would affect our exposure techniques. Because we focus on producing high-quality radiographs, the use of more radiation exposure than needed could easily become a routine. As a radiographer, I have a moral and ethical obligation to understand the new equipment, use it properly, and limit the amount of radiation exposure during procedures. Attending educational seminars makes me more knowledgeable, and consciously thinking about the radiation exposures selected improves my ability to produce high-quality radiographs at reasonably low exposures.

Taking professional responsibility for each patient, including the quality of procedures, privacy, confidentiality, and limits on radiation exposure, must be foremost in my daily activity as an imaging professional. As an important member of the team, the radiographer plays a critical role in setting and maintaining high ethical and legal standards for health care.

Terri L. Fauber, EdD, RT(R)(M)
Radiography Program Director
VCU Medical Center
Richmond, Virginia

ETHICAL ISSUES

Health care decision-making processes require the consideration of all aspects of a problem. When the health care team and patient must decide whether to proceed with an invasive imaging procedure or drastic surgery, the team must intend good for the patient. Moreover, they must consider whether this good outweighs the risks of evil consequences.

Two integral components of decision making in medical ethics are beneficence, or the performance of good acts, and nonmaleficence, or the avoidance of evil. These two

IMAGING SCENARIO

A 4-year-old boy with Down syndrome is scheduled for a cardiac catheterization. The completed test shows a defect that will drastically limit his life expectancy if left untreated. The pediatric cardiologist does not recommend surgery because of the child's low intelligence quotient (IQ).

The child's parents are afraid their son will outlive them if he has the surgery. A vascular imaging technologist who assisted with the cardiac catheterization is horrified when she finds out the young child will not be operated on because of low IQ and quality-of-life decisions made for the child by others. She wonders whose good the parents and physician are considering and in what way they arrived at such a decision.

Discussion question
- In what various ways do law, custom, relationship, and contract interact in this scenario?

definitions may sound similar, but a closer examination reveals distinctions between the two.

This chapter explores beneficence and nonmaleficence and the ways they relate to the roles of the imaging professional and patient. It also considers justice and patient autonomy and the ways in which pursuit of those values may conflict with the ideals of beneficence and nonmaleficence.

Society expects health care professionals to "do good" and thus aid patients. This has long been an expectation of health care professionals; indeed, the Hippocratic Oath begins with the exhortation, "First, do no harm."

This good encompasses proper behavior within "law, custom, relationship, and contract."[1] State and federal laws, which presumably have been based on moral and culturally virtuous processes, may give the health care professional defined guidelines within which to do good as society sees matters. For example, society perceives caring for sick people and supplying high-quality imaging services as inherently good. Custom further helps define good behavior based on repeated patterns within the society. Relationships between individuals, individuals and institutions, and individuals and society also contribute to a definition of good within a society. In addition, the contractual process may indicate an individual's conception of a good act.

PROPORTIONALITY

The avoidance of all evil is impossible. Because of this, society tends to value the utilitarian theory described by philosopher John Stuart Mill in which the ideal is to do the most good for the most people. In the achievement of good, however, people may be subjected to its opposite—harm. For example, chemotherapy may achieve its goal of curing cancer only after causing pain, nausea, and hair loss. Individuals and society therefore need to determine the amount of harm or evil that may be tolerated. To make this determination, society often applies the **principle of double effect,** which states that a person may perform an act that has evil effects or risk such effects as long as four conditions are met:

1. The action must be good or morally indifferent in itself. For example, a proposed imaging procedure must help the patient or at least not cause harm.

PRINCIPLE OF DOUBLE EFFECT
A person may perform an act that has evil effects or risk such effects as long as four certain conditions are met.

2. The agent must intend only the good effect and not the evil effect. That is, the imaging technologist must intend for the imaging to aid in the health care process, not injure the patient or cause pain.
3. The evil effect cannot be a means to the good effect. This condition may be complicated for the imaging technologist. The patient may believe the imaging procedure to be an evil effect; however, to gain a diagnosis, or good effect, the patient may have to undergo an unpleasant examination.
4. Proportionality must exist between good and evil effects. The good of the procedure must at least balance with the unintended pain or discomfort.

To conform to the principle of proportionality, "the action should not infringe against the good of the individual. There also has to be a proportionate good to justify the risk of an evil consequence."[1] The following questions may be used to define proportionality:

- Are alternatives with less evil consequences available? Might another procedure produce the same diagnosis with less pain? For example, might magnetic resonance imaging (MRI) be used instead of mammography?
- What are the levels of good intended and evil risked? What will be gained from the procedure? For example, can a contrast media fluoroscopic examination of a first-trimester pregnant woman be justified?
- What is the probability that the good or evil intended will be achieved, and what action and influence do the health care team and patient have? What gains to the patient are possible, and will the imaging specialist have to convince the patient or surrogate that the patient should undergo the procedure?

BENEFICENCE

The term **beneficence** may encompass many aspects of goodness, promoting good action and preventing evil or harm. Beneficence requires the action of an imaging professional to do good or prevent harm. For example, a patient scheduled for an invasive imaging examination may have determined that he or she does not wish to risk the possibility of the complications resulting from the procedure. The imaging professional may then have to share these concerns with the radiologist and speak on behalf of the patient. A clear definition of nonmaleficence, or the avoidance of evil, may therefore aid in the critical consideration of beneficence.

NONMALEFICENCE

Nonmaleficence, or the avoidance of evil, hinges on a system of weighting. Nonmaleficence does not require individual action. It only requires that the imaging professional do no harm. The good desired must outweigh the risk of evil. For example, the performance of a balloon angioplasty offers the patient the great good of opening the coronary artery and enhancing the patient's quality of life. However, the health care team and patient must consider the risk that plaque will dislodge within the artery and produce myocardial infarction, stroke, or death. The team weighs the possible good and evil outcomes of the procedure by assessing the patient's physical condition and his or her mental and emotional ability to understand the risk and significance of the possible harm. If the patient is otherwise healthy, the intended good usually outweighs the unintended evil; if the patient already has suffered heart damage or has serious respiratory disease, however, the evil consequences may overshadow the intended good. Both the performance of good and the avoidance of evil benefit the patient. A decision must be made by weighing both good and evil.

TABLE 2-1 **DIFFERENCES BETWEEN NONMALEFICENCE AND BENEFICENCE**

Nonmaleficence	Beneficence
Goal is to do no harm	Goal is to do good
Achieved through passive omission	Achieved through active process
Primary responsibility of the health care provider	Secondary in importance to nonmaleficence

From Creasia J, Parker B: *Conceptual foundations of professional nursing practice,* ed 2, St Louis, 1996, Mosby.

DIFFERENCES BETWEEN BENEFICENCE AND NONMALEFICENCE

Beneficence and nonmaleficence differ in the degree of force each possesses. The stronger action of the two is nonmaleficence, or the avoidance of harm; beneficence, or the performance of good, is weaker. Although the interest of imaging professionals is in doing good, they must not cause harm while doing so. This is a vital consideration in the practice of imaging. For example, an elderly patient may have arrived in the imaging department for a thoracic spine image. The patient has a kyphosis and is crippled with degenerative arthritis and finds lying on the table intolerable. The guiding principle in this case may be to do no harm, even at the expense of the patient's receiving the good of the diagnostic image. Decisions in health care should be made after consideration of both beneficence and nonmaleficence.

Although beneficence and nonmaleficence are both important considerations in patient autonomy, they differ in the way they are practiced. Beneficence is an active process, whereas nonmaleficence is passive (Table 2-1). This difference is evident in the scenario on p. 32.

MEDICAL INDICATIONS INVOLVING PRINCIPLES OF BENEFICENCE AND NONMALEFICENCE

Jansen, Siegler, and Winslade[2] provide six points to consider when dealing with issues of beneficence and nonmaleficence. With some modifications to suit imaging situations, these are the points:

1. What is the patient's medical problem (what brings the patient to the imaging department)? History? Diagnosis? Prognosis?
2. Is the problem acute? Chronic? Emergent? Reversible? How will this affect the imaging procedure?
3. What are the goals of the treatment or imaging procedure?
4. What are the probabilities of a successful imaging exam?
5. What are the plans in case of therapeutic failure or the inability to complete the exam?
6. In sum, how can this patient benefit by the medical and imaging care? How can the imaging professional avoid harm to the patient?

JUSTICE

For imaging professionals, justice, or the principle of fairness, requires the performance of an appropriate procedure only after informed consent has been granted. Informed consent is permission, usually in writing, given by a patient agreeing to the performance of a procedure. (Issues of informed consent are discussed more fully in Chapter 4.)

| Resources | + | Needs | = | Limited choices |

FIGURE 2-1 The needs of patients and care providers can conflict because of limited resources, making ethical decisions part of a professional's daily tasks.

IMAGING SCENARIO

A female patient is scheduled for a lumbar spine imaging series. The imaging professional in charge of the examination is interrupted and called to the emergency room to care for victims of a massive accident. Another imaging professional arrives to take over the examination before the initial exposure is taken. When asked if everything is ready, the first technologist says yes and hurries to the emergency room. The second imaging technologist surveys the patient, who is covered with a sheet, introduces himself, and performs the lumbar spine series. The processed images reveal that the woman is in her first trimester of pregnancy. Obviously, an injustice has been done, and a lawsuit may possibly result.

Discussion question
- Was the injustice active, that is, did the first or second imaging professional deliberately not shield the patient and ask about possible pregnancy? Or was the injustice an unintentional error of omission resulting from the confusion caused by the first technologist's leaving to attend to accident victims in the emergency room?

Discussion
If the case is decided in court, the ruling may be affected by whether the injustice was a result of active intent or passive omission. The obligation not to harm is the strongest motivator in medicine, but the avoidance of evil is also essential.

Conflicts among beneficence, nonmaleficence, and autonomy (the state of independent self-government) may arise during consideration of principles of justice. The general belief in the right to health care brings beneficence and nonmaleficence into conflict with autonomy and justice. Although most people believe that the good of health care should be available to all, health care resources are limited and hard decisions must be made about their allocation. Limited resources reduce the overall quality of care and may lead to less avoidance of evil. When quality of health care is reduced, the patient's autonomy suffers from loss of freedom of choices. When choices are limited, the obligations of the patient and health care giver may conflict with resources and justice for the patient (Figure 2-1).

The performance of good and the avoidance of evil often come into conflict when medical indication principles or the proportionality of consequences is judged by the health care provider. The medical indication principle states that, "granted informed consent, the physician should do what is medically indicated such that from a medical point of view, more good than evil will result."[1]

The conflict between beneficence and nonmaleficence on the one hand and informed consent and patient autonomy on the other may be explored further by asking how, if the health care professional cannot make quality-of-life decisions concerning patients but must make recommendations concerning good and evil, decision making can lead to patient autonomy. For example, an imaging professional may be asked to give an imaging examination to a neonate in intensive care. The infant has the majority of its organs outside the abdomen, including a massive spina bifida. The imaging professional wonders why the infant's life is being maintained by artificial methods. This question, however, is an issue for the family. It is not the imaging professional's responsibility to make quality-of-life decisions for others.

CONTRACTUAL AGREEMENTS

Verbal and written contractual agreements help provide patient autonomy. Patients requiring imaging services enter into contractual agreements when they agree to enter a hospital and undergo a series of diagnostic imaging studies. Usually such contracts take the form of blanket statements of informed consent. They are general agreements; other processes of informed consent may be required as specific procedures are scheduled. The processes of informed consent and the procedures employed in providing it are discussed at length in Chapter 4.

SURROGATE OBLIGATIONS

Surrogate obligations present another area of conflict. The interactions among patient autonomy, beneficence, and nonmaleficence become even more complex in these situations. If the patient is incompetent, either the best interests of the patient or the rational choice principle should be used. The rational choice principle "commands that the surrogate choose what the patient would have chosen when competent and after having considered all available relevant information and the interests of the relevant others."[1] In a determination of the best interests of the patient, the proportionality between good and evil may be different for patient and surrogate; this may interfere with patient autonomy. In this situation the surrogate must consider the patient's and perhaps significant others' attitudes regarding good and evil consequences.

IMAGING SCENARIO

A 6-year-old boy arrives in the emergency room (ER) after being found floating face down in the neighbors' pool. The ER imaging professional is called in to take a portable chest x-ray. The child has been receiving cardiopulmonary resuscitation. No one knows how long he was without oxygen. He is nonresponsive, and the staff continues to work on the child. The radiograph is completed. When the radiographer returns, the child has a heartbeat and is receiving mechanical ventilation. He does not regain consciousness for a month. When he does awaken, he cannot communicate and is believed to have severe brain damage.

Discussion questions
- In a situation such as this, how does the imaging professional reconcile issues of "to do good" and "to do no harm"?
- Has the imaging professional actually done harm by participating in the diagnostic examination?

IMAGING SCENARIO

A young boy who has fallen from a tree is brought to the emergency room (ER), and x-rays of his shoulder and humerus are ordered. He is in pain and cannot move his arm. The student radiographer hesitates to move the youngster's arm because she knows it will cause significant pain. The ER doctor is waiting for the film and is becoming vocal about the time it is taking to complete the exam.

Discussion questions
- Can the student "do no harm"?
- What has to be considered in regard to risk, harm, and benefit for the child?
- How should this problem be handled?

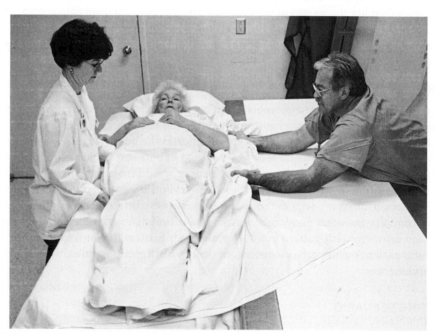

FIGURE 2-2 Safe transport of patients to, from, and within the imaging department is one way of showing both beneficence and nonmaleficence.
From Ehrlich RA, Daly J: *Patient care in radiography,* ed 6, St Louis, 2004, Elsevier.

IMAGING PROFESSIONAL'S ROLE

The imaging professional must be aware of the obligations to do good and avoid harm. Every imaging procedure has the potential to harm the patient; invasive procedures, radiation, and equipment malfunction all pose dangers to the patient. Maintaining a high quality of patient care and technologic skills helps ensure that procedures achieve good for the patient, and practicing protective measures aids in the avoidance of harm (Figure 2-2). Each imaging professional must be responsible for daily contact with patients undergoing diagnostic health care procedures.

PATIENT'S ROLE

Patients participate in protecting their own good and avoiding their own harm by gathering information about the imaging procedure they will be undergoing. If the patient is unable to understand this information, a surrogate should be appointed to guarantee that appropriate informed consent is given, which will lead to the avoidance of harm and the doing of good. If in doubt about a procedure, the patient or surrogate should seek a second opinion.

LEGAL ISSUES

The ethical concepts of beneficence and nonmaleficence may not generally be thought of as connected with legal theories involving health care. However, these concepts—the doing of good and avoidance of harm—are incorporated into the duty of a health professional to do no harm and provide reasonable care to the patient. This section explores the legal concept of **standard of care**. The reasonable care that is expected is defined and the negative results when less than reasonable care is provided are discussed.

STANDARD OF CARE
The degree of skill or care practiced by a reasonable professional practicing in the same field.

This section provides some methods to ensure that reasonable patient care is provided and litigation risk is decreased. Included in these methods are documentation, technical detail issues, radiation protection, and safety issues.

STANDARD OF CARE

The law provides many parameters for the delivery of imaging services. These parameters have evolved from statutes (laws written and enacted by state or federal legislatures) and court decisions. The most basic legal parameter in health care is the standard of care, which encompasses the obligation of health care professionals to do no harm and their duty to provide reasonable patient care. Each profession establishes standards of care to define the parameters within which that profession is obligated to practice. Standards of care are not limited to the imaging services but exist for all other health care providers in the facility, the physicians, and the facility itself.

The legal standard is the degree of skill or care employed by a reasonable professional practicing in the same field.[3] Lack of training or experience is not an excuse for the failure of a health care professional to perform a duty to the patient adequately. For example, imaging professionals working as nuclear medicine technologists are held to the same standard of care as trained and certified nuclear medicine technologists. If the appropriate standard of care is violated, liability may be imposed on both health care professionals and medical facilities.

Professional Standard of Care

Practice standards, educational requirements, and curricula developed for the medical imaging sciences all help to establish the standard of care to which imaging professionals must hold themselves. The practice standards for health care specialists are set forth by that discipline's national professional organization. Practice standards are important because they are recognized as the authoritative basis of a profession. Specific practice standards exist for each subspecialty of imaging, including cardiovascular-interventional technology, computed tomography, magnetic resonance imaging, mammography, nuclear medicine, radiation therapy, radiography, and sonography.[4] These standards may be found on the website of the American Society of Radiologic Technologists (www.asrt.org).

The practice standards may be used to define what radiologic technologists do and how they do it. For example, health care facilities use professional standards to develop job descriptions, departmental policies, and performance appraisals. If there is a question as to whether an activity falls within the professional duties of the radiologic technologist, a radiology manager may consult the practice standards. Practice standards may also be used to hold the radiologic technologist to a certain standard of care. In the case of medical malpractice or negligence, a lawyer may use the practice standards to establish the generally accepted standard of care and show whether the professional met that level of care.[4]

Standards for accreditation for educational programs in radiologic sciences as defined by the Joint Review Committee on Education in Radiologic Technology (effective January 1997)[5] or other regional accreditation agencies with similar standards must be met for graduates to be recognized by the American Registry of Radiologic Technologists (ARRT). ARRT recognition, as well as state licensure, is generally a requirement for reimbursement by Medicare, Medicaid, and many private insurers. In fact, the Consumer Assurance of Radiologic Excellence Act, introduced in the U.S. Congress in February 2006 (as it had been in some form, with the support of the imaging professionals, in each Congressional session since 1999), would require medical imaging and radiation therapy professionals to have state licensing in order to receive federal payments for these services.[6]

Imaging professionals must maintain knowledge of the current standard of care. This becomes particularly important as an imaging professional's time out of the educational program increases. The radiologic sciences are changing rapidly. Professionals in these fields have an obligation to update their knowledge and remain current. Attending appropriate continuing education programs and reading professional publications are ways to keep abreast of the current standard of care. Every patient receiving imaging services is entitled to expect the same level of care as the standard of care recognized by the law.

Additional Sources of Standards

In addition to the professional standard of care to which imaging professionals are held, other standards apply that come from a variety of sources. One source is institutional and departmental policies and procedures. If written guidelines exist, professionals need to be aware of them and follow them. Liability can be found based on the failure to follow the written policies of the institution. An example is a claim of negligence in credentialing against an Illinois hospital, which resulted in a $7.7 million award after a podiatrist negligently performed surgery.[7] The hospital failed to follow their own bylaws in granting privileges to the podiatrist when he did not meet their criteria.

Federal and state statutes also create standards that must be followed. The prime example is HIPAA, which is discussed in Chapter 5, but others are also discussed throughout the book. These guidelines should be conveyed from the employer to health care professionals, who must follow them to avoid liability. Another source of standards is the Joint Commission on Accreditation of Healthcare Organizations (JCAHO), which has provided guidelines governing almost every aspect of hospital operation.

A facility must follow JCAHO guidelines to be accredited and therefore eligible for payments by the federal government and other insurance sources.

National Patient Safety Goals

On May 25, 2005, JCAHO approved the 2006 National Patient Safety Goals (Box 2-1). Almost every one of these goals has a place in the imaging profession. Examples include the following:
- Patient identification
- Communication among caregivers
- Medication safety (with regard to contrast media, radiopharmaceuticals, and other medications used in the imaging department)
- Elimination of wrong site, wrong patient, wrong procedure surgery (this goal was designed for surgeries, but the principles apply to imaging, particularly digital radiography, since marking of orientation is sometimes done after exposure, although this is not recommended)
- Reduction in the risk of health care–associated infections
- Reduction in the risk of patients' falls
- Encouragement of the active involvement of patient care as a patient safety strategy

BOX 2-1	NATIONAL PATIENT SAFETY GOALS

Goal 1   Improve the accuracy of patient identification.

Goal 2   Improve the effectiveness of communication among caregivers.

Goal 3   Improve the safety of using medications.

Goal 4   Eliminate "wrong site, wrong patient, wrong procedure" surgery.

Goal 5   [Goal was retired in 2006]

Goal 6   Improve the effectiveness of clinical alarm systems.

Goal 7   Reduce the risk of health care–associated infections.

Goal 8   Accurately and completely reconcile medications across the continuum of care.

Goal 9   Reduce the risk of patient harm resulting from falls.

Goal 10 Reduce the risk of influenza and pneumococcal disease in institutionalized older adults.

Goal 11 Reduce the risk of surgical fires.

Goal 12 Implement applicable National Patient Safety Goals and associated requirements at the component and practitioner site levels [Networks].

Goal 13 Define and communicate the means for patients to report concerns about safety and encourage them to do so [Assisted Living, Disease-Specific Care, Home Care, Laboratory].

Goal 14 Prevent health care–associated pressure ulcers (decubitus ulcers).

From Joint Commission on Accreditation of Healthcare Organizations: *Facts about 2006 National Patient Safety Goals*, Oakbrook Terrace, Ill, 2006, Author.

NEGLIGENCE

Negligence is an unintentional tort resulting from actions not intended to do harm. It occurs in situations in which a duty to use reasonable care is owed to another person and an injury results from a failure to use reasonable care. **Reasonable care** is the degree of care a reasonable person, similarly situated, would use. Reasonable care may be determined by the applicable standard of care, by statute, or by previous judicial decisions, called precedents.[8] If a duty is not performed with reasonable care, liability may be imposed.

Negligence requires a duty, a breach of that duty, injury, and causation. For example, if a driver falls asleep at the wheel, crosses the center line, strikes another car, and injures its driver, the driver has been negligent. Statutes and precedents have established that all drivers have a duty to share the road reasonably with other drivers. The driver who fell asleep and crossed the center line was not acting reasonably. The other driver's injuries were a direct result of the first driver's failure to act reasonably. The driver who crossed the center line was negligent and is liable for damages.

Medical Negligence

A special relationship exists between health care providers and patients. This special relationship entails a duty on the part of the health care professional to provide patients with reasonable care. Whether reasonable care is provided is determined by the standard of care for whatever is done to the patient. A health care provider's failure to follow the appropriate standard of care is therefore a special type of negligence called **medical negligence**. This type of negligence is sometimes referred to under the general term *medical malpractice.*

A medical imaging professional owes a duty to the patient to ensure that procedures are performed according to the applicable standard of care. That standard of care requires the imaging professional to follow accepted guidelines for the procedure. A deviation from those guidelines that causes harm to a patient may form the basis for a judgment of liability. Although variations exist between jurisdictions, generally a plaintiff must provide evidence establishing an applicable standard of care, demonstrate that the standard has been violated, and prove a causal relationship between the violation and the alleged harm.[9]

The applicable standard of care is generally established through the testimony of a medical expert practicing in the same field as the defendant. A plaintiff must offer proof that the defendant breached this legally required standard of care and thus was negligent. Expert testimony is needed to establish both the proper standard of care and a failure by the defendant to conform to that standard.[10] An expert witness may not be required in a medical malpractice suit, however, when the facts to be decided are such that a layperson can understand them and determine the question of fact without the aid of an expert witness.[11]

If a lawsuit proceeds to trial, the imaging professional may have an opportunity to provide his or her personal recollections of the events. Written documentation, however, is extremely important; attorneys, judges, and juries may take the position that if an event was not documented, it did not happen. An example is a case in Nevada when a hospital was sued for an alleged near fall from a gurney in the imaging department, allegedly resulting in a broken hip. The jury returned a verdict for the defense, based on the fact that the incident was never documented in the medical record.[12] The patient care documentation was complete and detailed, and therefore the lack of documentation of this alleged event led the jury to believe that since this event was not documented, it did not occur.

Medical imaging professionals have an obligation to perform examinations in a manner consistent with policies and procedures, never vary from accepted standards of care, and provide appropriate documentation. These and other methods to decrease risk are discussed thoroughly later in this chapter.

The legal doctrine of ***res ipsa loquitur*** (Latin for "the thing speaks for itself") may have a significant impact on medical malpractice cases. It is applicable in situations in which a particular injury would not have occurred in the absence of negligence and is often used as a basis for lawsuits arising when sponges or instruments are left in a patient after surgery.

When *res ipsa loquitur* is claimed as the basis for a lawsuit, all parties involved in the procedure are defendants because obviously at least one of them was negligent. Therefore they all must try to prove that they were not negligent. The doctrine may apply to many situations in the medical imaging practice. For example, a confused elderly patient left alone on a cart in the hall after a procedure may fall and suffer a broken hip. The fall and injury would not have happened if the patient had not been left alone in the hall without being appropriately restrained. Therefore all health care professionals who worked with the patient, including the imaging professionals, may be called on to prove absence of negligence. Expert testimony may be used to prove that the standard of care was violated. If a clear breach of duty is evident to a layperson after the presentation of the facts of the case, however, expert testimony may not even be needed.

RES IPSA LOQUITUR
Latin term meaning "the thing speaks for itself." It is a legal concept invoked in situations in which a particular injury could not have occurred in the absence of negligence.

METHODS TO DECREASE RISK

Documentation

The type of information to be documented (see Appendix B) and incorporated into the medical record is a crucial consideration for medical professionals. From the risk management perspective, the medical record is the most important element in preventing and minimizing adverse consequences of malpractice suits. The record will serve as the basis for the defense of the suit. Poorly maintained, incomplete, inaccurate, illegible, or altered records create questions as to the treatment given the patient and may be used to show liability. Proper documentation creates a medical record that accurately and completely reflects the patient's care and can be used to correlate the facts related by witnesses. From a legal perspective, certain information is mandated by statutes, regulations, and institutional requirements. The Code of Ethics adopted by the ASRT[13] and ARRT[14] requires that the radiologic technologist act as an agent through observation and communication to obtain pertinent information that will aid in the diagnosis and treatment of the patient. JCAHO regulations require that pertinent patient histories be taken before all procedures performed in the medical imaging sciences.[15] Departmental policies generally mandate that this information be recorded on every patient record, which becomes a part of the patient's medical record. (See Appendix B for a sample patient data sheet and incident report.)

Other than the basic information mandated by statutory, regulatory, ethical, and institutional requirements, no steadfast rules govern the documentation of additional information in the medical imaging sciences. An examination of the purposes of documentation, however, may help the imaging professional make decisions regarding the inclusion of additional patient information.

High-quality patient care in the imaging sciences, particularly accurate diagnosis in diagnostic procedures and correct application of therapeutic radiography, depends

IMAGING SCENARIO

An imaging professional and a radiologist perform an arteriogram to evaluate peripheral vascular disease of the right leg. Significant narrowing is found, and a stent is placed to open the artery. Almost 2 years later a lawsuit is filed alleging that the arteriogram and stent placement were improperly performed. The specific allegation is that the stent placement was incorrect and caused further deterioration of the leg and foot to the point at which the patient had constant pain in his leg and was barely able to walk. The imaging professional is told that she is likely to be deposed, and the hospital's legal department gives her a set of questions she will probably be asked to answer under oath:

How much do you remember about the procedure?

Did you document the procedure?

How thorough was your documentation?

Did you document the stent placement and location?

Did you document any patient complaints at the time?

Did you document any report of patient status at the conclusion of the examination indicating the patient had no complaints?

Did you document your observations on a form that became a permanent record along with the patient's images?

Did the images you took include the stent placement site and the area of diagnostic interest?

Is documentation available to prove that the risks of the procedure were explained to the patient and that the patient understood?

largely on the interpreting physician's receiving pertinent information about the patient. The imaging professional must communicate with the patient, observe the patient, and interpret responses and observations. This process helps the professional formulate the patient's pertinent history. Often judgments regarding examinations to be performed and specific positioning to be used are based on the patient's history. Moreover, the interpreting physician may not be able to analyze images correctly or make accurate diagnoses without the information contained in an accurate and pertinent patient history.

Even the information necessary to ensure that the correct procedure is performed properly and interpreted accurately may not be adequate to protect health care professionals and the medical facility from liability. Thus imaging professionals must consider ways to obtain enough information to minimize the litigation risks.

As the scenario above indicates, remembering all the details of the particular procedure performed is extremely difficult. Written and radiographic documentation is a great aid in the defense of an unfounded medical negligence case. Imaging professionals have the opportunity and obligation to document thoroughly and thus avoid or minimize the effects of unfounded medical negligence claims (Box 2-2).

Patient Data Sheet

A uniform patient data sheet or computerized form should be developed for use in each facility (Box 2-3). Input from the department administrator, risk manager, physicians, and legal counsel in the drafting of this form is advisable.

BOX 2-2	**DOCUMENTATION BASICS**

Never alter or falsify a record. You will lose all credibility if alteration or falsification of records is discovered.

If you make an error, draw a line through it and write "error." Never use correction fluid or put a sticker over an error. Others must be able to see clearly the information you have changed in order for you to maintain credibility.

Know and adhere to your department's policies and guidelines. They help define expectations of reasonable care in your facility and may be evaluated in a lawsuit to determine whether your actions complied.

Document clearly and in chronologic order. If comments are necessary, make them in chronologic order. Do not leave blanks to fill in later. Blank spaces give the impression that the documentation was altered or sanitized. All corrections, late entries, entries made out of time sequence, and addenda should be clearly marked as such in the record and should be dated and timed on the day they are written and signed.

Do not document irrelevant details.

Provide objective, factual information. Avoid subjective, conclusory terms such as well, good, fine, and normal.

Document all instances of patient noncompliance or refusal of recommended treatment.

Sign your legal name and title and always make your documentation legible. Illegible writing can only hurt you if litigation results.

Keep records in a safe place and respect confidentiality. The maintenance of patient confidentiality is a duty of each member of the health care team. Documentation in a medical imaging department carries the same obligation of patient confidentiality as does the information in the patient's chart.

Use incident reports to report unusual circumstances. Do not refer to incident reports in routine documentation. The incident report is for use in quality assurance and risk management to improve patient care. Acknowledgment of it in routine documentation may change it from a patient care improvement tool to a discoverable document in a lawsuit.

Modified from McMullen P, Philipsen N: Charting basics 101, *Nurs Connect* 6(3):62, 1993; and Creasia JL, Parker B: *Conceptual foundations of professional nursing practice: charting basics*, St Louis, 1996, Mosby.

BOX 2-3	**ITEMS TO BE INCLUDED IN THE PATIENT DATA SHEET**

Basic patient identification information
Pertinent patient history
Answers to questions regarding pregnancy and last menstrual period
Signature line
Time of patient arrival and departure
Name of technologist performing examination
Comment section

Generally the form should include basic patient identification information, questions to assess for pregnancy, and pertinent patient history. A signature line for the patient and a line to note the time the patient arrived in and departed from the medical imaging department may also be included. In addition, the form may indicate the imaging technologist who performed the examination and provide space for additional comments. This comment section should be used to note and explain any variance from written procedure such as the patient's refusal or inability to cooperate during part or all of the examination. If data are collected in a computer, a comment section should be available on the computerized form or an alternative method should be available to document any variance from standard procedure. If computerized patient data documentation is used, an alternate system must be in place for the inevitable "computer-down" situations. The patient data sheet should be part of the permanent patient record.

Every page of a patient's record should be clearly labeled with the patient's name and medical record number. Electronic systems should require a password, and if paper records are used, these should be hospital-approved forms only and should be written only with pen, never pencil. Associated records, such as films, reports, requisitions, contrast forms, consent forms, and any other documents used in the imaging department, must also be labeled with the patient's name and medical record number and the time and date the action took place.

Inappropriate Documentation

Because proper documentation is so crucial, the imaging technologist must understand what type of information is inappropriate for documentation and the reason for this determination. Because medical records are business documents, they must reflect only factual information regarding patients and their care and treatment. Documentation of personal opinions or derogatory statements regarding the patient is inappropriate and may result in liability for the imaging professional, medical facility, or both. Mention of the preparation of an incident report should never be included in the medical record. An objective description of the incident should be reported in the medical record along with follow-up information.

Incident Reporting

The incident report is a valuable risk management tool. It allows the hospital to immediately investigate the circumstances of the incident and, if necessary, institute corrective action to prevent similar future occurrences. Although procedures may vary by facility, health care facilities generally require incident reports on occurrences involving patients and visitors that have resulted or may result in hospital liability or patient dissatisfaction. Examples include sudden deaths; falls; drug, contrast, and radiopharmaceutical errors and reactions; injuries caused by faulty equipment; injuries to employees or visitors; threats of legal action; and unexplained requests from attorneys for medical records. Department heads and supervisors are usually responsible for filing incident reports, but imaging professionals should know the procedures in their facilities before the need arises, as well as what circumstances necessitate the filing of an incident report.

Incident reports are generally directed to the risk manager, who investigates as necessary. The risk manager also informs appropriate administrative and medical staff and, if necessary, the facility's insurer. The incident report is a valuable tool because it allows compilation of data to identify problem areas and thus prevent future errors and injuries. Incident reporting should not be done on the patient data sheet. Instead, the incident reporting procedures set up by the facility's risk management department should be followed. The reasons for this are twofold:

1. The risk management department has put specific incident reporting procedures in place because the incident report is a valuable tool for assessing risk and tracking problems in a facility. The ultimate goal of such reports is to improve patient care.

2. From a legal perspective, the patient chart, including all imaging department documentation, is discoverable in a lawsuit. Incident reports generally fall into a different category and may not be as easily discoverable. However, acknowledgment of an incident report in routine documentation may make it more easily discoverable.

Documentation of the Introduction of Intravenous Contrast Material and Radiopharmaceuticals

Any procedure performed in an imaging department that involves the intravenous (IV) administration of contrast material carries with it the risk of allergic reaction. Although these reactions may range from mild, such as an itchy nose, to severe, such as anaphylactic shock, the risk is great enough to mandate extensive documentation.

Procedures involving the introduction of contrast material or radiopharmaceuticals present special documentation needs. Forms for documenting the type of material administered during the examination and other important information are very useful. A standardized form with spaces for each piece of information makes the regular recording of this information much more likely (Box 2-4). A form is useful, however, only if it is properly and consistently used. Imaging professionals performing risky procedures have a responsibility to ensure such proper and consistent documentation.

A form for documenting procedures involving injection of contrast medium or radiopharmaceuticals should include a place for allergies to be noted. For risk management purposes a notation should always be entered in that space, such as "NKA" (no known allergies) if the patient denies having allergies. Strict adherence to this requirement ensures that the question is asked and answered every time IV contrast material is

BOX 2-4	ITEMS TO BE INCLUDED IN THE DATA SHEET FOR INTRODUCTION OF CONTRAST MATERIAL AND RADIOPHARMACEUTICALS

Documentation of the obtaining of informed consent
Allergies
Material used
Amount (volume and radioactivity if using radiopharmaceutical)
Time of administration
Path of administration (oral, IV, through catheter, rectal)
Injection sites
Name of person administering material
Reaction
Time of reaction
Symptoms of reaction
Treatment of reaction
Physician treating
Time and condition on leaving department

administered. The form should include a space for recording that informed consent was obtained and the proper documentation is in the patient chart.

The form should include space for documentation of basic information about the material used, including identification, amount used, time administered, path of administration (oral, IV, through catheter, rectal), name of the person administering the material, and injection site or sites.

Documentation of the injection site is important for several reasons. The delivery of high-quality patient care, especially continuity of care, requires this documentation because problems with the injection site may develop. Risk management requires the information because infiltration of contrast material may raise litigation issues. Questions on the form that prompt the entering of required information and spaces for responses are helpful in ensuring adequate documentation.

Space should be provided to note any reaction the patient exhibits to the contrast material. This documentation should include all reactions: nose itching not requiring treatment, hives requiring treatment with diphenhydramine (Benadryl), or full-blown anaphylactic shock reactions. Documentation of reactions should be chronologic and include the symptoms observed, actions taken in response to the reaction, and detailed descriptions of treatments initiated. The condition of the patient on leaving the radiology department and the transfer of care to other health care providers such as the nursing floor or emergency department should also be documented, with signature, date, time, and to whose care the patient was transferred.

As with pharmaceuticals given on the nursing floor, pharmaceuticals given in an imaging department must be charted. Each facility should have a facility-wide system of charting in place. All individuals authorized to record information on patient charts (including imaging professionals) should be educated regarding the charting style, including accepted abbreviations. This will ensure that charting is performed uniformly by all health care providers.

Technical Detail Issues

Correct Film Identification and Care with Films

Although the concept of correctly identifying films and using care in filing films seems second nature, it is worth mentioning as a risk management tool. Liability has been imposed in cases based on the incorrect identification of films and mix-ups of films.

Film identification as to both patient identity and right and left orientation is extremely important and has become more troublesome with the advent of computerized radiography and digital radiography. Films must be correctly identified as to the patient. The imaging professional has the sole responsibility for ensuring that this is done, often by selecting the correct name from a computerized list of patients. The imaging professional is also responsible for ensuring that films are marked correctly for right and left orientation. With the advent of the new technologies, particularly digital radiography, the radiologist has virtually no way to know whether the orientation as to right or left is correct. It is the sole responsibility of the imaging professional to correctly mark digital radiographs, whether before or after exposure. Use of a uniform, consistent system to identify films will help eliminate errors that can lead to litigation in this area.

The mix-up of films is another area in which there is much litigation. This seems particularly important when films are removed from the department, often to be used as a guide during surgery. In Mississippi a $1.4 million verdict was awarded when brain surgery was done on the wrong patient because the MRI was switched with that of another patient.[16] A habit of routinely looking at the patient's identification each time the imaging professional views a film will help to prevent mix-ups and decrease risk in this area.

Timely Distribution of Reports

The delay or failure of a report to get to the appropriate physician is a common source of litigation in the radiology arena.[17,18] The imaging professional may play a variety of roles in the delivery of information, depending on how the department or facility is structured. In many small facilities and physicians' offices, the imaging professional helps with the process of distributing reports and makes the necessary phone calls regarding positive results to physicians. In almost every facility the radiologist sometimes asks the imaging professional to notify a physician by phone about an abnormal result and the need for further tests. Another issue in this area is the delivery of oral reports to other departments such as the emergency department, the operating room, or intensive care. The most effective way for the imaging professional to decrease risk in this area is documentation. The professional should always record that the report was delivered, to whom it was given, and the time and date and should initial this notation. If an oral report is being delivered, the contents of that report should also be documented in writing. This small step will prove valuable if litigation looms on the horizon.

Radiation Protection

The National Council on Radiation Protection and Measurements (NCRP) establishes policies and procedures regarding radiation exposure based on the phrase "as low as reasonably achievable" (ALARA). The NCRP states, "The primary goal is to keep radiation exposure of the individual well below a level at which adverse effects are likely to be observed during the individual's lifetime. Another objective is to minimize the incidence of genetic effects."[19] When ordering a radiographic procedure, the physician must weigh the benefits to be obtained against the risk of exposure.

Because radiation exposure is a risk, an important task for imaging professionals is the use of proper radiation protection to provide high-quality patient care and reduce litigation risk. Radiation protection education is essential in keeping exposures to patients ALARA.[19]

Methods of radiation protection are use of proper exposure factors, filtration, collimation, and shielding devices. Other methods that can be used to reduce the number of repeat exposures include restraining devices, technique charts, and a quality control program that ensures proper equipment performance. Repeat film analyses and clear policies concerning pregnant patients are also essential to keep radiation exposure ALARA.[19]

Instruction in radiation protection is part of the curricula of accredited educational facilities and is documented in student records. In addition, many states and medical facilities require continuing education in radiation protection on an established schedule.

Preventive maintenance and calibration performed routinely on equipment ensure that the radiation dose emitted is accurate and appropriate. State and federal agencies also inspect equipment periodically to verify that each piece has been properly maintained and calibrated and meets acceptable standards. Calibration of therapeutic radiation equipment is important and is performed by qualified radiation physicists in

IMAGING SCENARIO

A patient comes to the medical imaging department for a chest x-ray for suspected pneumonia. The routine questions regarding pregnancy are asked, and the patient says that she is sure she is not pregnant but does not remember the date of her last menstrual period. On the patient data form, she answers no to the pregnancy question but leaves the last menstrual period space blank. She signs the signature line. Posteroanterior (PA) and lateral chest x-rays are taken. Later the patient finds out that she was approximately 4 weeks pregnant when she underwent radiography. Her obstetrician calls the radiologist, concerned that the woman has had radiography and worried about possible harm to the fetus. The radiologist requests that the imaging technologist pull the films. The films demonstrate the collimation line, which shows that the beam was collimated to approximately ½ inch within all edges of the film. The documentation includes the patient's response to the pregnancy question.

Discussion questions
- Is the radiation dose to the fetus likely to be significant? Why or why not?
- Is the technologist or facility liable for negligently exposing a fetus to ionizing radiation?
- What else could have been done to protect the fetus? Would those measures have limited the risk of litigation?

accordance with state and federal agencies. Records of all preventive maintenance, calibration, and government inspections should be kept in the department.

Quality control and assurance programs are implemented in the imaging department to make certain that patients do not receive unnecessary radiation. These programs include repeated examination analysis, tracking of results, and measures to correct noticed problems. They also ensure that processing equipment is performing correctly and consistently. Consistently following policies and procedures for shielding and collimation helps to protect patients against unnecessary radiation. Pregnancy poses the greatest risk in this area. For this reason an imaging professional should always ask a female patient whether she may be pregnant and question her about the date of her last menstrual period.

If radiography of a pregnant patient is necessary, informed consent should be obtained and additional shielding should always be used. The informed consent procedure must include an explanation by a physician of the risks involved in exposing the fetus to ionizing radiation. This consent must be documented. (For further information about obtaining informed consent, see Chapter 4.)

Imaging professionals and therapeutic technologists must be diligent about radiation protection, both for the patient's benefit and from a risk management standpoint. Litigation arises from exposure issues. Two recent reported cases involved radiation overexposure. In one case a 300-pound man sustained a radiation burn on his lower back after fluoroscopy during a cardiac catheterization. The plaintiff was awarded $300,000.[20] The other case involved external beam therapy for anal cancer, which resulted in total fusion of the vagina. The defense denied any deviation from the standard of care, and the jury found for the defense.[21]

IMAGING SCENARIO

A patient falls on an uneven floor between the emergency and sonography departments. The sonographer tells the patient, "We keep waiting for them to fix that spot. Several other people have fallen, and we keep telling them to fix it." The sonographer takes the patient to the ultrasound room, performs the study, and returns the patient to the emergency department without relating the incident to anyone or filling out an incident report. The patient had complained only of a little swelling in her ankle.

Discussion questions
- Was the standard of care regarding incident reports followed?
- Were other standards not met?
- Did the statement by the sonographer have any impact on any liability issues?

Discussion

Any statement made regarding previous incidents resulting from the same hazard has a legal impact because such a statement establishes that the facility knew about the hazard and therefore breached its duty by failing to warn of the hazard or remedy it. If the patient was indeed injured in the fall, the facility would be liable for negligence. In addition, the facility would be liable for failing to follow policies and procedures for incident reporting and safety and for violating those standards of care.

Safety

Safety is an important concern in any health care facility, both in the provision of good-quality patient care and in the reduction of litigation risks. Larger facilities generally have comprehensive safety programs that include written policies and procedures regarding handling of hazardous materials, fire and electricity safety, emergency codes, back safety, patient transport and lifting techniques, infection control, occurrence reporting, and loss prevention. Most facilities use risk management guidelines as they develop these policies and procedures. JCAHO guidelines exist for safety programs, and institutional policies and procedures generally follow these guidelines.

Special attention should be paid to the transporting of patients from wheelchair or cart to the x-ray, MRI, CT, ultrasound, or radiation therapy table. Litigation commonly arises because one technologist attempts to perform the transfer alone when two people are needed. In one recent case, transfer to an MRI table was blamed for brain damage and lumbar spine injury, resulting in a $200,000 judgment,[22] and in another the failure to provide a two-person lift to an x-ray table was alleged to cause a leg fracture and eventual death from pneumonia.[23]

Although smaller facilities may have fewer staff members to provide education regarding safety issues, the same safety standards must be met as those expected of larger facilities. Imaging professionals should know their facility's programs and be familiar with policies and procedures. If a safety issue arises while a patient is in the imaging department, the imaging professional is responsible for knowing the correct action to take. The department should keep records of attendance at safety instruction and in-service meetings.

If imaging professionals do not know whether their facilities offer safety programs, they should find out by asking supervisors until they get an appropriate answer. If no safety program exists, JCAHO guidelines EC1, 1.1-1.9 and EC2, 2.1-2.14 are excellent starting points.[15]

SUMMARY

- The values of beneficence and nonmaleficence have been respected since the time of the earliest health care providers who tried to provide a good by aiding the sick and injured. These values provide a system of checks and balances for providers and patients to aid in making decisions concerning medical care. To facilitate this decision-making process, the principle of double effect helps weigh the proportionality between good and evil consequences.
- Although both beneficence and nonmaleficence are necessary to patient autonomy, some differences exist between them. Beneficence is active, whereas nonmaleficence is passive; further differences are evident in the importance of the ways they are practiced.
- Conflict may arise between beneficence and nonmaleficence, and this often affects patient autonomy. Conflicts may occur when good intentions have negative consequences. They also may result from friction between the notion that all people deserve good health care and the reality of limited resources, power struggles, quality-of-life decisions, and surrogate obligations.
- By examining the medical indications, including the medical problem, its severity, the goals of the examination, the success probability, options for imaging procedures, and how the patient will benefit from the examination, the imaging professional will gather information needed for problem solving.
- The imaging professional and patient are both responsible for encouraging good and avoiding harm in the imaging process. Continuing education enhances the imaging professional's skills, and obtaining information concerning the procedure aids the patient in appropriate decision making.
- In any pluralistic society, the many interpretations of beneficence and nonmaleficence ensure that patient autonomy remains a source and cause of conflicts. These conflicts must be addressed to provide society with appropriate health care.
- The ethical concepts of beneficence and nonmaleficence, which are integrated into the legal standard of care for health care professionals, define the duty to do no harm and provide reasonable medical care.
- The legal standard of care is the degree of skill or care practiced by a reasonable professional practicing in the same field. The standard of care for imaging professionals is established through practice standards, educational requirements, and curricula developed for imaging professionals. It is an important consideration if negligence is alleged. If the appropriate standard of care is violated, liability may be imposed on both health care professionals and medical facilities.
- Negligence is an unintentional tort resulting from actions not intended to cause harm. For negligence to be proved, a duty to use reasonable care must exist, this duty must be breached, and harm must result from this breach. The existence of a duty and the determination of reasonable care may be established by statutes, previous judicial decisions, or appropriate standards of care.

- Health care providers have a special relationship with patients that involves a duty to follow the appropriate standard of care. If that standard is not followed, liability may ensue for the health care provider and medical facility. This is called *medical negligence* or *medical malpractice.* To establish medical negligence, a plaintiff must provide evidence of an applicable standard of care, demonstrate that the standard has been violated, show that an injury occurred, and prove that the injury was caused by the violation of the standard of care.

- Methods to ensure quality patient care and decrease risks include thorough and consistent documentation, attention to technical detail issues, radiation protection, and dedication to safety. Documentation forms are useful tools in ensuring consistent documentation; examples of information to be included on these forms have been provided in this chapter.

- Care must be taken in technical detail issues such as correct film identification with regard to patient identification and proper orientation, tracking of films to avoid mix-ups between films, and timely distribution of reports. Radiation protection must be diligently practiced, and safety issues must be a constant concern.

- The principles of beneficence and nonmaleficence also have an impact on patient consent, informed consent, advance directives, and surrogate decision makers. Legal issues concerning consent and informed consent are discussed in Chapter 4 in the context of patient autonomy. Legal issues regarding advance directives and surrogate decision makers are addressed in Chapter 6 in the context of choices about death and dying.

REFERENCES

1. Garrett TA, Baillie HW, Garrett RM: *Healthcare ethics, principles and problems*, ed 2, Englewood Cliffs, NJ, 1993, Prentice Hall.
2. Jonsen AR, Siegler M, Winslade WJ: *Clinical ethics: a practical approach to ethical decisions in clinical medicine*, ed 5, New York, 2002, McGraw-Hill.
3. *Bruni v. Tatsumi*, 346 N.E. 2d 673 (Ohio 1976).
4. American Society of Radiologic Technologists: *Practice standards for medical imaging and radiation therapy*, Albuquerque, 2006, Author.
5. Joint Review Committee on Education in Radiologic Technology: *Standards for an accredited educational program in radiologic sciences*, Chicago, 1996, Author.
6. *House of Representatives Bill 1426.* March 17, 2005.
7. Laska L (Ed): Bunionectomy performed on foot of diabetic, *Medical Malpractice Verdicts, Settlements & Experts*, no 37, May 2005.
8. Schwartz V, Kelly K, Partlett D: *Prosser, Wade, and Schwartz: cases and materials on torts*, ed 10, Westbury, NY, 2000, Foundation Press.
9. *Kennis v. Mercy Hospital Medical Center*, 491 N.W. 2d 161 (Iowa 1992).
10. Furrow BR, Greaney TL, Johnson SH, et al: *Health law: cases, materials and problems*, St Paul, Minn, 2004, West.
11. *Smith v. Weaver*, 407 N.W. 2d 174 (Neb. 1987).
12. Laska L (Ed): Man claims hip fracture from near-fall from gurney, *Medical Malpractice Verdicts, Settlements & Experts*, January 2005, p 37.
13. American Society of Radiologic Technologists, *Code of ethics*, Albuquerque, 2006, Author.
14. American Registry of Radiologic Technologists: *Code of ethics*, St Paul, Minn, 2005, Author.
15. Joint Commission on Accreditation of Healthcare Organizations: *Accreditation manual*, Chicago, 1994, Author.
16. Laska L (Ed): Man undergoes unnecessary brain surgery due to mix-up of MRI films, *Medical Malpractice Verdicts, Settlements & Experts*, April 2005, p 27.
17. Laska L (Ed): Failure to timely communicate finding of mass on spine from MRI, *Medical Malpractice Verdicts, Settlements & Experts*, July 2005, p 30.

18. Laska L (Ed): Failure to properly communicate MRI finding of stroke and blocked blood vessels, *Medical Malpractice Verdicts, Settlements & Experts*, January 2005, p 7.
19. Gurley LT, Callaway WJ: *Introduction to radiologic technology*, ed 6, St Louis, 2006, Mosby.
20. Laska L (Ed): Radiation burn from fluoroscopy used during cardiac catheterization, *Medical Malpractice Verdicts, Settlements & Experts*, November 2005, p 4.
21. Laska L (Ed): Fused vagina blamed on external beam radiation treatment for anal cancer, necessitating reconstruction, *Medical Malpractice Verdicts, Settlements & Experts*, October 2005, p 34.
22. Laska L (Ed): Collapse during transfer from bed to MRI table blamed for brain damage and lumbar spine injury, *Verdicts, Settlements & Experts*, June 2005, p 18.
23. Laska L (Ed): Failure to provide two-person lift to x-ray table, *Medical Malpractice Verdicts, Settlements & Experts*, September 2005, p 21.

REVIEW QUESTIONS

1 Beneficence involves which of the following?
   a. Active participation of the imaging professional
   b. Doing good
   c. Preventing harm
   d. All of the above

2 Nonmaleficence occurs when which of the following takes place?
   a. Good is done
   b. Evil is avoided
   c. Evil is done
   d. Good is avoided

3 Which of the following is a contractual agreement?
   a. Demonstration of a procedure
   b. Good intentions
   c. Informed consent processes
   d. None of the above

4 The strongest action is _____, or the avoidance of harm; _____ is weaker and concerns the doing of good.

5 What four conditions are used in the principle of double effect to assess the proportionality of good and evil in an action?
   a. _____
   b. _____
   c. _____
   d. _____

6 **True or False** Taking part in continuing education and performing risk management procedures help ensure high-quality imaging procedures for the patient.

7 Gathering information about imaging procedures is a method of participation for _____ in their health care.

8 Conflicts arise between _____ and _____ and may affect patient autonomy.

9 Explain why beneficence and nonmaleficence are important to the imaging professional. Explain the differences between them.

10 Give an example of an act of beneficence and an act of nonmaleficence in imaging services.

11 Which is more important: the doing of good or the avoidance of harm? In what way did you arrive at that conclusion?

12 In what way does the patient exercise personal responsibility over the proportionality of beneficence and nonmaleficence involved in the imaging procedure?

13 _____ and _____ agreements help provide patient autonomy.

14 If in doubt, the patient should seek a _____ _____.

15 **True or False**   Medical indications involving the principles of beneficence and nonmaleficence include the goals of the imaging procedure and the probabilities of success.

16 The standard of care for professionals is:
   a. Their yearly job evaluation
   b. The degree of skill or care employed by a reasonable professional practicing in the same field
   c. Their job description
   d. The average amount imaging professionals are paid

17 The standard of care for imaging professionals is established through:
   a. Educational requirements
   b. Curricula for the imaging sciences
   c. Practice standards
   d. All of the above

18 **True or False**   If you are asked to do an imaging job you have not been trained for, you do not need to worry about liability.

19 In a lawsuit, decisions regarding the appropriate standard of care and violations of those standards are made:
   a. By the testimony of the injured party
   b. By the judge
   c. By the testimony of the alleged negligent actor
   d. By expert testimony

20 **True or False**   A mistake by an imaging professional that harms a patient can create liability for negligence.

21 For negligence to be proved, which of these elements must be proved?
   a. A duty is owed
   b. A duty owed is breached
   c. Harm resulted from the duty being breached
   d. All of the above

22 For medical negligence to be proved, which of the following elements must be proved?
   a. The standard of care for the health care provider was breached
   b. The patient sustained harm
   c. The harm resulted from the breach of standard of care
   d. All of the above

23 **True or False**   The special relationship between health care providers and patients eliminates the need for a plaintiff to prove that a duty of care exists.

24 Which of the following is not a source of the standards of care?
   a. Institutional guidelines
   b. Federal and state statutes
   c. Advice of co-workers
   d. JCAHO guidelines

25 National Patient Safety Goals include the following:
   a. Patient identification
   b. Communication among caregivers
   c. Medication safety
   d. All of the above

26 **True or False**   Imaging professionals do not need to pay attention to the National Patient Safety Goals because they do not pertain to imaging.

27 Documentation is done to:
   a. Create a record of an event
   b. Help witnesses remember the events of an occurrence
   c. Assist in defending a medical malpractice case
   d. All of the above

28 Documentation can decrease litigation risks by:
   a. Providing an accurate record of what occurred
   b. Correlating facts related by witnesses
   c. Holding damages down
   d. a and c

29 Which of the following is not a method to decrease risk?
   a. Marking films correctly
   b. Following safety regulations
   c. Taking your lunch break on time
   d. Using proper collimation

30 **True or False**   Quality-of-life determinations, patient autonomy, and justice in health care delivery all require decisions involving beneficence and nonmaleficence.

31 **True or False**   The imaging professional and the patient are not both responsible for health care decision making.

CRITICAL THINKING *Questions & Activities*

1 Cite two or three routinely performed imaging procedures that involve the weighing of good and evil. Why do these procedures require this consideration? Ask other imaging professionals whether they agree.

2 Create a table of specific imaging procedures (e.g., barium enemas, intravenous pyelography) that have good and evil consequences. List these goods and evils and determine situations in which one outweighs the other. Discuss this system with your classmates.

3 Discuss the active and passive omission that occurred in the imaging scenario concerning the pregnant patient. Who bears the fault in this situation? Where would you place the blame? Discuss this scenario with your imaging manager.

CRITICAL THINKING *Questions & Activities —cont'd*

4 Consider an imaging situation in which ethical principles seem to conflict with one another. How would you determine the correct action? To initiate this activity, one person should present to the group an imaging situation offering possible good and bad consequences for the patient. Each person should then list the good and bad consequences. After all the individual lists are completed, the participants should read their lists aloud; a facilitator can record each good or bad consequence. The goods and bads should then be weighed, and a discussion of proportionality should follow. Do the goods outweigh the bads or vice versa? This exercise may help you develop a method of decision making concerning ethical dilemmas.

5 List several factors involved in determining the imaging professional's obligation to the patient. Compare with classmates' lists.

6 Discuss ways in which you can limit the chance of making mistakes that could cause liability for medical negligence.

7 Discuss the venogram legal scenario. Does the documentation form in your department cover these issues?

8 Discuss the different outcomes in the pregnancy legal scenario if the collimation lines were not visible on the film.

9 Discuss whether you are well informed about safety issues. If a fire were to break out in your department and you had a patient on the table and several waiting, what should you do? What if the fire is in another area of the hospital? What do you do if a patient slips and falls while in your care? What should you do if you notice a leaking ceiling while on your way out of the hospital?

3 CARING AND COMMUNICATION

Your character is constantly radiating, communicating. From it, in
the long run, I come to instinctively trust or distrust you and
your efforts with me.

STEPHEN COVEY

Chapter Outline

Ethical Issues
Definition of Caring
Professional Care
Examples of Caring and Communication

Legal Issues
Health Literacy
Caring

Learning Objectives

After completing this chapter, the reader will be able to perform the following:

- Identify the nature of care and its ethical and legal implications.
- Provide examples of the impact of communication on imaging.
- Define human care, professional care, and communication.
- Explain care and communication as a context for imaging practice.

- Develop a more caring and communicative demeanor.
- Identify what health literacy is and how it affects imaging.
- Implement the legal aspects of caring and communication.

Key Terms

caring
existential care
health literacy
professional care

Professional Profile

While practicing and teaching radiologic technology for more than four decades, I have observed the results of both ethical and unethical conduct. We are not perfect; mistakes occur. But an informed commitment to ethical principles greatly diminishes the likelihood of errors.

I have served as an expert witness in several cases of medical malpractice that involved unfortunate incidents in medical imaging departments. In one case a patient suffered permanent, incapacitating brain damage because of administration of the wrong intravenous fluid in an emergency situation. This could have been avoided if the technologist had followed orders and obtained the correct solution. A second opportunity to avoid this same error was missed because of incomplete and unvalidated communication between the technologist and the physician.

It is clear that communication is both vitally important and potentially perilous in the practice of health care. Those who are guilty of gossip, thoughtless sharing of confidential information, inaccurate reporting, or incorrect medical recording often cause serious consequences for the patient as well as professional or legal problems for themselves. I participated in another case in which the family of a patient who died of natural causes sued the hospital based on careless, unfounded remarks by a technologist, which were overheard in the imaging department.

We are all tempted to take shortcuts when we are in a hurry, but lack of compliance with safety procedures places both the patient and the imaging professional at risk. I have been called to consult in two cases where patients were injured in imaging departments because of falls. In both situations, injuries occurred when technologists were rushed and failed to make the effort to be careful. Because they were preoccupied with their own concerns, they did not place a high value on the well-being and protection of their patients.

When providing testimony about the actions of an imaging professional, I compare the person's actions to the code of ethics of the applicable professional organization. I also review the organizational policies and procedures that relate to the situation. Patients rightfully expect their health care providers to be educated in ethical principles and aware of the rules that apply to their care. When principles and rules are not conscientiously applied, unmet expectations raise concerns and resentments, even when no harm is done. These resentments increase the likelihood of a lawsuit. When patients have confidence in those who care for them, lawsuits are rare.

Ruth Ann Ehrlich, RT(R)
Senior Instructor, Radiology
Western States Chiropractic College
Portland, Oregon

ETHICAL ISSUES

Caring and communication are essential for life and growth; they are crucial ingredients in the imaging professional's ability to serve the needs of self and others. Caring and communication require the developmental strengths of trust, autonomy, initiative, identity, justice, industry, and intimacy, all of which play a role in discussions of ethics and ethical problem solving for the imaging professional.[1]

Health care professionals, including imaging professionals, refer to the therapy and other services they provide in their practices as *care. Care is shown to the patient through appropriate communication.* Therefore caring and communication are the primary tasks of the imaging professional. A caring attitude should influence the imaging professional's feelings and ethical problem solving arising from interactions and communication with patients. This chapter defines caring and communication, describes their ethical implications for imaging practice, and provides methods to help the imaging professional develop a more caring and communicative demeanor.

Eleanor McMartin explains that the imaging professional plays an important role in maintaining patient autonomy by projecting a caring attitude through appropriate communication.

DEFINITION OF CARING

CARING
Caring is a function of the whole person in which concern for the growth and well-being of another is expressed in an integrated application of the mind, body, and spirit that seeks to maximize positive outcomes.

Caring is defined as a function in which a person expresses concern for the growth and well-being of another in an integrated application of the mind, body, and spirit designed to maximize positive outcomes. Expressions of caring include feelings of compassion and concern, a philosophy of commitment, an ethical approach to problems, altruistic acts, conscious attention to the needs and wishes of others, protection of the well-being of others, nurturing of growth, and empathy and advocacy. Because caring plays such a vital role in human interaction, an appreciation of caring is fundamental to an understanding of human nature.[2]

Such activities as listening, providing information, helping, communicating, and showing respect are expressions of caring.[3] Other caring activities include touching, nurturing, supporting, and protecting (Box 3-1).[4] Caring is a universal phenomenon, although expressions, processes, and patterns may vary among cultures.[5]

EXISTENTIAL CARE
Existential care is compassion arising from an awareness of common bonds of humanity and common expressions, fates, and feelings.

Caring is essential in the development of the imaging professional.[6] Radiographers must be caring individuals, part scientist and part humanist. Humanism entails the provision of **existential care**, a more abstract form of care arising from an awareness of common bonds of humanity and common expressions, fates, and feelings.[7] Care may occur as a product of the rapport between imaging professionals and patients. Unfortunately, this is not always the case[8]:

> In radiology, particularly, the administrative focus is on reducing costs by increasing productivity. The efficiency of virtually every radiology department in this country is based on how many exams its technologists can complete per hour. This emphasis on speed means that radiologic technologists often must spend less time than they would like getting to know each patient. This can have a detrimental effect on patient satisfaction. Patients who are treated like bodies on a mechanized production line are bound to go somewhere else the next time they need health care. Patients who perceive a lack of genuine concern and empathy are the first to complain about their care and ask for their records to be transferred to another facility.

BOX 3-1	**EXPRESSIONS OF CARING**
Advocacy	Courage
Altruism	Ethical behavior
Commitment	Monitoring
Compassion	Nurturing
Concern	Protection

Empathy and Empathetic Care

The empathetic imaging professional is sensitive to the needs of others and strives to meet those needs. Building a respectful rapport between the health care provider and the patient portrays the ability of the provider to connect as a human being.

The connection must not merely be a reaction to the patient's distress. Empathy is not sympathizing or feeling sorry for the patient. It is a constructive and objective response that allows the imaging professional to provide high-quality patient care.

Communication

Communication is a symbolic interaction: when one person says something to another and that person responds. There has to be at least one response to one initiation, creating a tie of communication. Human communication is how an individual interacts with another. This may be through symbolic interaction or language or both. It is transactional and affective in nature. Human communication is not static, and it involves human feelings and attitudes, as well as the delivery of information. Health communication is narrower in scope than human communication. It is a subset of human communication that is concerned with how individuals in a society seek to maintain health and deal with health-related issues.

The key elements of communication regarding imaging are the speaker or sender (the imaging professional), the language spoken or body language (explaining the procedure and asking for information), the environment (the imaging department), listening (to the patient or to peers, physicians, etc.), and feedback from the receivers.

Care as an Ideal

Philosophically, care is an ideal analogous to beauty, truth, and justice; although it is sought after, it can never be fully attained or perfect in human expression. Imaging professionals are not capable of providing perfect care. In striving for the ideal, however, the imaging professional may occasionally come close to achieving it and in so doing provide great benefits for the patient. One danger in discussing ideals is viewing them as achievable and measurable commodities; this leads to the idea that those who fall short of achieving ideal care should be ashamed.[7] This misperception may lead imaging professionals who consider caring to be a vital part of their professional practice to feel guilty, selfish, or discouraged when they are unable to give more time to their patients.[9]

Obstacles to Caring

Imaging professionals face a variety of obstacles to providing caring treatment:
- Scarcity of time
- Technical priorities
- Impact of personal life
- Lack of training in caring for patients who are critically or terminally ill
- Lack of communication
- Societal pressures
- Lack of faith in self

All these obstacles lend themselves to personal and professional ethical dilemmas. Imaging professionals who feel inadequate as a result of any of these obstacles may have difficulty feeling or expressing caring.

EMPATHY
Empathy is the ability to recognize and to some extent share the emotions and state of mind of another and to understand the meaning and significance of that person's behavior.

IMAGING SCENARIO

A patient who has a family history of breast cancer and has found a lump in her breast arrives at a mammography imaging center. She is frightened and emotional. She has read a great deal of literature about breast cancer and knows it is one of the leading causes of death in women. Her mother and sister died painful deaths at early ages, and she is frantic to learn her diagnosis. The breast imaging center has been informed that it needs to complete procedures more rapidly to allow a greater number of mammograms to be performed per day. This pressure for speed has elevated the stress of the mammographers. Moreover, unexpected emergencies and procedures that call for additional views have been causing backups in the waiting room, increasing the anxiety of patients anticipating their examinations. Such a backup occurs on the day the patient arrives, and by the time her procedure begins, she is almost hysterical and has difficulty following the mammographer's directions. Her inability to hold still and endure the compression necessitates retakes of the films. By the time the woman is finished with the examination, she is angry and vows never to return to the breast imaging center. Her anger may even prevent her from following through with future mammograms.

Discussion questions
- What problems have occurred in this scenario?
- Whose problems are they, and what are the possible solutions?
- What impact has caring and communication or the lack of either had on the ethical dilemma facing the mammographer?

Obstacles to Communication

Obstacles to communication also exist and are intertwined with the obstacles to caring. Some obstacles may come from the sender or the receiver. If the patient or the imaging professional is thinking about other things, this may interrupt the flow of communication in the information-gathering process. Noise, temperature, or other distractions in the imaging environment may present an obstacle in the communication process. Distance and the inability to see or hear are obvious obstacles between the imaging professional and the patient. The relationship between the patient and imaging professional as it is affected by roles, personalities, values, and ethical differences may also influence the communication process.

PROFESSIONAL CARE

PROFESSIONAL CARE
Professional care is the application of the knowledge of a discipline, including its science, theory, practice, and art.

Professional care is characterized by the application of the knowledge of a professional discipline, including its science, theory, practice, and art. It is complementary to human caring. Imaging professionals must possess human caring before they are able to provide professional caring. Human and professional caring are both activities of the whole person (although activities are only a portion of caring). The interaction of compassion, knowledge, and the experiences and emotions of the whole person gives rise to human and professional caring.[7]

Clearly, professional expertise unaccompanied by human compassion is not enough to serve all the needs of the patient: "If we fail to motivate that feeling (empathy and compassion) and the earnest desire within our student to help our fellow man, we will have created the equivalent of human robots."[10] Such an emphasis on skill at the expense of caring and empathy produces a "patient care gap" in which the patient is ignored as the "scale tips toward science and technique."[11]

Caring in the Imaging Sciences

The professional and human caring practiced by imaging professionals is based on individual and institutional values. Adherence to a set of values and the use of ethical problem solving help the imaging professional to develop a more caring demeanor. The three strengthen one another. Without values, caring and ethics in the imaging health care environment are without foundation and force. In turn, a strong commitment to caring requires a fusion of feeling, thought, and action, all of which aid the technologist in coping with stress and solving problems ethically. Taken together, caring, values, and ethical problem solving give meaning to professional practice, create the possibility of ever-improving care, and enhance patient comfort and feelings of safety.[2] For example, cardiac ultrasonographers who have the ability to make their patients comfortable find them more willing to comply with directions, leading to an examination with greater diagnostic success.

Caring brings together all the resources of the imaging professional. When imaging professionals care for patients by performing imaging procedures, monitoring equipment, and meeting patient needs, they do more than provide therapy; they become a part of the patient's life.

Caring in the imaging sciences also involves an appreciation of the universal patterns of human experience. As imaging students enter educational programs, they are exposed through their patients to the universality of pain, loneliness, suffering, fear, and looming death. Human caring and professional caring require compassion for the suffering endured by patients and an understanding of the ways in which people construct and draw meaning from their lives. This unending activity of inventing, restructuring, and reinterpreting is universal, even though the outcomes are personal. Compassionate imaging professionals respond to the universal appeal made by suffering human beings by caring. The potential for this response is also universal.[7]

Imaging professionals see patients in all phases of life and all conditions of health and disease. Because the nature of their practice requires care for a diverse patient population, imaging educational programs incorporate classes to develop skills in caring. Professionals in other modalities, however, may not have as much continued and direct contact with a wide variety of patients and therefore may not be as prepared to care. This disparity may be an obstacle to providing the safe, comfortable environment patients require.

Careful monitoring of radiologic equipment is an activity that shows caring by ensuring the autonomy, comfort, and safety of the patient. Quality control specialists exhibit caring by spending as much time as necessary monitoring imaging machinery. Imaging professionals also show caring for their patients by ensuring confidentiality, obtaining informed consent, thoroughly explaining procedures, and taking complete and accurate histories. Nuclear medicine technologists exhibit human and professional caring

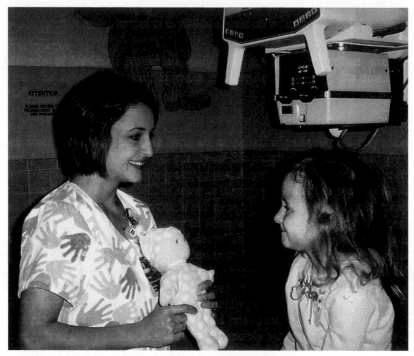

FIGURE 3-1 A caring demeanor can be expressed through helping, nurturing, and offering support.
From Gurley L, Callaway W: *Introduction to radiologic technology*, ed 6, St Louis, 2006, Elsevier.

by explaining the significance of the radioactive material being injected into a patient receiving a therapeutic dose.

Developing a More Caring Demeanor

Caring is an attitude that may be developed and learned (Figure 3-1). Courses in professional caring have been part of the radiologic sciences curriculum for some time. Education in human caring and human relations skills, however, is a somewhat newer addition. To enhance caring, imaging professionals must strengthen and integrate their mental, physical, and spiritual capacities. By learning all they can about professional practice and human interaction, loving more, and being more creative and generous in spirit, imaging professionals can improve their ability to evaluate and solve ethical and technical problems. Self-analysis and rating of caring abilities provide further insights into strengths and weaknesses in caring.

Imaging programs can use a variety of means to instill a desire to increase caring skills in students:

- Communications classes that address body language and the importance of listening
- Critical thinking classes that focus on recognizing, analyzing, and evaluating ethical dilemmas
- Discussions of films that illustrate caring scenarios (e.g., *The Doctor*)
- Empathy rotations that require students to become patients for a day and participate in a variety of imaging patient activities

- Role modeling by instructors and staff technologists, including student evaluation
- Discussions among classmates about experiences with hospitalization and health care providers, emphasizing the ways in which caring influences outcomes
- A review of patient interviews in which care needs are identified and the department's response to those needs is evaluated
- Review and discussion of educational and professional materials dealing with issues of caring

Improving Communication

Not only must imaging professionals evaluate their caring and improve this all-important ability, they also must continue to improve their communication skills. To do this, they must want to objectively evaluate and change their communication styles. The next step is trying to change. Active listening is an important key to improving communication between the imaging professional and the patient. Active listening requires not only hearing the patient, but also watching the patient's body language, observing the patient's physical presentation, asking open-ended questions, and waiting for responses and feedback from the patient. The true active listener strives to recognize and understand the patient's needs. Investment of time and effort is imperative in the ongoing improvement of communication in imaging.

EXAMPLES OF CARING AND COMMUNICATION

Each of the following scenarios provides an illustration of caring and communication. They demonstrate the ways in which this essential human quality is finely honed by professional training and expressed humanly rather than perfectly. The scenarios depict imaging professionals engaged with the whole of their professional knowledge, as well as their human spirit.[12]

IMAGING SCENARIO

Jane Smith is a radiographer in charge of portable imaging, and one of her patients is a young man who is an illegal immigrant. He was in a car accident and has a serious head injury. He has no family in the United States. The patient has been unconscious since his accident. Smith is quite concerned about the well-being of this patient, and though she does not condone his illegal status, she does not feel it is relevant to the situation. She realizes that she must monitor every change in the patient's condition when she is taking his radiographs. She watches all the monitoring equipment carefully. She also uses all her physical assessment skills to detect any complications that may arise. She talks to him in an attempt to stimulate his mind and penetrate his coma while performing radiographic procedures. He cannot talk to her, however, and may not even be aware of her care. Nonetheless, the imaging professional feels it is her duty to use her whole person on behalf of the patient's well-being ... to care.

Discussion questions
- What else could the imaging professional do to communicate with the patient?
- How could she provide the maximum support for the patient's autonomy?

Modified from Creasia JL, Parker B: *Conceptual foundations: the bridge to professional nursing practice,* ed 3, St Louis, 2001, Mosby.

IMAGING SCENARIO

Mike Jones, a radiation therapist, is the primary therapist for a 53-year-old grand-mother who has advanced cancer. She is in pain and aware that her prognosis is poor. While Jones is positioning her, she says to him, "Are you a religious man, Mike?" Actually, Jones does not consider himself a particularly religious man, and furthermore he has a great deal to do this morning. He is inwardly annoyed at being called on to enter into this patient's suffering. This morning, at least, he would rather attend to other things. He is a human being and not capable of providing perfect care. However, he recognizes that religion is not the issue here; rather, the patient is seeking a human connection and comfort in her fear.

Jones sits down beside the patient to signal his intention to be fully present for her and enter into her experience, not because he plans to stay a long time. Human interaction need not always take a long time. Speaking truthfully, he says, "My own religion has its ups and downs—does yours provide you some comfort now?" The question is gentle and undemanding. The patient may choose to speak briefly about her religion and remain silent about other concerns. However, she may also choose to accept and respond to his gentle acknowledgment of her need for comfort. She replies, "I know that I haven't much longer to live. I long to watch my grandson grow up a bit longer and offer more support to his parents. My comfort is in knowing that the Lord does things in His own good time and that He will provide for my children." Jones takes her hand for a moment and says, "Your faith that the Lord will provide for your children seems a comfort to you now indeed." His answer is brief and tacitly accepting of everything she has said. He waits to see if she needs any further support, and she pats his hand and says, "Well, you have others to take care of. Thank you so much."

Discussion questions
- If the radiographer is not a religious person, how can he comfort and communicate with this patient concerning her situation?
- What other hospital personnel could be called on to help this patient?
- What types of educational activities could help prepare a student imaging professional for this type of situation?

Modified from Creasia JL, Parker B: *Conceptual foundations: the bridge to professional nursing practice,* ed 3, St Louis, 2001, Mosby.

LEGAL ISSUES

Caring and communication are the cornerstone of the art of medicine. When the relationship between care provider and patient is marked by mutual trust and open communication, a major step has been taken toward patient satisfaction. Evidence shows that clear, two-way conversation is a key element in the prevention of patient dissatisfaction and malpractice claims. This section discusses health literacy, the lack of which causes almost half the population to be unable to understand what their health care provider is telling them. Once imaging professionals understand health literacy and its impact on the profession, they will understand that inability to communicate health care information effectively to patients has implications for risk management and litigation.

HEALTH LITERACY

A serious and growing problem is affecting the ability of health professionals to deliver care: low levels of **health literacy**. To quote the movie *Cool Hand Luke*, "What we have here is a failure to communicate."

Health literacy is the ability to read, understand, and act on health care information in order to make effective health care decisions and follow instructions for treatment. Many factors contribute to a person's health literacy, but the most common is the individual's general literacy, or ability to read, write, and understand written material. Other factors include the person's amount of experience with the health care system, the complexity of the information being presented to the person, cultural factors that may influence decision making, and the way the material is communicated.[13]

Research in adult literacy has been done mainly in general literacy. The most recent data available come from the 2003 National Assessment of Adult Literacy (NAAL), which measured the English literacy of America's adults.[14] Participants in this assessment were scored at four levels according to their ability to understand prose, documents, and quantitative data (Table 3-1).

At the lowest level of literacy skills, termed Below Basic, individuals possess only the most simple and concrete literacy skills. This level, when averaging the components of prose, document, and quantitative testing, represents 16% of the adult population.

At the second level, termed Basic, individuals possess only skills necessary to perform simple and everyday literacy activities. This level, when averaging the components of prose, document, and quantitative testing, represents 28% of the adult population.

Together, the Below Basic and Basic Levels include 44% of the population, almost half of U.S. adults. What this means is that one out of five American adults reads at or below the fifth-grade level and the average American reads at the eighth- to ninth-grade level. Yet most health care materials are written above the tenth-grade level. In contrast, persons at NAAL levels of Intermediate or Proficient have sufficient literacy skills to permit full functioning in society.

Imaging professionals commonly see patients who have trouble reading and understanding health information. If almost half of the adult U.S. population has limited or marginal general literacy skills, these individuals are likely to have limited health literacy skills as well. Even persons with adequate literacy skills may have trouble understanding and applying health care information, especially when it is explained in unfamiliar technical terms. Patients may be articulate and appear well educated and knowledgeable, yet fail to grasp disease concepts or understand how to carry out medication regimens properly.[13] The patient's inability to understand may not be obvious to the health professional. Patients are generally under stress and concerned about their health when receiving medical information, which exacerbates their inability to take in this information.

The Institute of Medicine, in their 2003 report "Priority Areas for National Action: Transforming Health Care Quality,"[15] has identified health literacy and self-management as a priority area for national action in transforming health care. John Nelson, MD, then president-elect of the American Medical Association, said, "Limited health literacy is a huge obstacle standing between millions of America's patients and the health care they need."[16] Because low health literacy has been identified as a barrier to good care, the American Medical Association Foundation and other organizations have done much work to improve the way health care providers communicate with patients.

HEALTH LITERACY
Health literacy is the ability to read, understand, and act on health care information to make effective health care decisions and follow instructions for treatment.

TABLE 3-1 **OVERVIEWS OF THE LITERACY LEVELS IN THE NATIONAL ASSESSMENT OF ADULT LITERACY**

Level and Definition	Key Abilities Associated with Level	Sample Tasks Typical of Level
Below Basic Indicates no more than the simple and concrete literacy skills Average score 215*	Locating easily identifiable information in short, commonplace prose texts Locating easily identifiable information and following written instructions in simple documents such as charts and forms Locating numbers and using them to perform simple quantitative operations, such as addition, when the mathematical information is very concrete and familiar	Searching a short, simple text to find out what a patient is allowed to drink before a medical test Signing a form Adding the amounts on a bank deposit form
Basic Indicates skills necessary to perform simple and everyday literacy activities Average score 242*	Reading and understanding information in short, commonplace prose texts Reading and understanding information in simple documents Locating easily identifiable quantitative information and using it to solve simple one-step problems when the arithmetic operation is specified or easily identifiable	Finding in a pamphlet for prospective jurors an explanation of how people were selected for the jury pool Using a television guide to find out what programs are on at a specific time Comparing the ticket prices for two events
Intermediate Indicates skills necessary to perform moderately challenging literacy activities Average score 304*	Reading and understanding moderately dense, less commonplace prose texts as well as summarizing, making simple inferences, determining cause and effect, and recognizing the author's purpose Locating information in dense, complex documents and making simple inferences about the information Locating less familiar quantitative information and using it to solve problems when the arithmetic operation is not specified or easily inferred	Consulting reference materials to determine which foods contain a particular vitamin Identifying a specific location on a map Calculating the total cost of ordering specific office supplies from a catalog

Modified from Hauser RM, Edley CF, Koenig JA, Elliott SW (Eds): *Measuring literacy: performance levels for adults, interim report,* Washington, DC, 2005, National Academics Press; and White S, Dillow S: *Key concepts and features of the 2003 National Assessment of Adult Literacy (NCES 2006-471),* Washington, DC, US Department of Education, National Center for Educational Statistics.

*Average score is the average of the Prose, Document, and Quantitative scores for each level.

TABLE 3-1   **OVERVIEWS OF THE LITERACY LEVELS IN THE NATIONAL ASSESSMENT
OF ADULT LITERACY—cont'd**

Level and Definition	Key Abilities Associated with Level	Sample Tasks Typical of Level
Proficient Indicates skills necessary to perform more complex and challenging literacy activities Average score 420*	Reading lengthy, complex, abstract prose texts, as well as synthesizing information and making complex inferences Integrating, synthesizing, and analyzing multiple pieces of information located in complex documents Locating more abstract quantitative information and using it to solve multistep problems when the arithmetic operations are not easily inferred and the problems are more complex Stating in writing an argument made in a lengthy newspaper article	Comparing viewpoints in two editorials Interpreting a table about blood pressure, age, and physical activity Computing and comparing the cost per ounce of food.

Imaging professionals must communicate with patients to obtain maximal results. They can benefit from tips to communicate better and be assured that patients understand (Box 3-2).[13] These ideas are simple to implement and can make a huge difference in patients' level of understanding. In addition to the suggestions in the box, others include sitting down to talk with the patient, making eye contact, and establishing that the patient can hear the health professional. When the teach back method is used, it should be done in a way that does not intimidate the patient. Examples of questions to ask are, "When you get home, what are you going to tell your wife you have to do to get ready for this exam?" and "Can you tell me when you are to come back for your next film?" The professional can also note his or her responsibility for the communication by saying something like, "I'm not sure I did a very good job explaining. Why don't you tell me what you understand?" Patients should never be asked, "Do you understand?" because they will always say yes and the health provider will have no idea what it is they understood.

Legal Side of Health Literacy

Poor communication between patients and clinicians is a major factor leading to malpractice lawsuits. In fact, attorneys estimate that a clinician's communication style and attitude are important factors in nearly 75% of malpractice suits.[17] The most frequently identified communication errors are inadequately explaining diagnosis or treatment and communicating in such a way that patients feel that their concerns have been ignored (Box 3-3).[13]

Although the data in the preceding paragraph were gathered for physicians, they hold true for all health care providers who deal with patients. Few hospitalized patients complete their stay without having some contact with the imaging department. In addition, a steady flow of outpatients go through the imaging department. Imaging professionals have the opportunity and the responsibility to improve interpersonal communication with patients. By doing so, they will also be decreasing risk for themselves and their facility.

BOX 3-2	SIX STEPS TO IMPROVE INTERPERSONAL COMMUNICATION WITH PATIENTS

1. Slow down. Communication can be improved by speaking slowly and by spending just a small amount of additional time with each patient. This will help foster a patient-centered approach to the clinician-patient interaction.
2. Use plain, nonmedical language. Explain things to patients as you would to a family member.
3. Show or draw pictures. Visual images can improve patients' recall of ideas.
4. Limit the amount of information provided, and repeat it. Information is best remembered when it is given in small pieces that are pertinent to the tasks at hand. Repetition further enhances recall.
5. Use the teach back or show me technique. Confirm that patients understand by asking them to repeat back your instructions.
6. Create a shame-free environment. Make patients feel comfortable asking questions. Enlist the aid of others (patient's family, friends) to promote understanding.

From Weiss B: *Health literacy: a manual for clinicians,* Chicago, 2003, American Medical Association Foundation and American Medical Association.

BOX 3-3	CLINICIAN-PATIENT COMMUNICATION PROBLEMS INVOLVED IN MALPRACTICE LAWSUITS

Explanation of diagnosis is inadequate.
Explanation of treatment is inadequate.
Patient feels ignored.
Clinician fails to understand perspective of patient or relatives.
Clinician discounts or devalues views of patients or relatives.
Patient feels rushed.

Data from Vincent C, Young M, Phillips A: Why do people sue doctors? A study of patients and relatives taking legal action, *Lancet* 343:1609, 1994; Hickson GB, Clayton EW, Githena PB, Sloan FA: Factors that prompted families to file medical malpractice claims following perinatal injuries, *JAMA* 267:1359, 1992; and Hickson GB, Clayton EW, Entman SS, et al: Obstetricians' prior malpractice experience and patient satisfaction with care, *JAMA* 272:1583, 1994.

CARING

Caring may not appear to be a topic with many legal implications, and strictly speaking this is true. A review of the many legal issues previously discussed, however, reveals that patient care does indeed have legal aspects. No federal or state statutes define or mandate caring; no complainant will attempt to make a prima facie case of "not caring." Because of this lack of legal guidance, imaging professionals must use a commonsense approach when caring for patients. Patients are more likely to file a malpractice suit when they are unhappy with the "care" they received, so caring has a practical aspect.

Researchers from Harvard University reviewed more than 31,000 New York hospital records from 1984 to determine the incidence of injuries resulting from medical negligence.[17] This study found that the incidence of adverse events caused by negligence during hospitalizations in New York in 1984 was 3.7%. In studying the litigation data for the same year, the researchers also found that 8 times as many patients suffered an injury from negligence as filed a malpractice suit, and that about 16 times as many patients suffered an injury from negligence as received compensation. Another study of 645 physicians from 1992 to 1998 found a direct correlation between malpractice suits and unsolicited patient complaints, indicating patient dissatisfaction.[18]

The preceding data indicate that most patients injured as a result of negligence do not file malpractice claims. Patient dissatisfaction, however, is a major factor linked with the filing of medical malpractice claims. In general, patients do not consult an attorney unless they are unhappy with the "care" they receive.

Caring, then, may be the single most important thing the imaging professional can do to minimize the risk of litigation. Imaging professionals can do their best to ensure that their patients understand the procedures and are able to give truly informed consent. Imaging professionals can also do their best to follow procedures with the goal of obtaining maximal studies, providing minimal radiation exposure, and keeping patients safe.

Probably the most important benefit gained in caring for patients is the patient's knowledge of the professional's care. As stated earlier in this chapter, imaging professionals must be part scientist, part humanist. Imaging professionals who share their humanist side with patients by caring not only communicate compassion but also go a long way toward minimizing the risks of litigation.

IMAGING SCENARIO

A 40-year-old man who was injured on the job is brought to the emergency room with a fractured pelvis and internal injuries. He is conscious and is scheduled to have a vascular examination. The radiologist speaks to the patient and obtains informed consent. The imaging professional, in trying to explain exactly what the patient will be experiencing, has some reservations about whether the patient really understands what is happening. However, the schedule that day is swamped, the patient is obviously severely injured and needs a diagnosis for treatment, the special procedure room is open, the consent form has been signed, and the radiologist and staff are ready to begin the procedure. During the vascular examination the patient suffers heart failure and cannot be revived.

At a later date the family questions the informed consent process and brings suit against the hospital and the imaging professional. It is brought into evidence that the deceased patient was hard of hearing and could not read. The family believes that his inability to understand and recognize the danger of the vascular procedure was a deciding factor in his death. They also believe that the persons involved in the consent process should have recognized this and dealt with the informational procedure in another manner.

Discussion questions
- How does health literacy enter into this situation? Were there signs the physician and imaging professional should have seen indicating that the patient did not understand?
- What were the obstacles to caring and communication?
- What ethical and legal dilemmas were involved in this unfortunate situation?
- What should the imaging professional have done?

Apology Statutes

When errors happen, studies indicate that it is not necessarily the medical error itself that causes patients and families to sue, but the response to it.[19] A study published in the *Journal of the American Medical Association* in 2003 reported that after an error occurs, patients want information about why it happened, how the consequences will be mitigated, and what is being done to prevent recurrence. They also want emotional support—including an apology.[20]

Sixteen states have passed legislation giving a physician the right to provide a compassionate statement or say "I'm sorry" to patients at the time of an adverse outcome without threat of litigation.[21] These statutes allow an honest and open dialog when a medical error, accident, or unanticipated outcome occurs without the apology being taken as an admission of guilt. Open communication between patients and their health care professionals about their care decreases the likelihood that a patient will file a lawsuit.[21] Empirical evidence shows that the use of a compassionate statement has lowered the litigation costs at the University of Michigan Hospital System, the Children's Hospitals and Clinics of Minnesota, and the Veterans Affairs Medical Center in Lexington, Kentucky.[21] Because not all states have this legislation, imaging professionals should ask their facility's risk management department whether their state has such a statute and how they should handle situations when errors occur.

SUMMARY

- Caring and communication are crucial in the development of the imaging professional. They are essential to the treatment provided in the imaging environment and the ethical problem solving required to provide high-quality imaging services.
- Caring is a function of the whole person in which concern for the growth and well-being of another is expressed in an integrated application of the mind, body, and spirit that seeks to maximize positive outcomes. Existential care is compassion arising from an awareness of common bonds of humanity and common expressions, fates, and feelings. Professional care is the application of the knowledge of the discipline, including its science, theory, practice, and art.
- Human and professional caring in the imaging sciences provides safety and comfort for patients, involves imaging professionals in their patients' lives, and enhances patient autonomy, confidentiality, and informed consent.
- Empathy is the ability to recognize and to some extent share the emotions and state of mind of another and to understand the meaning and significance of that person's behavior. It is not the same thing as sympathy or feeling sorry for the patient. It is an objective response that allows the imaging professional to provide high-quality patient care.
- Communication is a symbolic interaction. It is not static, and it involves human feelings and attitudes as well as information. Health communication is a subset of human communication that is concerned with how individuals in a society seek to maintain health and deal with health-related issues.
- Education to enhance caring and communication may be incorporated into the imaging curriculum through a variety of methods. By developing a more caring

and communicative demeanor, imaging professionals become better able to provide patients with compassionate treatment and high-quality imaging services. Caring and communication are therefore ethical imperatives in the imaging sciences.

- Caring and communication are cornerstones of medicine, since mutual trust and open communication are major factors in patient satisfaction.
- Health literacy is the ability to read, understand, and act on health care information to make effective health care decisions and follow instructions for treatment.
- Low health literacy is a barrier to open communication. Unfortunately, almost half of the adult population suffers from low health literacy. Imaging professionals see patients every day who have trouble understanding and applying health care information.
- Health care professionals can make simple changes in the way they communicate to help their patients understand. These include slowing down, choosing less technical terms, having eye contact with patients, and using the teach back technique to ensure patient understanding.
- Better communication can decrease litigation risks. Attorneys estimate that the clinician's style and attitude are major factors in 75% of malpractice suits.
- Imaging professionals also decrease litigation risks through caring. Patient dissatisfaction is linked to the filing of medical malpractice claims. Caring may be the single most important thing an imaging professional can do to minimize risk.
- Legislation in place in 16 states allows physicians to apologize when an error or adverse outcome has occurred without the apology being taken as an admission of guilt. When errors occur, it is not necessarily the medical error that causes families and patients to file suit, but rather the response to it and the failure to provide communication and emotional support. Not all states have apology statutes, so imaging professions should consult their risk management team to learn how error communication is handled in their state and facility.

REFERENCES

1. Erikson EH: *The life cycle completed*, New York, 1982, Norton.
2. Griffin AP: A philosophical analysis of caring in nursing, *J Adv Nurs* 8:289, 1983.
3. Warren L: Review and synthesis of nine nursing studies on care and caring, *J NY State Nurs Assoc* 19(4):17, 1988.
4. Gaut D: Development of a theoretically adequate description of caring, *West J Nurs Res* 5(4):311, 1983.
5. Leininger M: The phenomenon of caring: importance, research questions and theoretical considerations. In Leininger M (Ed): *Caring: an essential human need*, Thorofare, NJ, 1988, Slack.
6. Dowd S: The radiographer's role: part scientist, part humanist, *Radiol Technol* 63(4):240, 1992.
7. Younger J: Literary works as a mode of knowledge, *Image: J Nurs Scholar* 22(1):39, 1990.
8. Stumpfig K: Caring can't be scheduled, *Radiol Technol* 66(3):208, 1995.
9. Dowd S: Do we care? *RT Image* 3:16, 1990.
10. Ohnysty J: *Aids to ethics and professional conduct for student radiographers*, Springfield, Ill, 1968, Charles C Thomas.
11. Fengler K: The patient care gap, *Radiol Technol* 49:599, 1978.
12. Creasia JL, Parker B: *Conceptual foundations: the bridge to professional nursing practice*, ed 3, St Louis, 2001, Mosby.
13. Weiss B: *Health literacy: a manual for clinicians*, Chicago, 2003, American Medical Association Foundation and American Medical Association.
14. National Center for Education Statistics, US Department of Education, Institute of Education Sciences: *National assessment of adult literacy: a first look at the literacy of America's adults in the 21st century*, NCES 2006-470, Washington, DC, 2003, Author.

15. Institute of Medicine: *Priority areas for national action: transforming health care quality*, Washington, DC, 2003, Author.
16. Landers SJ: Low health literacy is pervasive barrier to care, *AMA News,* April 26, 2004.
17. Furrow B, Greaney TL, Jost TS, et al: *Liability and quality issues in health care,* St Paul, Minn, 2004, West.
18. Hickson GB, Federspiel CF, Pichert JW, et al: Patient complaints and malpractice risk, *JAMA* 287:2951, 2002.
19. Robeznieks A: The power of an apology: patients appreciate open communication, *AMA News,* July 28, 2003.
20. Gallagher THG, Waterman AD, Ebers AG, et al: Patients' and physicians' attitudes regarding the disclosure of medical errors, *JAMA* 289:1001, 2003.
21. Iowa Medical Society: *Medical Liability Reform 2006*, West Des Moines, Iowa, 2006, Author.

REVIEW QUESTIONS

1 Define human caring.
2 Define professional care.
3 Define existential care.
4 Define communication.
5 Define health communication.
6 Imaging professionals must provide _____ _____ in addition to professional caring and communication to satisfy the needs of the patient.
7 Caring is an _____ analogous to truth and justice.
8 List three of the obstacles to caring.
9 List three of the obstacles to communication.
10 The human caring practiced by professionals is based on _____ and _____ values.
11 List three methods of developing caring skills.
12 List three methods of improving communication skills.
13 Explain the ways in which advocacy influences care for the imaging patient.
14 **True or False** Caring involves initiative.
15 **True or False** A more caring demeanor cannot be developed.
16 **True or False** An ethical approach to problem solving is an expression of caring.
17 **True or False** Time constraints may have a detrimental effect on patient satisfaction.
18 **True or False** Caring can be fully attained with perfect human expression.
19 **True or False** The lack of training in caring for critically ill patients is an obstacle to caring.
20 **True or False** Most patients do not consult an attorney unless they are unhappy with the "care" they received.
21 **True or False** Trust and open communication between care provider and patient are major steps toward patient satisfaction.
22 **True or False** Very few of the patients you see have trouble with reading.
23 Health literacy is:
   a. Being able to understand medical journals
   b. Part of the medical librarian curriculum
   c. The ability to read, understand, and act on health care information
   d. Being able to read your chart

24 The percentage of U.S. adults who are functionally illiterate is:
   a. 15%
   b. 85%
   c. 30%
   d. 48%
25 **True or False** There is nothing we can do to help patients with low literacy understand heath care information.
26 Tips to change the way health care professionals communicate with patients include:
   a. Slow down.
   b. Avoid medical terms and use words that everyone understands.
   c. Ask your patient to tell you what they understand.
   d. All of the above.
27 **True or False** "Caring" has no relationship to minimizing the risk of litigation.
28 **True or False** Federal and state statutes define and mandate caring.
29 **True or False** Most patients injured as a result of negligence file malpractice suits.
30 **True or False** Patient dissatisfaction has been linked to the filing of malpractice claims.

CRITICAL THINKING *Questions & Activities*

1 Is involvement in the universal conditions of life experienced by patients an important aspect of caring? Defend your answer.
2 The technical aspects of providing imaging services for patients may adversely affect the human caring delivered by the imaging professional. Give an example of this and justify your reasoning.
3 In what way does the appropriate taking of a patient's history enhance caring? Why?
4 List the resources of the imaging professional that enable caring for the patient. In what way do they enable caring?
5 Why is caring the foundation of the imaging services?

4 PATIENT AUTONOMY AND INFORMED CONSENT

The last of the human freedoms [is] to choose one's attitude in any given set of circumstances, to choose one's own way.

VIKTOR FRANKL

Chapter Outline

Ethical Issues
Definition of Autonomy
Patient Care Partnership
Information Delivery
Complications of Autonomy, Informed Consent, and Right of Refusal
Verification of Informed Consent
Competence and Incompetence Surrogacy
Obstacles to Autonomy and Informed Consent
Respect for Autonomy

Therapeutic Privilege
Emergency Situations
Competence and Advance Directives
Application of Ethical Theories to Autonomy
Legal Issues
Tort Law
Simple Consent
Intentional Torts
Unintentional Torts
Informed Consent

Learning Objectives

After completing this chapter, the reader will be able to perform the following:

- Describe the relationship between autonomy, the respect for autonomy, and informed consent.
- Identify the stresses involved in granting informed consent and autonomy.
- List methods of verifying informed consent.
- Define surrogacy.
- Compare and contrast competence and incompetence.
- Correlate coercion, paternalism, and therapeutic privilege.
- Explain why emergency situations and certain facilities may alter informed consent processes.
- Identify ethical theories that may be implemented to facilitate problem solving.

- Give examples of the difference between intentional and unintentional torts and ways the perception of intent rather than the actual intent may be the basis for allegations.
- Provide examples of simple consent as it relates to assault, battery, and false imprisonment.
- Define informed consent.
- Differentiate standards of care with regard to the duty of informed consent.
- Define and contrast the roles of the physician and the imaging professional in informed consent.
- Identify the important but limited role of the consent form.

Key Terms

advance directives
assault
autonomy
battery
competence
consent forms

false imprisonment
informed consent
intentional torts
simple consent
unintentional torts

A client with cancer comes to the radiotherapy clinic at a most challenging time in his or her life. For many, it is a time filled with emotional anxiety, social disruption, physical strain, and uncertainty. My primary role as a radiation therapist is to deliver a precise amount of radiation to the cancer, and in doing so try to bring about a positive change and a return to normalcy for the client. How my goal is achieved depends on many ethical and legal issues that provide the framework for all of my professional responsibilities.

Within my scope of practice I need to be intimately familiar with the protocols, codes, guidelines, and legislation that outline the specific techniques I perform as a radiation therapist but also what I ought to do as a health care provider. There are many scenarios in radiation therapy where there are ethical and legal concerns. These issues may be very clear but at times may be elusive and complex. Here are some situations from my experience that demonstrate these concerns:

- Signing my initials in a logbook for a daily quality assurance procedure that was performed on a treatment unit
- Ensuring that I have the correct client when retrieving him or her from the waiting room
- Asking a client for permission for a student to participate in his or her simulator planning procedure and then balancing the needs for student learning, client comfort, and efficiency
- Reporting unusual or unexpected variances in the treatment process
- Counseling a client at his or her level within my scope of practice, such as educating a client on the anticipated side effects, offering emotional support, and providing referrals to other departments
- Covering up all patient lists and hospital records when the family of a client watches the client on a CCTV monitor in the control area during treatment
- Deciding during portal imaging if a field border deviating 3 mm away from the expected position is acceptable and whether or not to proceed with irradiation
- Communicating with the family members of a client from a non-Western culture who does not speak English and is unaware that he or she is being treated for cancer
- Treating a comatose client for an oncologic emergency without having prior written consent for treatment from either the client or a substitute decision maker (in radiotherapy it is rare not to have written consent at the time of treatment)

These situations are related to concepts of informed consent, client confidentiality, or professional practice, all of which have ethical and legal considerations. As an instructor, I emphasize to students that poorly made decisions can potentially have serious implications. To the client, these consequences could be disastrous: breach of confidentiality, physical harm, severe and debilitating radiation side effects, and radiation-induced death. To the hospital, damage to its reputation could be irreparable. To the therapist, it could mean the end of a professional career, loss of income, and criminal convictions. Health care workers are fully accountable for their actions (or inactions) and must always exercise diligence and vigilance in the care of the client.

The perspectives of care can vary, and I have learned that what is important to me as a radiation therapist may be much less important to the client. For example, I value the client's compliance in attending daily treatments because daily fractions help to increase tumor cell kill. However, for some clients, visiting the clinic every day for treatment may not be a priority because of other competing interests such as work obligations, family schedules, and transportation issues. Having cancer is only another part of the client's life. The ethical and legal considerations become more apparent when the standard policies and procedures do not fit the needs or expectations of the client. I have a moral obligation to ensure not only that the client is being cared for, but also that the client feels cared for.

While I work within a multidisciplinary team of highly trained health care workers and support staff, the clients are the leaders of the team. They rightfully demand superb health care while expecting good outcomes and positive experiences. For the health professional, this comes about through exercising good judgment, employing the appropriate skills, and carefully reflecting upon one's own limitations and strengths.

Martin J. Chai, MRT(T), BSc, MTS
Faculty,
Medical Radiation Sciences,
Department of Radiation Oncology

Faculty of Medicine,
The Michener Institute for Applied Health Sciences and
The University of Toronto, Toronto, Ontario

ETHICAL ISSUES

INFORMED CONSENT
Informed consent is the
written assent of a patient
to receive a proposed
treatment; adequate
information is essential for
the patient to give truly
informed consent.

AUTONOMY
Autonomy is the concept
that patients are to be
treated as individuals and
informed about procedures
to facilitate appropriate
decisions.

Informed consent is a common concern in all the imaging modalities. Imaging professionals must be proficient in the recitation of facts and figures required to inform the patient. Health care providers, however, should also be able to provide patients with a process that renders them truly knowledgeable about procedures and their alternatives.

During the early stages of development within the medical community, the patient's **autonomy** was not a serious consideration. Physicians were expected to be omniscient and were rarely questioned. They acted as the "fathers" of their clientele. This paternalism and the invocation of therapeutic privilege were standard professional philosophies. As years passed and patients became more aware of their rights and privileges, however, the medical community developed new methods of informing patients. The emphasis on patient autonomy and informed consent has come from many areas (Box 4-1).

Some physicians still find the model of patient education difficult because they believe that the informational process complicates health care and brings their expertise into question. Fortunately, however, most physicians and institutions understand the relevance of informed consent and patients' rights.

Maintaining patient autonomy and obtaining valid informed consent are vital in the vascular imaging laboratory. Imaging professionals routinely visit patients before procedures and explain the processes, contrast media involved, and physical sensations to which the patient will be subjected. They may also discuss imaging procedures with patients during transportation and preparation. These are important parts of the informational process and are vital to the maintenance of patient autonomy. Occasionally the imaging professional may be required to witness the signing of a written informed consent form. Other imaging procedures, including fluoroscopic studies, vascular studies, and a variety of other noninvasive and invasive examinations, often require the technologist to facilitate the informed consent process. Imaging professionals must decide on the basis of personal and professional parameters whether this is appropriate, and they must remember that the physician is ultimately responsible for the informed consent process.

BOX 4-1	**CRUCIAL ELEMENTS IN PATIENT AUTONOMY AND INFORMED CONSENT**

Maintenance of patients' rights
Provision of education to facilitate consent
Promotion of human dignity
Determination of incompetence
Advocacy of surrogates
Elimination of attitudes of paternalism
Clarification of unclear communication involving therapeutic privilege
Strategies for dealing with emergency situations
Use of compatible parameters for consent in specific health care facilities
Education regarding the ethical theories involved in patient autonomy
   and informed consent

DEFINITION OF AUTONOMY

Autonomy means that "one human person, precisely as a human person, dares not have the authority and should not have power over another human person. In a medical sense, a patient will not be treated without informed consent of his or her lawful surrogates, except in narrowly defined emergencies."[1]

PATIENT CARE PARTNERSHIP

The patient's right to information is important in considerations of autonomy. The American Hospital Association has established a patient care partnership document (see p. 255),[2] which is to be given to hospitalized patients to help them understand the expectations, rights, and responsibilities regarding their health care.

Expectations should include high-quality hospital care delivered with skill, compassion, and respect. Patients have the right to know the identity of physicians, nurses, and other health care providers. They also have the right to know if they are being treated by students, residents, or other trainees. Patients should expect a clean and safe environment, including special policies and procedures to avoid mistakes in care and ensure freedom from abuse or neglect.

Patients should expect to be involved in decision making regarding care. This includes discussing medical conditions and information about medically appropriate treatment choices. Patients should be informed of the benefits and risks of each treatment, whether that treatment is experimental or part of a research study, what can reasonably be expected from the treatment, and any long-term effects it might have. The financial consequences of using noncovered services or out-of-network providers should be explained. Patients should expect to be informed of what they and their families will need to do upon leaving the hospital.

When entering the hospital, the patient signs a general consent-for-treatment form. Specific treatments such as surgery, invasive procedures, or experimental treatments may require specific consent, called *informed consent,* which confirms in writing what is planned and the patient is agreeing to as part of that plan. This process protects the patient's right to consent to or refuse a treatment. The physician must also explain the consequences of refusing recommended treatment.

To make good decisions regarding care, caregivers need complete and correct information from patients about their health and coverage. The patient is responsible for delivering this information, which includes past medical history, past allergic reactions, medicines and dietary supplements, and specific health plan information, as well as health care goals, values, or spiritual beliefs important to the patient's well-being. Patients should make available to the physician and the hospital any documents such as a living will or advance directive regarding health care decisions.

Patients' privacy is protected by state and federal laws, as well as hospital operating policies. Patients receive a notice of privacy practice document that outlines the way information is used, disclosed, and safeguarded. This also explains how a patient can obtain a copy of the information regarding care.

Patients can expect assistance with treatment plans when leaving the hospital, including arrangement of follow-up care and disclosure of any financial interest in any such referrals. They can also expect hospitals to file claims with health insurers, Medicare, and Medicaid, as well as provide help with needed documentation, explanation of hospital bills, and insurance coverage.

INFORMATION DELIVERY

The way in which information is given depends on the criteria used to inform the patient. The following four potentially conflicting rules may guide the physician or other health care provider in explaining information to patients[1]:

1. Patient preference rule
2. Professional custom rule
3. Prudent person rule
4. Subjective substantial disclosure rule

Institutional rules must also be taken into account.

Patient Preference Rule

The patient preference rule requires health care professionals to tell patients what they want to know. For example, the patient may prefer to know how the procedure may aid in the diagnostic process or may ask a radiation therapy professional how the treatment will affect the patient's quality of life. The health professional will then do his or her best to communicate this information in the patient education process.

Professional Custom Rule

The professional custom rule states that the health care professional should give the patient the information normally given to patients in similar situations. For example, a patient may have no specific requests for information concerning scheduled ultrasonography. This does not necessarily indicate the patient's lack of concern. He or she may just not know what to ask. The ultrasonographer would then provide the patient with the typical information concerning the examination. Patient education that enables the patient to comply with the requests of the imaging professional will also make the examination more understandable to the patient.

Prudent Person Rule

The prudent person rule, or reasonable patient standard, measures the physician's disclosure to the patient based on the patient's need for information to make decisions regarding treatment.[1] The imaging professional must consider the information the patient needs to make informed decisions concerning a procedure. In the previous examples, the imaging professional or physician would have to decide how much the patient needs to know before he or she can make an adequate informed consent decision.

Subjective Substantial Disclosure Rule

The subjective substantial disclosure rule encourages the physician to disseminate all information important to the individual patient. In responding to the previous examples, the physician would feel obliged to explain *all* the possible ramifications of the examinations to the patient.

The prudent person rule addresses many of the important elements of informed consent. A combination of the prudent person rule and the subjective disclosure rule, which requires the physician to communicate meaningfully with the patient, provides the information the patient needs to make an informed decision. Such a combination ensures that the physician has adequate knowledge about the patient and the patient has adequate knowledge about the procedure (Box 4-2).

BOX 4-2	**RULES FOR EXPLAINING PROCEDURES**

Patient preference rule—provides information patients want to know
Professional custom rule—provides the information normally given to patients
Prudent person rule—provides the information patients need to know to consent
  to or refuse treatment
Subjective substantial disclosure rule—provides patients with all information
Combination of rules—provides information without overburdening the patient

Institutional Rules Regarding Informed Consent

Imaging professionals must consider institutional rules concerning a variety of ethical issues, including informed consent. During the interview process before employment, they should investigate issues of institutional ethics and values before making choices concerning their abilities to function and provide patient care within the parameters provided by the institution.

COMPLICATIONS OF AUTONOMY, INFORMED CONSENT, AND RIGHT OF REFUSAL

After examining the issues included in defining patient autonomy and protecting patient rights, imaging professionals should be able to recognize the dilemmas involved in ensuring informed consent. Whether a patient may ever give truly informed consent is open to question. To be totally informed, the patient would need to be educated in many areas from anatomy to imaging procedures. Imaging professionals may consider whether this is possible or whether informed consent is simply an idealistic (although necessary) ritual. They must also recognize their responsibility in the process of obtaining informed consent. Even if the procedure is complicated to explain, imaging professionals should make every effort to help patients become more knowledgeable. Until patients become responsible for providing and obtaining information concerning their medical procedures, a truly informed, educated consent that ensures autonomy may never be realized.

The Patient Self-Determination Act of 1991 helps ensure patient autonomy[3]:

> Heeding the principle of autonomy … means that imaging professionals should respect a patient's choice to refuse treatments. The basic human right of all patients to refuse treatment was formally legislated by the Omnibus Budget Reconciliation Act (1990). The Patient Self-Determination Act became effective December 1, 1991, and requires all health care institutions receiving Medicare or Medicaid funds to inform patients that they have the right to refuse medical and surgical care and the right to initiate a written advance directive (i.e., a written or oral statement by which a competent person makes known his or her treatment preferences and/or designates a surrogate decision maker in the event he or she should become unable to make medical decisions on his or her own behalf [Box 4-3]). Hospitals, home health care agencies, and managed care organizations are required to make this information available, in writing, at the time the patient comes under an agency's care.

VERIFICATION OF INFORMED CONSENT

One ethical challenge inherent in many imaging procedures is the appropriateness of the verification of informed consent. Imaging professionals should always be available to answer patients' questions concerning their procedures. However, questions concerning

BOX 4-3	**REQUIREMENTS OF THE PATIENT SELF-DETERMINATION ACT**

Provision of written information to adult patients about their rights to make medical decisions, including the right to accept or refuse treatment and the right to formulate advance directives

Documentation in each patient's record regarding whether the patient has executed an advance directive

Implementation of written policies regarding the various types of advance directives

Ensuring of compliance with state laws regarding medical treatment decisions and advance directives

Elimination of discrimination against individuals regarding their treatment decisions made through an advance directive

Provision of education for staff members and the community on ethical and legal issues concerning advance directives

From the Omnibus Budget Reconciliation Act of 1990, Sections 4206 and 4751, Public Law 101-508, November 5, 1990.

specifics of informed consent such as alternative therapies, failure rate, risks, or other subjects should always be directed to the patient's physician.

The physician has a crucial role in the process of obtaining informed consent. Because of their knowledge and expertise, physicians bear the responsibility for informing patients concerning procedures. To facilitate the informed consent process, the imaging professional should refer the patient to the physician if the professional feels questions about the procedure are out of his or her field of expertise.

An important ethical consideration is whether imaging professionals should allow themselves to be placed in the position of witnessing the patient's signature on the informed consent form. Imaging professionals are commonly given the responsibility of getting the patient to sign the imaging procedure consent form. If they are not present when the patient's physician presumably gives the necessary instructions and explanations to the patient, they are qualified only to witness the fact that the patient has signed the form.

Many imaging professionals involved in carrying out informed consent procedures find themselves in the difficult situation of determining how much of the responsibility for informed consent is theirs. Nevertheless, probably few have ever questioned this process. Many student imaging professionals are required to explain the injection of contrast media and possible reactions to patients as part of their clinical objectives. Although students must learn this skill, imaging professionals may need to consider whether this important patient education duty should be left to students and whether this is conducive to the patient's truly informed consent and the imaging professional's protection from liability.

An example of the difficulties inherent in ensuring patient autonomy and eliciting truly informed consent may be observed in a fluoroscopic imaging suite in which gastrointestinal procedures are performed. The patient may have been informed, but can anyone ever be ready for an air contrast colon examination? Patients subjected to this procedure are already afraid, sick, and in pain and may feel as though they have no control over their care. Imaging professionals need to consider ways of facing this challenge and informing patients as fully as possible about an often dehumanizing procedure without completely discouraging them from an examination that may have enormous diagnostic benefits. Throughout all of this, the dignity and autonomy of the patient must be preserved.

An imaging professional may overhear a co-worker speaking disrespectfully about an unconscious or deaf patient. Because respect for freedom and privacy is ultimately rooted in the dignity of each person, the maintenance of autonomy requires health care providers to respect all individuals, even those who are not currently capable of free choice.[1] In short, people do not lose their dignity because they are unconscious, in a coma, or out of contact with reality. Such patients present special difficulties, but they must nevertheless be respected. Dignity and autonomy do not stem from a person's ability to function in an imaging suite; instead, the clinical area should accommodate itself to the individual's limitations.

COMPETENCE AND INCOMPETENCE SURROGACY

Competence is a necessary element in informed consent. In the medical setting, competence entails the ability to make appropriate choices and consider their consequences. A patient's competence may be temporarily compromised by prescription or over-the-counter drugs. In this condition of short-term incompetence, the patient may require a surrogate or postponement of the procedure until the patient is competent. Incompetence is difficult to prove. An evaluation of the patient's ability to make decisions is an important component in determining competence.

Imaging professionals should consider methods of dealing with patients who are temporarily incompetent or rendered permanently incompetent by brain damage, developmental disabilities, dementia, or Alzheimer's disease. Such patients do not have less dignity or less right to be informed. Even the most incompetent person has basic human dignity, and imaging professionals must keep this in mind.

Questions regarding methods for determining competence and adequately informing patients who are incompetent often lead to a consideration of surrogacy, or the appointment of a person or persons to make decisions regarding care in the name of the patient. A surrogate may be a parent, an individual named by the patient while competent, or a person or persons appointed by the courts. Surrogates may be involved in the determination of competence and in the informed consent process. As such, they may pose an obstacle to autonomy, especially if the patient did not give advance directives regarding personal wishes. No person can ever truly know the wishes of another; nevertheless, surrogates must do their best to surmise the patient's wishes.

OBSTACLES TO AUTONOMY AND INFORMED CONSENT

Undue influences that may restrict the patient's choices are a hindrance to autonomy. Ill patients may feel pushed into decisions out of concern for their health, future, and family members. A patient's family members or physician may pressure the patient because of personal or professional feelings concerning the patient's welfare. Imaging professionals must be careful not to add influences that may render patients, who have already experienced a loss of personal freedom, unable to make decisions concerning their care. The imaging suite environment itself may negatively influence the patient; its intimidating atmosphere may frighten the patient past the point of sound decision making. Imaging professionals must therefore make every effort to calm and reassure the patient. At the same time, they should recognize that no person is ever completely free from outside influences and that truly informed, educated consent and autonomy may be impossible.

COMPETENCE
Competence is the ability to make choices.

Given the increased diversity of the patient population, language and culture are often barriers to autonomy and informed consent. These issues are discussed thoroughly in Chapter 9.

A lack of time can influence the completeness of the informed consent process. Imaging professionals often face this problem, but they cannot sacrifice proper patient communication because of time constraints.

Lack of communication on the part of the patient or professional may interfere with the informed consent process. In this situation the professional should elicit feedback from the patient to verify that the information was understood.

Serious obstacles to autonomy and informed consent may spring from health care providers, including physicians, nurses, and allied health professionals. Because of their education and experience, they often believe they know what is best for patients. They become confused and sometimes angry when patients refuse treatment or question their explanations. An attitude of paternalism is unhealthy for autonomy. Patients who perceive such an attitude on the part of the health care provider may come to distrust the provider. An irritated, know-it-all imaging professional may frighten or annoy a patient out of the examination room and past the point of diagnosis. Clear communication between the provider and patient is crucial, and the imaging professional has an obligation to communicate properly and not merely spout facts. If the patient does not understand, informed consent is not possible. Imaging professionals should remember to talk *to* patients, not *at* them.

Imaging professionals may become so accustomed to the repetition of information that they do not truly listen to patients. Students especially may be so involved in covering all the information that they sound like waiters explaining the catch of the day, not professionals describing the possible complications of a medical procedure. Patients are usually frightened, and when asked if they understand, they may nod yes with heads empty of actual understanding.

RESPECT FOR AUTONOMY

Autonomy, surrogacy, informed consent, and the obstacles to each should continually remind imaging professionals that they must have an ongoing respect for the self of the patient. Jonsen, Siegler, and Winslade[4] provide seven points to enable the health care professional to maintain respect for autonomy. They have been modified below for imaging professionals:

1. Is the patient mentally capable and legally competent? Is there any evidence of incapacity that would affect the imaging procedure?
2. If competent, has the imaging patient expressed any preferences for the imaging procedure?
3. Does the imaging patient understand the benefits and the risks, and has he or she given consent?
4. If the patient is in need of a surrogate, is the surrogate using the appropriate standards for decision making?
5. Has the imaging patient expressed prior preferences (e.g., advance directives)?
6. If the imaging patient is unable or unwilling to cooperate with the imaging procedure, is there a specific reason?
7. After a consideration of the first six points, is the patient's right to choose being respected to the extent possible both ethically and legally?

The use of these points of respect for autonomy is a valuable tool in ethical and legal problem solving.

THERAPEUTIC PRIVILEGE

Physicians and imaging professionals must decide what the patient needs to know. These difficult decisions may raise the issue of therapeutic privilege, a narrowly construed prerogative invoked when health care providers withhold information from patients because they believe the information would have adverse effects on the patients' conditions or health. The physician must have reason to believe that the patient would become unusually emotionally distraught if the information was disclosed.[5] Physicians and other health care providers may believe they are knowledgeable about what the patient can tolerate. They may use this belief as a reason to omit information if they think it may have an adverse effect on the patient. Imaging professionals who believe they know the way the patient feels better than the patient does should reevaluate their omission of information. Therapeutic privilege is used less often by caregivers who realize that patients are becoming much more aware of their rights. When their autonomy is denied, their ability to give informed consent is impaired. Most patients want to be told the truth about their condition. When imaging professionals omit necessary information, the result may be deceit, mistrust, and very possibly harm to the patient.

EMERGENCY SITUATIONS

In emergency situations the informed consent process may have to be abandoned to save the patient's life. Imaging professionals may find themselves in such situations in the emergency department. According to the laws of many states, three conditions must be present for the omission of informed consent to be justified:

1. The patient is incapable of giving consent, and no lawful surrogate is available.
2. Danger to life or risk of a serious impairment to health is apparent.
3. Immediate treatment is necessary to avert these dangers.

Providing treatment without the patient's consent may be considered a denial of autonomy; however, autonomy is not relevant if the patient dies. In this case autonomy becomes a consideration of the patient's family or surrogate. If the family feels the patient's rights have been denied, they may take legal action. Many emergency room physicians are faced with this difficult situation and the quick but vital decisions it requires. Informed consent and autonomy are not always possible in emergency situations.

COMPETENCE AND ADVANCE DIRECTIVES

Certain facilities and situations may pose serious threats to autonomy and informed consent. Mental health facilities and nursing homes may compromise the autonomy processes. Many patients in these institutions are considered incompetent as a result of mental illness or age, although neither of these factors necessarily renders the patient incompetent. Many mental health and nursing facilities are now asking competent patients to give written **advance directives** or assign a surrogate to provide protection for the patient and provider if the patient becomes incompetent at a later date.

APPLICATION OF ETHICAL THEORIES TO AUTONOMY

The imaging professional may experience further difficulty in choosing a theory of ethics to apply when considering patient autonomy. The theory of consequentialism (utilitarianism) requires the greatest good to be done for the greatest number. Deontology

ADVANCE DIRECTIVES
An advance directive is a predetermined (usually written) choice made to inform others of the ways in which the patient wishes to be treated while incompetent.

IMAGING SCENARIO

A 90-year-old patient with terminal cancer who is mentally limited, hard of hearing, and visually impaired is scheduled for a double contrast barium enema. Even a healthy 20-year-old patient may have difficulty with this procedure, which is embarrassing and often uncomfortable. The imaging professional wonders why this terminally ill, feeble, geriatric patient should be forced to endure the procedure. The professional is not sure that the patient truly understands what it entails. The patient may have been influenced by a physician concerned with doing everything possible to avoid legal repercussions, and informed consent may have been given by a family member who wants to hang on to this elderly relative no matter what. If the patient had made himself clearer concerning his wishes before the illness became invasive, all the involved parties would not be struggling with the implications and consequences of the procedure.

Discussion question
- In what way do the three ethical theories address the difficult decisions involved in this scenario?

holds that the motives for an action are the most important considerations. Virtue ethics invokes practical wisdom and right reason. (See Chapter 1 for a more detailed review of ethical theories.)

Utilitarianism is not very relevant in considerations of autonomy and consent because it is generally applied to large numbers of persons. Although the informed consent process may affect other persons, the patient has a more immediate interest in understanding the process. The deontologic viewpoint, with its emphasis on motives instead of consequences, is difficult to apply in considerations of the maintenance of a patient's autonomy because in this situation the consequences are crucial. Both utilitarianism and deontology assume that people use ethical constructs to address the difficulties involved in encouraging the individual's autonomy while obtaining genuinely informed consent. Because moral significance and other factors vary with each individual, however, even those using similar constructs may come to differing conclusions.

Virtue ethics relies on virtues, practical wisdom, and an appreciation of the consequences of actions. This theory is the most adaptable for dealing with the difficulties of patient autonomy because it promotes the dignity of patients and their freedom of choice.

LEGAL ISSUES

Patient autonomy is crucial to many legal theories applicable to imaging professionals. Consent and informed consent are the two legal issues in which patient autonomy is most obvious and necessary. Failure to obtain consent may result in allegations of torts such as assault, battery, false imprisonment, and negligence with regard to lack of informed consent. These torts and the legal issues regarding consent, informed consent, and the imaging professional's role in both are discussed at length in this chapter.

TORT LAW

A tort is a civil wrong for which the law provides a remedy.[5] A tort action is filed to recover damages for personal injury or property damage occurring from negligent conduct or intentional misconduct. Tort law may be divided into two categories—intentional torts and unintentional torts. Intentional torts result when an act is done with the intention of causing harm to another.[6] The intentional torts that are most likely to have an impact on the provision of medical imaging services are assault, battery, false imprisonment, and defamation. Assault, battery, and false imprisonment are discussed in this chapter. Defamation is discussed in Chapter 5, which covers truthfulness and confidentiality.

SIMPLE CONSENT

Justice Cardozo stated in the 1914 case *Schloendorff v Society of N.Y. Hospitals* that "every human being of adult years and sound mind has a right to determine what shall be done with his own body; and a surgeon who performs an operation without his consent commits an assault for which he is liable in damages."[7] This court decision provided the basis for the concept of consent and established that violation of consent constitutes assault and battery.

A patient must consent to any procedure. This **simple consent** does not require knowledge of the procedure. It simply means that a patient's permission must be obtained before the procedure can be performed. Consent may be given simply by the patient's getting on the table or stepping up to the chest board. If a patient is in an emergency situation, consent need not be asked for or given. Instead, the situation is evaluated legally by assessing what a reasonable person would do in a similar situation. Again, the applicable standard of care prevails.

Most problems with simple consent arise when consent is withdrawn by a patient or when the boundaries to which the patient has consented are exceeded. This may be a difficult situation to address, because although an imaging professional cannot continue a procedure without the patient's consent, the patient often may be reassured by a more thorough explanation of the procedure, and consent can and must again be obtained.

INTENTIONAL TORTS

Although the concept that a provider of medical imaging services would intend to harm a patient is bizarre, if the patient feels the tort was intended, the determination of intent may well be left to a jury. Communication with patients to ensure their understanding is the best tool to lessen or decrease the risk of allegations of **intentional torts**.

Assault and Battery

An **assault** is a deliberate act wherein one person threatens to harm another person without consent and the victim perceives that the other has the ability to carry out the threat.[5] **Battery** is touching to which the victim has not consented, even if the touching may benefit the patient.[8] For example, assault may be alleged if an imaging professional threatens to perform a portable chest x-ray examination on a competent person against his or her will. Battery occurs if the x-ray examination is actually performed on the competent, unwilling patient.

SIMPLE CONSENT
Simple consent is the assent required of a patient for any procedure.

INTENTIONAL TORTS
Intentional torts are wrongs resulting from acts done with the intention of causing harm to another.

ASSAULT
Assault is a deliberate act wherein one person threatens to harm another without consent and the victim feels the attacker has the ability to carry out the threat.

BATTERY
Battery is touching to which the victim has not consented.

BOX 4-4	**LEGAL CRITERIA FOR THE USE OF RESTRAINT**

Touching or restraint to which the patient has not consented is needed to protect the patient, health care team members, or the property of others.
The restraint used is the least intrusive method possible.
Regular reassessment of the need to restrain occurs.
The restraint is discontinued as soon as practicable.

Modified from Harper F, James F, Gray O: *The law of torts,* ed 3, Boston, 1996, Little, Brown.

In situations involving patients who are incompetent or those requiring restraint, the law allows providers to touch patients without consent. In these situations consideration must be given to four important conditions, as listed in Box 4-4.

Medical immobilization is often needed in the imaging department. This immobilization includes mechanisms usually and customarily applied during diagnostic and therapeutic procedures and is considered a regular and usual part of such procedures and based on standard practice. Such immobilization to perform effective treatment is not considered restraint.

Restraints are rarely used in the medical imaging department. If the need arises, however, imaging professionals must keep in mind that they should be able to justify use of restraints according to the four criteria in Box 4-4.

When dealing with children, which often necessitates immobilization, imaging technologists must communicate clearly with parents. This communication not only increases parental confidence in the imaging professionals but also minimizes the risk of litigation. Adequate communication should include an explanation of the necessity for immobilization to decrease radiation exposure and obtain optimal studies, reassurance that the immobilization equipment used is the least intrusive, and a guarantee that immobilization will be used only when necessary and discontinued as soon as possible.

False Imprisonment

FALSE IMPRISONMENT
False imprisonment is the unlawful confinement of a person within a fixed area.

Although **false imprisonment** seems to be a ridiculous allegation to make against an imaging professional, certain circumstances in the medical imaging setting may give rise to such allegations. False imprisonment occurs when a person is unlawfully confined within a fixed area.[7] The confined person must be aware of the confinement or must be harmed by the confinement. Even if the health care provider does not intend harm, these allegations can be made if the patient perceives the acts to be done with the intent of harm.

For false imprisonment to be found, plaintiffs must prove that they were restrained either physically or by threat or intimidation and that they did not consent to the restraint. Because restraints are often important and necessary tools in obtaining successful medical images or therapeutic treatment, a successful false imprisonment suit would require the jury to find that an imaging professional acted in an unreasonable, unjustified, and unprivileged manner. Again, the applicable standard of care would be used.

UNINTENTIONAL TORTS

UNINTENTIONAL TORTS
Unintentional torts are wrongs resulting from actions that were not intended to do harm.

Unintentional torts result from actions that were not intended to cause harm. The unintentional tort most commonly encountered in medical imaging is medical malpractice, a broad term that in most jurisdictions encompasses negligence, failure to obtain informed consent, and breach of patient confidentiality. All these causes of action are alleged based on the fact that a duty is owed, the duty is breached, and harm results from the breach.

In the health care setting, duties are owed to patients by physicians, hospitals or other health care facilities, and all health care providers, including imaging professionals. If a duty is not performed adequately, in violation of a statute or as judged by the appropriate standard of care, and harm results from the failure to perform the duty adequately, liability may be found.

Medical negligence is discussed in Chapter 2 and breach of confidentiality in Chapter 5. Medical malpractice cases alleging failure to obtain informed consent are discussed here because patient autonomy is the ethical principle underpinning informed consent.

INFORMED CONSENT

Case law concerning informed consent was established in the 1957 case of *Salgo v Leland Stanford Jr. University Board of Trustees*[9] and the 1972 case of *Canterbury v Spence*.[5] All 50 states have now recognized a legal duty for physicians to obtain informed consent.[10] While the basis of this duty may differ by jurisdiction, generally physicians are required to give patients enough information to enable them to make informed decisions.[11] This information includes risks, benefits, alternative treatment options, and expected outcomes if they choose not to undergo the proposed diagnostic testing or treatment.

According to the *Canterbury* case, informed consent is necessary to allow the patient to determine the direction of treatment.[5] The amount of information needed for this determination varies depending on the patient, the procedure, and the applicable standard of care in the particular jurisdiction. Basically two standards of care are applied throughout the states. One standard is the professional standard, in which a physician is required to disclose those risks that a reasonable and prudent medical practitioner would disclose under the same or similar circumstances.[10] In contrast, under the lay standard the physician's disclosure duty is measured by the patient's need for information rather than by the standards of the medical professional.[11] Generally under the lay standard the physician is required to describe the benefits of the procedure and the accompanying risks, including the risk of death or paralysis.[11]

Two basic exceptions exist in which informed consent need not be obtained—emergency situations and cases in which therapeutic privilege is invoked. The emergency exception occurs only if the patient is unconscious or otherwise unable to give consent and harm from failure to treat is imminent and outweighs any harm inherent in the proposed treatment. Therapeutic privilege applies only if risk of disclosure poses such a threat to the patient that it will lead to further harm. The physician must have reason to believe that the patient would become unusually emotionally distraught if the information was disclosed.[5]

To prove lack of informed consent, a plaintiff must prove that a material risk existed that was unknown to the patient, the risk was not disclosed, disclosure of the risk would have led a reasonable patient to reject the medical procedure or choose a different course of treatment, and the patient was injured as a result of the lack of disclosure.[12]

As discussed previously, the basis of informed consent can vary in different jurisdictions. One source of the standard of care with regard to informed consent is statutes that regulate informed consent. In many states statutes have established panels that determine which procedures require written informed consent and define exactly what must be disclosed, including the wording to be used. Facilities and physicians are free to establish more stringent requirements of disclosure for patients.

In many cases the jury does not find liability because it cannot determine that a reasonable patient who had been informed would have rejected the procedure. Whether or not liability is imposed on this basis, a great deal of time (on the part of lawyers, employees, and physicians), money, and emotional distress is expended in litigation. Therefore consistently obtaining informed consent is a valuable risk management tool.

State of Informed Consent Law

The following cases demonstrate the legal issues inherent in informed consent and the state of the law at publication of this book. Virtually all jurisdictions impose the duty of informed consent only on physicians. However, some jurisdictions, with limited success, have attempted to impose such a duty on the hospital. It is important for imaging professionals to find out the law in their state, as well as department and facility policies regarding this issue.

The 1987 Iowa Supreme Court decision in *Pauscher v Iowa Methodist Medical Center* clarified the elements necessary to prove lack of informed consent.[12] Six days after delivering her first child, Becky Pauscher was scheduled for an intravenous pyelogram because of fever, pain in her right side, and blood in her urine. No physician told Mrs. Pauscher that severe reactions to the procedure included the possibility of death, nor did anyone ask if Mrs. Pauscher consented to the procedure. The requisition could not be found after the procedure, but the technologist stated that Mrs. Pauscher had denied having allergies. Her chart, however, noted an allergy to bee stings and a history of asthma as a child.

After the injection of some of the contrast medium, Mrs. Pauscher began to scratch her face. The technologist stopped the injection but continued after seeing no further distress signs. When Mrs. Pauscher complained of chest pain, the technologist again stopped the injection and called the radiologist. Mrs. Pauscher died of anaphylactic shock despite resuscitation attempts.

Mrs. Pauscher's husband sued the urologist and radiologist for failing to disclose the risk of death, stating that his wife could not make an informed choice without that knowledge. He charged the hospital with failing to have an established policy for informed consent.

The Iowa Supreme Court found that the physicians were responsible for informing the patient of the risks but determined that Mrs. Pauscher would not have refused the test based on the "extremely remote" risk of death.

The Pauscher case did not find the hospital to have a duty to inform the patient of risks or to obtain informed consent. This is still generally the state of the law regarding hospitals and informed consent. However, such a duty has been recognized in at least one jurisdiction.

The 1992 Kentucky Supreme Court case of *Keel v St. Elizabeth Medical Center* found the hospital liable for failure to obtain informed consent.[13] In this case, Leslie Keel came to the St. Elizabeth Medical Center for a computed tomography (CT) scan with contrast injection. Before the test, Mr. Keel was given no information concerning risks. Whether Mr. Keel responded to questions regarding allergies and previous history of reactions to contrast injections is uncertain. A thrombophlebitis later developed at the injection site.

The Kentucky Supreme Court separated the issue of informed consent from the issue of negligence. Although the issue of whether the injection was negligently performed was not explored, the court found that the hospital had a statutory duty to disclose the risks of the procedure and failed to perform that duty.

More recent case law in numerous jurisdictions indicates a refusal to impose a duty on hospitals to inform patients of the material risks of a procedure prescribed by the patient's physician or to obtain informed consent. Some of these courts refused to find such a duty for a hospital based on statutes that impose this duty only on the physician.[14] Other courts refused to extend the duty of informed consent to hospitals even when the statute defining informed consent used the term "health care providers," which can include both hospitals and physicians.[15-17] These courts held that to impose a duty of informed consent on all entities meeting the statutory definition of "health care providers" would result in an unwarranted imposition on the physician-patient relationship and would be far more disruptive than beneficial to the patient.[15] Other courts followed previous authority in refusing to find such a duty for hospitals.[16] *Goss v Oklahoma Blood Institute* cited authority from Washington, Iowa, Florida, Texas, North Carolina, New Mexico, North Dakota, Colorado, Michigan, West Virginia, and Illinois for support in its refusal to recognize a duty for the hospital to disclose risks and obtain informed consent.[18] Other courts have held that even when the hospital provides the consent form and encourages physicians to obtain informed consent, the responsibility of obtaining informed consent lies with physicians because of the skill and experience they possess.[19]

While the overwhelming state of the law is that physicians are responsible for obtaining informed consent, imaging professionals should be aware of the state of the law in their jurisdiction and the policies and procedures of their facility.

Obtaining Valid Informed Consent

The patient's capacity to consent to or refuse the procedure must be evaluated. The primary issue to be considered is whether the patient is capable of understanding the medical condition and the risks, benefits, alternative treatment options, and expected outcomes if treatment is not commenced (Box 4-5).

Although the physician bears the ultimate responsibility for obtaining valid informed consent, imaging professionals must often make subjective judgments of patients' capacities to make decisions. This is particularly true if the patient is in severe pain.

BOX 4-5   **ELEMENTS IN INFORMED CONSENT**

The consent must be given voluntarily by a mentally competent adult. The patient should not be coerced into giving consent.

Patients must understand exactly to what they are consenting. If a patient speaks a foreign language or is deaf, an interpreter must explain the procedure requiring consent.

The request for consent should include a description of the risks and benefits of the procedure, alternative treatment options, and expected outcomes if treatment is not commenced.

The consent should be written, signed by the patient or representative, witnessed, and dated.

Consent to treat a minor patient is usually given by a parent or guardian, but if the minor patient is at least 7 years old, he or she should be included in the decision-making process.

Modified from Deloughery GL: Key elements for informed consent. In Deloughery GL (Ed): *Issues and trends in nursing*, St Louis, 1995, Mosby.

If imaging professionals, after consulting with radiologists, do not feel that patients have the capacity to give valid informed consent, surrogate consent should be sought. If such consent is impossible to obtain, the involved parties should consider invoking the emergency exception to the informed consent doctrine. If that exception does not apply, the procedure should not be performed.

Patients who are minors are another problematic population for informed consent. Historically, consent was obtained on behalf of a minor by a parent or guardian (most states define *minor* as a person less than 18 years of age). Because important limitations and problems in the application of informed consent with regard to pediatric patients have been identified, however, the American Academy of Pediatrics (AAP) has revisited this issue. The AAP recognizes two concepts, parental permission and patient assent.[20] The AAP believes that in most cases physicians have an ethical and legal obligation to obtain parental permission before undertaking recommended medical intervention. In many circumstances the physician should also solicit a patient assent when the patient is of an appropriate age and developmental level. In cases of emancipated or mature minors with adequate decision-making capacity, or when otherwise permitted by law, informed consent should be obtained directly from the patient.[20]

Because laws vary, imaging professionals should know the state of the law in their own jurisdiction. Inclusion of the minor in the decision-making process is advisable, however, both because it nurtures a cooperative relationship and because it allows the minor to indicate a difference of opinion from the parents. If a conflict develops between the wishes of the two parties, the imaging professional should seek help from the hospital's risk management department or legal counsel to determine the correct action to take.

Role of Imaging Professionals in Informed Consent

As has been discussed, informed consent is absolutely necessary for many procedures in the imaging department, including any contrast injection. The facility must establish and follow policies and procedures identifying when informed consent is needed. Although legal responsibility for obtaining consent lies with the physician, most facilities have also adopted policies and procedures requiring imaging professionals to ensure that informed consent is obtained. Imaging professionals should recognize this responsibility as part of any procedure they perform that requires written consent. Because the imaging professionals perform the study, they have a duty to ensure that procedures are explained and consent is obtained before beginning the procedure.

Imaging professionals have excellent opportunities to explain procedures to patients. They spend much more time with patients than do physicians, and their communication with patients helps build a good imaging professional–patient relationship that not only makes the patient more comfortable about asking questions concerning the procedure, but also is likely to result in a better outcome.

Consent Forms

Forms are useful tools to help inform patients about procedures and document consent. A general form adapted to include specifics of the particular procedure requiring consent or individual forms specifically designed for each procedure may be used. Because laws and rules differ among states and facilities, these forms should be carefully written with input from physicians, the technologists performing the studies, the risk management department, and legal counsel.

The forms should be written clearly in terms understandable by laypersons and must be used in conjunction with a thorough explanation to the patient that includes a discussion of risks, benefits, alternative diagnostic or treatment plans, and expected outcomes if the patient decides not to undergo the procedure. A **consent form** must never be used in place of an oral explanation.

CONSENT FORMS
Consent forms are useful tools to help inform patients about procedures and document consent.

IMAGING SCENARIO

The imaging department is swamped, and you find yourself relieving an imaging professional in the intravenous pyelography (IVP) room. He tells you everything is ready for you to inject the patient. You speak to the radiologist between other procedures, and she hurriedly comes in and injects the contrast medium without inquiring about informed consent or looking at the form. Just as you finish the IVP films, the patient begins to exhibit signs of anaphylactic shock. The appropriate emergency care is administered. As the activity in the IVP room slows down, you notice that the informed consent form is neither filled out nor signed. The patient ends up in intensive care and eventually dies, leaving behind a husband and a 3-month-old child.

Discussion questions
- Have you created liability for yourself?
- Have you created liability for the hospital?
- Have you created liability for the radiologist?
- What must the family prove to be successful in a lawsuit?

IMAGING SCENARIO

A man and his wife arrive at the emergency room (ER), the man complaining of severe pain in his left flank area. Upon their arrival they explain that they do not have insurance coverage. They are both fairly certain the problem is a kidney stone because the man has had three previous bouts with kidney stones. He is in significant pain, but quite capable of the informed consent process. The ER physician sends the man for a computed tomography (CT) scan and numerous other exams. The stone is located and removed, and the man and his wife return home. A few weeks later they receive a "hefty" hospital bill that includes the many exams. They contact the hospital billing department and explain that they have no insurance and did not give permission for the many exams. The hospital employee with whom they speak explains to them that the ER physician does not need permission to do these exams, but they continue to argue their case. Finally they contact the finance officer and question the hospital's informed consent process. The hospital drops the CT charges after the couple continues to state their case.

Discussion questions
- Was the informed consent process necessary in this case?
- Did the physician respect the autonomy of the patient?
- If the man had questioned the CT technologist about the exam, what should the technologist have done?
- Could this have been handled differently?

A consent form generally includes the name of the procedure; a brief explanation of the procedure, including benefits and risks; spaces for the patient's name and the name of the person performing the procedure; and signature lines for the patient or surrogate, the person explaining the procedure and obtaining consent, and at least one witness. The form must also be dated with the time recorded. Laws and facility regulations vary, but in general consent should be obtained within 24 hours before the procedure.

Policies and procedures should be developed regarding when written consent must be obtained. They should ensure that consent is obtained in writing whenever an invasive procedure is to be performed or when a procedure has associated risks and disclosure of these risks may be helpful to a patient in deciding whether to undergo the procedure. If informed consent forms are computerized, these forms and their accompanying patient signatures should become part of the permanent patient record.

SUMMARY

- The informed consent process seeks to provide the patient with enough information to make informed decisions about whether to undergo certain medical procedures. This consent process enables the patient to maintain dignity, independence, and autonomy.
- Physicians and other professionals attempting to obtain informed consent should provide patients with information concerning diagnosis, treatment, prognosis, risks, duration of incapacitation, alternatives, billing costs, hospital rules, and the names of persons performing the procedure. If a procedure requires informed consent, the physician if responsible for obtaining this consent.
- Four rules for providing the patient with information to make an informed decision are the patient preference rule, prudent person rule, subjective substantial disclosure rule, and professional custom rule. The prudent person rule and the subjective substantial disclosure rule are a good combination to use in the informed consent process.
- The patient's competence is a key concept in giving informed consent. If the patient is incompetent, an advance directive or surrogate may aid the process.
- Obstacles to autonomy and informed consent include undue influence on patients, paternalism, therapeutic privilege, and inept communication. Respect for the autonomy of the patient requires the imaging professional to evaluate patient competence, the informed consent process, surrogacy, patient preferences, and the patient's ability to make choices and cooperate.
- Emergency situations may necessitate dispensing with informed consent processes to save the patient's life. In rare circumstances, informed consent may also be superseded by therapeutic privilege if the physician believes the disclosure would cause the patient to become unusually emotionally distraught.
- Among the ethical theories that might be applied when issues of patient autonomy are considered, virtue ethics, involving practical wisdom and reason, may be the most adaptable.
- As education regarding health care becomes more prominent and individuals become more involved in all aspects of their health care, the maintenance of patient autonomy may become more achievable; however, the achievement of absolute patient autonomy and informed consent may be impossible.

- Patient autonomy is the ethical concept behind issues of consent and informed consent. Simple consent from the patient must be obtained before any procedure, but such consent does not require knowledge of the procedure. It may be given simply by the patient's getting on the table or stepping up to the chest board. Failure to obtain consent can result in allegations of assault, battery, or false imprisonment.
- Assault, battery, and false imprisonment are intentional torts, meaning that the acts are done with the intent of harming another. Even if the health care provider does not intend harm, these allegations can be made if the patient perceives the acts to be done with the intent of harm.
- Medical immobilization is considered a regular part of medical diagnostic or therapeutic procedures based on standard practice. The use of immobilizing devices to reduce radiation exposure and obtain optimal images or treatment is not considered restraint. When restraints are necessary, the imaging professional must be able to justify the restraint using specific criteria.
- Communication is the best tool imaging professionals have to prevent allegations of intentional torts. Obtaining consent and explaining necessary restraints to patients and parents limit the risk of these allegations.
- Unintentional torts, which result from acts not intended to cause harm, include negligence, lack of informed consent, and breach of patient confidentiality.
- Informed consent is required for invasive procedures and those for which disclosure of associated risks would help the patient determine whether to proceed with the procedure or treatment. Facilities must establish and follow policies and procedures for informed consent.
- The physician has the legal duty to obtain informed consent. Many facilities require the imaging professional to ensure that informed consent is obtained and the proper documentation is made in the patient's medical record. During preparation for the procedure, the imaging professional should talk with the patient to encourage communication and gauge understanding.
- Consent forms are helpful to inform patients about procedures and document consent. These forms, however, cannot substitute for the required explanation of the procedure and full disclosure of associated risks.
- The goal of informed consent is to allow patients to make determinations regarding the direction of their treatment. Two standards of care, the professional and the lay standard, are recognized by various U.S. jurisdictions in determining how much information a physician must give the patient to make this determination.
- Imaging professionals should be aware of statutes and procedures for written informed consent in their jurisdiction and facility. They should consistently ensure that informed consent is obtained when needed and is documented in the patient's medical record.

REFERENCES

1. Garrett TM, Baillie HW, Garrett RM: *Healthcare ethics, principles and problems*, ed 2, Englewood Cliffs, NJ, 1993, Prentice Hall.
2. American Hospital Association: *A patient's bill of rights*, Chicago, 1992, Author.
3. Mezey M, Evans LK, Golub ZD, et al: The patient self-determination act: sources of concern for nurses, *Nurs Outlook* 42(1):30, 1994.
4. Jonsen AR, Siegler M, Winslade WJ: *Clinical ethics: a practical approach to ethical decisions in clinical medicine*, ed 5, New York, 2002, McGraw-Hill.

5. *Canterbury v Spence*, 464 F.2d 772 (1972).
6. Schwartz V, Kelly K, Partlett D: *Prosser, Wade, and Schwartz: cases and materials on torts*, ed 10, Westbury, NY, 2000, Foundation Press.
7. *Schloendorff v Society of NY Hospitals*, 105 N.E.92 (NY 1914).
8. Aiken T: *Legal and ethical issues in health occupations*, Philadelphia, 2002, Saunders.
9. *Salgo v Leland Stanford Jr. University Board of Trustees* (Cal. 1957).
10. *Ketchup v Howard*, 543 S.E.2d 371 (Ga. App. 2000).
11. *Truman v Thomas*, 611 P.2d 902 (Cal. 1980).
12. *Pauscher v Iowa Methodist Medical Center, Jeff Watters, and John Bardole*, 408 N.W.2d 355 (Iowa, 1987).
13. *Keel v St. Elizabeth Medical Center*, 842 S.W.2d 860 (Ky. 1992).
14. *Boney v Mother Frances Hospital*, 880 S.W.2d 140 (Tex. App.—Tyler 1994); *Kelley v Kitahama*, 675 So.2d 1181 (La. App. 5 Cir. 1996).
15. *Giese v Stice, and Bishop Clarkson Memorial Hospital*, 567 N.W.2d 156 (Neb. 1997).
16. *Alexander v. Gonser*, 711 P.2d 347 (Wash. 1985)
17. *Howell v Spokane & Inland Empire Blood Bank*, 785 P.2d 815 (Wash. 1990).
18. *Goss v Oklahoma Blood Institute*, 856 P.2d 998 (Okl. App. 1990), Cert. Denied (1993).
19. *Bynum v Magno, Dang, Callan, and the Queen's Medical Center*, 125 F. Supp 2d 1249 (Haw, 2000).
20. American Academy of Pediatrics Committee on Bioethics: Informed consent, parental permission, and assent in pediatric practice, *Pediatrics* 95(2):314, 1995.

REVIEW QUESTIONS

1 Autonomy involves which of the following?
   a. Informed consent
   b. The self
   c. Patient rights
   d. All of the above

2 Informed consent should include the following:
   a. _____
   b. _____
   c. _____
   d. _____

3 Why is two-way communication between patients and imaging professionals important in imaging services?

4 Should the imaging professional be responsible for the informed consent process? Explain.

5 Define the following terms:
   a. Competence
   b. Surrogacy

6 Paternalism is defined as which of the following?
   a. Motherlike caretaking
   b. Fatherlike (God-like) caretaking
   c. Necessary
   d. None of the above

7 Define therapeutic privilege.

8 Describe three conditions in which emergency situations may alter the informed consent process:
   a. _____
   b. _____
   c. _____

 9 **True or False**   Combining the prudent person rule and the subjective substantial disclosure rule in most cases provides the information the patient needs to make informed decisions.

10 **True or False**   Respect for the autonomy of the patient includes the ability of the patient to make choices.

11 **True or False**   Surrogacy is not an issue in respecting the patient's autonomy.

12 **True or False**   Truly informed consent may not be possible.

13 **True or False**   Intentional torts can occur only if the perpetrator of the tort intends to do harm.

14 **True or False**   Assault occurs when the victim is touched without giving consent.

15 **True or False**   Battery cannot be found if the touching to which the patient has not consented is for the good of the patient.

16 **True or False**   Immobilization devices used in the imaging department are considered restraints.

17 **True or False**   Use of restraints of patients by imaging professionals is always an exception to the torts of assault and battery.

18 **True or False**   Communication is the imaging professional's best tool to decrease risk of litigation for assault, battery, and false imprisonment.

19 **True or False**   The legal duty to obtain informed consent lies with the imaging professional.

20 **True or False**   Informed consent need not be given if an imaging professional does not feel the patient wants to know about the procedure.

21 **True or False**   The duty of informed consent lies with physicians, so imaging professionals do not need to concern themselves.

22 **True or False**   Consent forms may be used to obtain consent instead of an explanation of the procedure and its risks.

23 List three reasons the seven points of respect for the autonomy of the patient are valuable tools in ethical and legal problem solving.

   a._____

   b._____

   c._____

24 **True or False**   For informed consent to be legally recognized, a patient's signature on the form is sufficient.

25 **True or False**   The professional standard of informed consent requires a physician to disclose the risks that a reasonable and prudent medical practitioner would disclose under the same or similar circumstances.

26 **True or False**   The lay standard of informed consent measures the physician's disclosure duty by the patient's need for information rather than by the standards of the medical professional.

27 **True or False**   An imaging professional does not need to be concerned with the law regarding informed consent in his or her jurisdiction, as long as the form is signed.

CRITICAL THINKING *Questions & Activities*

1 Is everyone in every situation entitled to autonomy in an imaging procedure? Why or why not?

2 What would you do in a critical situation if the patient was unresponsive and a surrogate was not available?

3 What would you do if you made the best decision you could in question 2 and were still involved in a lawsuit?

4 In what ways can imaging professionals promote the autonomy of patients in the imaging department?

5 Does the imaging professional's autonomy enhance or interfere with patient autonomy? In what way does this occur?

6 A 79-year-old woman arrives in the emergency department with severe chest pain and breathlessness. She has been treated previously for a minor stroke and had a breast removed 4 years ago. She is a nervous individual and does not want to deal with decision making; she would much rather have the physician make the decision concerning a cardiac catheterization. Her family wants her to proceed with the catheterization and consider surgery. She continues to fear the process and refuses to make a decision. Role play the various processes that may occur in this particular informed consent process and indicate ways of encouraging autonomy for the fearful patient (by one or more groups of players). As the situation is played, the observers should record the appropriate and inappropriate methods employed. These could include any of the following:

   a. Positive and negative methods for obtaining informed consent and delivering information

   b. Attempts to ensure autonomy

   c. Paternalism

   d. Invocation of therapeutic privilege

   e. Surrogacy

   f. Responses to emergency situations

   Include these elements in your evaluation.

7 Discuss whether a person who commits an intentional tort must have the intent to cause harm to be liable.

8 Discuss situations that may result in allegations of assault or battery.

9 Discuss whether a patient can feel imprisoned without consent in the imaging department.

10 Discuss the ways in which restraints may be used and justified by the criteria presented in this chapter.

11 Discuss situations in which the imaging professional is in a difficult situation because the radiologist or interpreting physician does not want to take the time to inform the patient adequately about risks, alternative procedures, and expected outcomes if the procedure is not performed.

5 TRUTHFULNESS AND CONFIDENTIALITY

Never esteem anything as of advantage to you that will make you break your word or lose your self-respect.

MARCUS AURELIUS ANTONINUS

Chapter Outline

Ethical Issues
Truthfulness and Veracity
Right to the Truth
Confidentiality
Obligatory Secrets
Exceptions to Confidentiality
Confidentiality and AIDS

Legal Issues
HIPAA
Patient Authorization
Statutory Disclosure
Duty to Warn Third Parties
AIDS and HIV
Patient Access to Medical Records
Torts Regarding Confidentiality

Learning Objectives

After completing the chapter, the reader will be able to perform the following:

- Define truthfulness, veracity, and confidentiality.
- Identify the three variables involved in expectations of truth.
- Cite circumstances in which a person has a right to the truth.
- List and define three types of obligatory secrets.
- Explain the importance of the professional secret.
- Cite exceptions to confidentiality.
- Identify and discuss the elements of defamation, including slander and libel per se.
- Specify situations that may trigger the duty to warn third parties.

- Identify the conflict between confidentiality and disclosure of HIV and AIDS.
- List the statutory obligations regarding AIDS and HIV.
- Define the patient's right of access to medical records.
- Identify ways that the patient's right of access may come into conflict with the ethical and legal principles by which the imaging professional must practice.

Key Terms

confidentiality
defamation
duty to warn third parties
HIPAA
lie
place of communication

role of communication
secret
statutory duty to report
truthfulness
veracity

Professional Profile

Ethical codes and the Health Insurance Portability and Accountability Act (HIPAA) are an important part of all health care professions. The Society of Diagnostic Medical Sonographers (SDMS) has adopted ethical codes and examination protocols specific for diagnostic ultrasound. These issues define how I as a sonographer interact with patients, family members, and colleagues. Consistent protocol guidelines help to maximize patient benefits while minimizing potential harm.

My approach to each patient is similar, whether it is an obstetrical or an arterial duplex examination. Patient privacy and dignity are forefront. Interpreters are requested when there is a language barrier. Questions regarding the patient's medical history are discussed in private. Explaining the procedure, answering questions, and alleviating fears prior to and during the examination are routine.

Diagnostic ultrasound is dependent on the education, knowledge, and clinical skills of the operator.

When pathology is encountered, I must broaden the minimum standard guidelines to achieve additional pertinent diagnostic information. Continuing to update my knowledge and skills is an important part of my ethical responsibility to both patients and colleagues.

The approach of health care professionals to medical care is defined by legal regulations and codes of conduct. These protections have been adopted in the interest of the patient to ensure fair and consistent medical care. As sonographers, we are responsible for continuing to update our knowledge and skills and treating every patient equally while respecting his or her individual rights and beliefs.

Sue Ovel, RT, RDMS, RVT
Staff Sonographer/Clinical Instructor
Radiological Associates of Sacramento
Sacramento, California

ETHICAL ISSUES

The struggle between confidentiality and truthfulness is a common one in medical imaging, as in all of medicine. Imaging professionals have to consider when they must tell the whole truth and in what situations the whole truth may compromise the patient's outcome. On the other hand, some truths must be kept confidential. The difficulty for the imaging professional is in knowing what may be ethically concealed and what must be revealed.

The information required during the informed consent process is discussed in Chapter 4. This chapter discusses issues regarding truthfulness and confidentiality in imaging professionals' dealings with patients, surrogates, and other health care professionals. For example, if an imaging professional overhears a physician telling a patient not to worry, the chest x-ray film looks fine, but she should have another x-ray film in 6 months, should the imaging professional indicate to the patient that she has a spot on her lung and may have a problem?

The chapter also discusses the principles covering situations in which the truth should be kept confidential. For example, must an ultrasonographer conceal from a mother that her 13-year-old daughter is pregnant and desires an abortion?

TRUTHFULNESS AND VERACITY

Definitions

Truthfulness is defined as conformance with fact or reality. However, the perception of fact and reality may change, so truthfulness is a somewhat fluid concept. **Veracity** is defined as the obligation to tell the truth and not to lie or deceive others. Veracity and

TRUTHFULNESS
Truthfulness is conformity with fact or reality.

VERACITY
Veracity is the obligation to tell the truth and not to lie or deceive others.

IMAGING SCENARIO

Several accident victims arrive at the emergency department, and the trauma imaging specialist assigned to perform portable x-ray examinations becomes involved in a family's fight for life. The mother is critically injured, and a strong possibility exists that she will not survive. Her husband is making good progress. The physician tells him his wife is dying. The man then insists that his wife and children be told, but the physician decides not to tell them because it would only cause them more pain. The wife dies the next day.

The trauma imaging specialist is aware of this interaction because he is busy with chest imaging when the husband requests that his wife be told about her condition. The imaging professional knows this physician has a history of determining patients' needs, often contrary to their wishes. During one of the imaging procedures, the man asks the imaging professional what he thinks about the physician, but the trauma imaging specialist declines to share any information with the husband.

Discussion questions
- Should the imaging specialist have explained the physician's previous style of paternalism to the patient?
- Did the physician have an obligation to tell the patient that she was dying?
- Did the physician have a right to tell the husband about the wife's condition even when she was competent and had no need for a surrogate?
- Did the children have the right to know that their mother was dying?

truthfulness have long been regarded as fundamental to the establishment of trust among individuals, and they have a special significance in medical imaging and other health care relationships. Imaging professionals and patients may have differing perceptions of veracity and truthfulness. Imaging professionals may believe in telling the whole truth, no matter how painful, but the patient's need to know the truth may be entirely different.

Circumstances for Expectations of the Truth

Truthfulness is summed up in two commands: "Do not lie, and you must communicate with those who have a right to the truth."[1] The first command leaves the imaging professional free to not communicate to avoid telling a **lie**, and the second constrains the professional to share information only with those who have a right to the truth.

A lie is a falsehood told to a person who has a reasonable expectation of the truth.[1] The ethics of lying is judged in terms of consequences for the individual and society. The expectation of truth varies with the following conditions:
- **Place of communication**
- **Role of communication**
- Nature of the truth involved

All three of these conditions are related to the obligation of confidentiality and the right to privacy (Figure 5-1).

If an imaging student, within earshot of a patient, asks a clinical instructor about pathologic changes on an image, he or she does not have a reasonable expectation of truth. The question asked in this place of communication may force the instructor to avoid telling the truth about the examination results if the patient might overhear the

LIE
A lie is a falsehood told to another who has a reasonable expectation of the truth.

PLACE OF COMMUNICATION
The place of communication is the environment of the expectation of truth.

ROLE OF COMMUNICATION
The role of communication is the relationship between the communicators, which may have an impact on the expectation of truth.

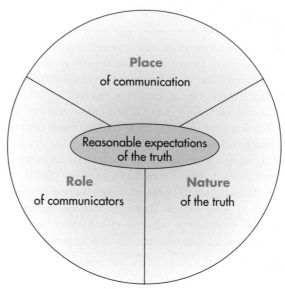

FIGURE 5-1 Components of a reasonable expectation of truth.

conversation and become distressed. Students do have an expectation of truth, however, if they ask the same question in the classroom during a film analysis class. This is an example of expectations varying with the place of communication.

If an imaging student asks the clinical coordinator for information about another student's performance on a clinical competency examination, the inquiring student has no reasonable expectation of truth because of the roles of the two communicators. The score of another student is not the student's concern, and the clinical coordinator has an obligation of confidentiality to all the students.

The nature of the truth involved alters the expectation of truth in questions concerning private matters. If an imaging professional asks a student or any other person about finances, sex life, or anything of a personal or private nature, the imaging professional should not expect a truthful answer.

Overly curious imaging professionals may be found in many imaging departments, just as overly curious people are found in every profession. Such people have unreasonable expectations of the truth. The temptation is to tell these people to mind their own business, but this is not always the wisest course in the hospital setting, where teamwork is imperative. "Snoopy" imaging professionals have no reasonable expectation of the truth and should be counseled about their unprofessional behavior.

Concealment of the truth is not necessarily a lie, and in certain situations the imaging professional does not have to tell the whole truth. Thus the question arises concerning the circumstances in which people have a right to the truth.

RIGHT TO THE TRUTH

A person has the right to truthful communication during the informed consent process, when making decisions about treatment, and when making important nonmedical decisions. If a patient's computed tomography (CT) scan reveals that lung cancer has spread to the liver and other vital organs, the patient needs to be informed of this terminal condition to make necessary plans. If the information is not provided, the patient may not make necessary arrangements or deal with family, psychological, and spiritual issues. In cases of terminal illness, such practical needs are often more important than medical needs to the patient.

In the previous section the patient's expectation of the truth was mentioned. This is an important consideration for the imaging professional because the patient may ask about the outcome of an imaging examination, fully expecting the truth. The truth about the examination, however, may entail information only a radiologist or the patient's physician can provide. Therefore the imaging professional in this situation cannot provide the whole truth to the patient. For example, if the patient expects a truthful answer to the question, "Has my cancer spread?", the imaging professional must deal with the patient's expectation of truth by being considerate and understanding but must explain to the patient that the radiologist or the patient's physician will provide this information. Imaging professionals do not have the authority to discuss pathologic findings with patients. In this type of dilemma they have to avoid the whole truth even if they are certain that the cancer has spread. Image interpretation for the patient is the purview of the physician, who is also qualified to answer follow-up questions.

CONFIDENTIALITY

Considerations of **confidentiality** are as important as truthfulness in the discussion of patients' rights and the imaging professional's obligations. Confidentiality concerns the keeping of **secrets**: "A secret is knowledge a person has a right or obligation to conceal. Obligatory secrets are secrets that arise from the fact that harm will follow if a particular knowledge is revealed....These are the natural secret, the promised secret, and the professional secret"[1] (Box 5-1).

OBLIGATORY SECRETS

Natural Secrets

Information shared in a natural secret is by its nature harmful if revealed. An imaging professional may know that a patient has acquired immunodeficiency syndrome (AIDS) but has the obligation to keep the knowledge confidential. If the information is made public, the person positive for human immunodeficiency virus (HIV) could have difficulty gaining employment and might be persecuted socially. Some situations are more complex. For example, a cardiovascular technologist is involved in a procedure that indicates a patient needs immediate cardiac surgery, but the patient decides not to have the surgery. Within a few days the technologist boards an airplane and realizes the pilot is the patient who chose not to have cardiac surgery. Should the technologist tell the

CONFIDENTIALITY
Confidentiality is the duty owed by health care providers to protect the privacy of patient information.

SECRET
A secret is knowledge a person has a right or obligation to conceal.

| BOX 5-1 | **OBLIGATORY SECRETS** |

An obligatory secret is a confidence that will result in harm if it is revealed. Obligatory secrets are of three types:
1. Natural—a secret that by its nature would be harmful if revealed
2. Promised—a secret the receiver has promised to conceal
3. Professional—a secret maintained to protect the patient, society, and profession

airline or some other authority of the pilot's medical condition? Does the harm that may come from concealing the natural secret outweigh the harm to the former patient?

Promised Secrets

Knowledge a person has promised to conceal is a promised secret. The harmful effects of breaking a promise complicate professional relationships and discourage the sharing of privileged information that may be vital to patient care. Imaging professionals who cannot be trusted to keep secrets about patients or co-workers not only breach confidentiality, but also lose trust as employees or friends. Proportionality must govern the imaging professional's decisions about divulging promised secrets. If the risk of keeping the secret outweighs the harm to the patient or friend, the imaging professional must make a decision. For example, if a student technologist knows another student has hepatitis (and has sworn not to tell because graduation is in a month and the student with hepatitis has already used the maximum sick time) and they are both scheduled to scrub for an invasive vascular procedure, the student may choose to confide in an instructor if concerned about the spread of infection, regardless of the degree of risk to the patient. The student's peace of mind is important when it may influence the successful completion of the procedure. The student who promises a classmate to keep such a secret may need to reevaluate the ethical implications of this kind of promise.

Professional Secrets

The most binding of the obligatory secrets is the professional secret. When professional secrets are revealed, both the patient and the imaging profession are harmed. This damage to the reputation of the imaging profession harms the community, which depends on a limited number of professionals for imaging services. If people lack faith in imaging professionals, they may choose not to have necessary imaging procedures performed. This in turn complicates the diagnostic process and endangers the health of patients.

The importance of professional secrecy has been recognized by society. A body of laws encourages privileged communication and the maintenance of confidentiality between health care providers and patients. The Patient's Bill of Rights of the American Hospital Association (AHA) describes the importance of professional secrecy in the hospital setting based on the nature of the knowledge, the implied promise of secrecy, and the good of society and the profession (see p. 255).

EXCEPTIONS TO CONFIDENTIALITY

Some exceptions to confidentiality are mandated by state law. They include mechanisms for the reporting of certain types of wounds, communicable diseases, automobile accidents, abuse, birth defects, drug addiction, and industrial accidents. State requirements may vary.

The AHA's Committee on Biomedical Ethics notes the following conditions in which confidentiality may be breached[2]:

> Also subject to state law, confidentiality may be overridden when the life or safety of the patient is endangered such as when knowledgeable intervention can prevent threatened suicide or self-injury. In addition, the moral obligation to prevent substantial and foreseeable harm to an innocent third party usually is greater than the moral obligation to protect confidentiality.

In many jurisdictions, imaging professionals are required to report suspected cases of child and adult abuse. Such situations may involve families with whom they are familiar.

BOX 5-2	EXCEPTIONS TO CONFIDENTIALITY
Wounds	Addictions
Abuse	Family's need to know
Communicable diseases	Public's need to know
Accidents	Third-party payers
Birth defects	

The family may urge them not to intercede because the abuser is in treatment and the reporting mechanism might deter continued treatment. Although this may be a difficult situation for the technologist, employers expect loyalty to the institution, which includes the reporting of abuse.

Exceptions to confidentiality may be debated in discussions of the family's need to know (as in the case at the beginning of this chapter), exceptions concerning children and adolescents (e.g., abortive processes, treatment for sexually transmitted diseases), medical condition of public figures (e.g., whether Americans have the right to know if the President is in critical condition), use of hospital records for research and billing purposes, and third-party payers (e.g., need for payment balanced against patient confidentiality). Exceptions to confidentiality are discussed further in the legal section of this chapter and are listed in Box 5-2.

CONFIDENTIALITY AND AIDS

Imaging professionals are not usually placed in situations in which they must inform a patient that they have HIV. Occasionally, however, patients ask imaging professionals if they are HIV positive. Imaging professionals must decide based on institutional rules and professional experience whether this information is necessary for the patient to give informed consent. Other situations may be just as difficult. An imaging professional may need to report a fellow technologist who has AIDS and does not take necessary protective measures with patients. Although the revelation may cause grief and loss of social contacts or even employment, the technologist must consider the good of patients and the profession.

Some professionals are deontologists and believe that stricter rules of right and wrong should be used in keeping information confidential. They believe that the act of keeping information confidential is more morally important than the consequences this act may cause.

Because of these differing and often conflicting viewpoints, questions concerning AIDS will continue to fuel public debate. The hope, however, is that a cure or vaccine will be discovered and the problem will no longer haunt the public and health care professionals.

LEGAL ISSUES

Ethical dilemmas often arise regarding conflict between truth, confidentiality, and secrecy. The law provides some definite parameters regarding patient confidentiality. One of the most important obligations a health care provider owes a patient is the protection of confidences revealed by the patient. Situations do exist in which this duty is not absolute, and at times the law actually imposes a duty to disclose confidential information. The law regarding the duty of confidentiality and the exceptions to these rules are discussed here.

HIPAA

HIPAA
Health Insurance Portability and Accountability Act, enacted by the federal government to enhance the rights of consumers regarding access to their records, limit access of others to those records, and improve quality, efficiency, and effectiveness of health care delivery through a national framework.

Concerns about the privacy of patient medical information have intensified with the growth of electronic recordkeeping and the Internet. In response to these concerns Congress enacted the Health Insurance Portability and Accountability Act of 1996 **(HIPAA)**. The major purposes of this regulation are (1) to protect and enhance the rights of consumers by providing them access to their health information and controlling the inappropriate use of that information; (2) to improve the quality of health care in the United States by restoring trust in the health care system among consumers, health care professionals, and the multiple organizations and individuals committed to the delivery of care; and (3) to improve the efficiency and effectiveness of health care delivery by creating a national framework for health privacy protection that builds on efforts by states, health systems, and individual organizations and individuals (Box 5-3).[3] A sample privacy notice appears in Appendix C.

HIPAA regulations have added some clarity and conformity to issues regarding electronic personal health care information and have mandated that patients receive a notice of the facility's privacy practices. HIPAA has also created a requirement that only the minimum necessary information for the purpose of disclosure be released, rather than the entire record as was assumed in the past. Disclosures allowed without permission from the patient include disclosures to the patient; to other health care providers for

---

BOX 5-3   HOW HIPAA WORKS

1. Patients gain more control over their own health information. Providers must inform patients how their information will be used and to whom it can be disclosed. The release of information is limited by patient authorization under many circumstances. Patients may access their own information and request correction of potentially harmful errors.

2. Boundaries are set on medical record use and release. The amount of information to be released is the "minimum necessary" for the purpose as opposed to release of the entire medical record, which was the standard in the past.

3. The security of personal health information is ensured by specific mandates on providers and others who may access health care information. Privacy-conscious business practices, with internal procedures including a compliance officer, must be in place to protect the privacy of medical records.

4. The rules create accountability for medical record use and release, with new criminal and civil penalties for improper use or disclosure.

5. The rules attempt to balance public responsibility with privacy protections, requiring the disclosure of information for only limited public purposes such as public health and research.

From Furrow BR, Greaney TL, Johnson SH, et al: *Health law: cases, materials and problems*, ed 5, St Paul, Minn, 2004, West.

treatment purposes; for payment of services; for health care operations, including quality assurance information; for appointment reminders, treatment alternatives, and health-related benefits; in the facility directory; for clergy; for individuals involved in payment of care; and for approved research projects. Under HIPAA, special circumstances also allow the disclosure of health information without patient permission. The most common of these are when required by law, including subpoenas or other court-ordered disclosures and law enforcement requests under certain conditions; to other entities for billing purposes; organ and tissue donors; and public health risks. See the sample privacy notice in Appendix C for more detailed information.

HIPAA also creates patient rights or in many jurisdictions reinforces existing patient rights. These rights include the right to inspect and copy their records; the right to ask for the information to be amended if the patient believes it to be inaccurate; the right to ask what disclosures have been made; the right to request restriction of information disclosure; the right to request the method of communication; and the right to a paper copy of the privacy notice of the institution.

HIPAA clarifies to some extent what may or may not be disclosed. Some of the exceptions are discussed further in the following sections. These include situations when patient authorization is required; statutory duties to disclose information; the duty to warn third parties of danger; and AIDS and HIV confidentiality and reporting.

HIPAA codifies and gives conformity to privacy regulations throughout the country. HIPAA does not provide a right to sue but instead provides a requirement to file a written complaint with the Secretary of Health and Human Services (HHS) through the Office of Civil Rights. The Secretary has discretion of investigation, and civil and criminal penalties may be imposed. However, according to the interim final rule by which HHS established procedures for imposing monetary penalties, the department "intends to seek and promote voluntary compliance."[3] This will probably mean that the HIPAA privacy rules will become a new standard of care for handling confidential patient information in negligence suits.

PATIENT AUTHORIZATION

Patients may explicitly consent to the release of medical information in their records. Presumed consent has always existed for access to treating providers, when a patient is transferred from one provider to another, and when emergency treatment requires access to records.[3] This has now been codified in HIPAA for electronic record disclosure. Under HIPAA, reasons for disclosure without consent include treatment, payment, health care operations, appointment reminders, treatment alternatives, and health-related benefits; fundraising activities; facility directory; clergy; disclosure to those involved in payment of care; and research. If permission is given for reasons other than these listed, that permission may be revoked in writing at any time. Special circumstances exist that do not require authorization for release of information, as discussed previously.

Much of the law regarding disclosure of health care information has not changed but has been codified by a federal statute. For example, patients have been found to have waived their rights to confidentiality when they put their mental or physical state at issue in a lawsuit. In the case of a lawsuit, a subpoena (a request signed by a judicial officer requesting records when a lawsuit is in progress) may be issued. The subpoena must specify the records to be disclosed. In addition, while most of this is now codified by HIPAA for electronic information, case law has found that patient consent for in-house

use of medical information (e.g., in-house quality assurance committees, Joint Commission on Accreditation of Healthcare Organizations [JCAHO] inspections, state institutional licensure reviewers) is implied by the patient's agreement to treatment, although some states have statutes expressly authorizing access.[3]

Release of patient information to outside reviewers is governed by state law as well as HIPAA, which supersedes state law in most respects and covers Veterans Administration (VA) hospitals and other federal facilities. Some statutes allow state boards to review patient records for evaluation of provider misconduct, and the Medicare program requires providers to allow peer review organizations access to records of Medicare patients. HIPAA regulations generally govern the release of electronic records for these purposes. Imaging professionals should consult the risk management department in their facility, however, since in the absence of statutory or judicial support for release of information to outside reviewers, the sharing of information from patient medical records poses liability risks.

Third-party payers are the most common outside requesters of medical information. Although patient consent has previously been necessary for this release, the HIPAA regulations now encompass this aspect for electronic information and do not require patient authorization. Regardless, most insurers require patients to authorize release of information when they file claims for payment.[3] Some states have also enacted statutes for disclosure to insurers without authorization to determine responsibility for payment. These regulations may seem confusing. The facility's risk management and privacy personnel should always be the imaging professional's guide for the procedures in the facility.

STATUTORY DISCLOSURE

STATUTORY DUTY
TO REPORT
The statutory duty to report is the legal obligation to report a variety of medical conditions and incidents, including venereal disease; contagious diseases such as tuberculosis; wounds inflicted by violence; poisonings; industrial accidents; abortions; drug abuse; and abuse of children, elderly people, and people with disabilities.

HIPAA reinforces the obligation to follow state public health laws that require medical professionals and institutions to report a variety of medical conditions and incidents, including venereal disease; contagious diseases such as tuberculosis; wounds inflicted by violence; poisonings; industrial accidents; abortions; drug abuse; and abuse of children, elderly people, and people with disabilities. The justification for overriding patient confidentiality is the state's interest in protecting public health.[3]

The **statutory duty to report** certain medical conditions or incidents may extend to the imaging professional. Because laws vary from state to state, imaging professionals should seek advice from legal counsel at their institution regarding conditions or incidents that must be statutorily reported.

DUTY TO WARN THIRD PARTIES

DUTY TO WARN THIRD
PARTIES
The duty to warn third parties is the obligation to disclose information to warn third parties of a risk of violence or contagious disease or some other risk.

The duty to maintain confidentiality may come into conflict with the duty to disclose information to third parties in order to warn them of a risk such as violence or contagious disease. Generally, the **duty to warn third parties** is based on statute (such as the venereal disease or child abuse reporting statute) and the duty established through case law to warn identifiable third parties threatened by patients. HIPAA also reinforces this duty. In recent years the most difficult conflict between confidentiality and duty to warn has arisen in cases in which AIDS or HIV information is involved; this dilemma is discussed in a separate section.

Case law imposes a duty to warn third parties regarding psychiatric dangerousness. The precedent-setting case was *Tarasoff v Regents of the University of California*[4] (Box 5-4). The duty to warn in *Tarasoff* involved a specific, identifiable third party.

IMAGING SCENARIO

A nuclear medicine technologist is performing a bone scan on a patient from the inpatient mental health center. Extra images are needed, and consequently the patient is in the imaging room for almost an hour, alone with the technologist for most of that time. The patient obviously wants to talk and starts telling the technologist about his brother-in-law, who the patient feels is responsible for his involuntary committal into the facility. The patient becomes increasingly upset and eventually tells the technologist about a plan to get even with the brother-in-law when he is released. The plan involves tampering with the brakes on the brother-in-law's car, which the patient assures the technologist he can do because he was formerly a mechanic.

Discussion questions
- Does the technologist have a duty to ensure that the brother-in-law is warned?
- Is the fact that disclosing this information will probably have an effect on the patient's continued hospitalization and treatment a consideration in this situation?
- Does a duty to disclose outweigh the basic duty to keep patient confidences?
- What should the technologist do if a statute mandates strict confidentiality regarding mental health treatment?

BOX 5-4	**CASE STUDY IN THE DUTY TO WARN THIRD PARTIES**

Tarasoff v Regents of the University of California involved an outpatient (Prosenjit Poddar) who was under the care of a psychologist (Dr. Moore) at the Cowell Memorial Hospital of the University of California. During the course of treatment, Dr. Moore learned from Poddar that he intended to kill Tatiana Tarasoff because she had spurned Poddar's romantic advances.

On the basis of this information, Dr. Moore had the campus police detain Poddar, apparently at the hospital. Poddar was released shortly afterward. Despite disagreement among the psychiatrists, the final decision was that no further action should be taken to confine Poddar. This judgment proved to be a mistake; 2 months later Poddar shot and then repeatedly stabbed Tarasoff.

The plaintiffs, Tarasoff's parents, brought a wrongful death claim against the four psychiatrists. The plaintiffs claimed that the defendants should be liable because they failed to confine Poddar and because they failed to warn Tarasoff or her parents about Poddar's threat. Liability was not found for failure to confine Poddar, but it was found for failure to warn the identifiable third person in danger.

This duty imposed by *Tarasoff,* to warn when an endangered third party is readily identifiable, has been accepted by most states. Only Texas and Virginia reject the Tarasoff duty.[5,6] Some jurisdictions have expanded the duty to include readily identifiable individuals who would be at risk of the patient's violence or even whole classes foreseeably at risk. Some cases attempt to identify third parties who must be warned, typically in situations of psychiatric dangerousness.[3]

Situations involving the duty to warn of psychiatric dangerousness are not routine to the imaging profession. Because this duty extends to all medical professions, however, imaging professionals may want to seek clarification on the extent of the duty imposed in their jurisdiction, particularly if their facility has a psychiatric or mental health component. Patients sometimes feel very comfortable with imaging professionals and volunteer information they have not shared with their physician, psychiatrist, or therapist. This situation is more likely to arise when the imaging procedure is lengthy and the imaging professional and patient are alone in the room throughout the procedure, as could occur during a nuclear medicine study.

Duties to disclose confidential information regarding contagious diseases have been imposed on physicians. Foreseeable third parties and parties at risk who must be warned in these situations have been held to include family members, neighbors, and anyone who is physically intimate with the patient. Generally, the standard for the imposition of liability is whether reasonable care was used.[3] This means that if a court was to find that a reasonable person would have found a duty to warn a particular third person, but the physician failed to warn, liability could be found. This duty extends to other health care professionals. However, situations in which an imaging professional would be required to disclose such information are rare. In reality, this issue would probably arise only if an imaging professional was also working in a clinic or physician's office as a medical assistant. In such a situation the imaging professional should become aware of the policies and procedures of the office or clinic regarding disclosure, ensuring that the duty to warn third parties is addressed. Generally, if accurate disclosure of information is made in good faith for a legitimate purpose, courts are reluctant to impose liability for that disclosure.[7]

AIDS AND HIV

Because of the special characteristics of AIDS and the AIDS epidemic, AIDS confidentiality and reporting present unique challenges to health care workers. A conflict often arises between the general duty to keep confidences and the specific obligation to disclose medical information as part of the duty to warn others. This is complicated by the fear of AIDS, the ignorance about the ways in which it is spread, and the history of prejudice and discrimination against gay men (among whom AIDS is most common).

Unlike many contagious diseases, the HIV virus cannot be spread by casual contact, which may limit the need for disclosure of information.[3] In addition, the rate of infection through heterosexual genital contact is very low (about 0.001 per exposure). The argument in favor of warning is that longer-term partners may not yet have been infected and so should be warned. Another argument for disclosure of HIV status is the transmission of the disease to unborn children. While mandatory testing of pregnant women is not required, the possibility of transmission to unborn children has justified implementation of U.S. Public Health Guidelines for universal counseling and

IMAGING SCENARIO

Mary Smith, a local dentist, is having a radionuclide ventriculogram this morning. The nuclear medicine technologist performing the examination has access to her chart and notices that she is HIV positive. The technologist uses universal precautions, and the examination is performed without event. At lunch in the cafeteria, the technologist tells a nurse friend who works in the emergency department that Mary Smith is HIV positive. This is not only overheard in the cafeteria but also spread in the emergency department as the friend tells several of her co-workers. When Mary Smith returns to her practice, she finds that many of her scheduled patients have canceled their appointments. She tracks down the cause of some of the cancellations to information regarding her HIV status, which her patients learned from various hospital employees.

Discussion questions
- Did the technologist breach patient confidentiality by telling a friend about Mary Smith's HIV status?
- Did the technologist also expose the facility to liability?
- What are possible origins of the duty to maintain this confidence?

voluntary HIV testing for pregnant women. As a result of testing and the use of medication to prevent perinatal transmission of HIV, the number of pediatric HIV cases diagnosed each year has significantly decreased since 1993.[8] Despite recent strides in treatment techniques, the strongest argument for warning is that at present AIDS is incurable and therefore prevention is essential.[3]

The conflict is evident. Strict confidentiality may encourage persons who could be infected to come forward to be tested and voluntarily modify their behavior to avoid infecting others, but limited disclosure may better protect persons who could be exposed to possible infection (Box 5-5).

The states have adopted a variety of legislative and administrative approaches to confidentiality and disclosure of information regarding HIV positivity, AIDS-related complex (ARC), and AIDS status.[3] All states now require physicians to report both HIV and AIDS to the state health department. Several states have mandated strict confidentiality by statute, and others have adopted statutes to permit disclosure, including some states that allow disclosure only after counseling and physician's warning of intent to disclose. In these states physicians are protected from liability whether they choose to disclose or not.[3]

Consider the AMA position on the subject:

Where there is no statute that mandates or prohibits reporting of seropositive (AIDS or ARC infected) to public health authorities and it is clear that the seropositive individual is endangering an identified third party, the physician should (1) attempt to persuade the infected individual to cease endangering the third party; (2) if persuasion fails, notify authorities; and (3) if authorities take no action, notify and counsel the endangered third party.[9]

Because of the differences in statutes among jurisdictions, imaging professionals may want to consult the risk management department or legal counsel at their facility to determine the law in their jurisdiction.

| BOX 5-5 | **CURRENT EVENTS IN AIDS CONFIDENTIALITY AND REPORTING** |

These recent news reports may support the argument for disclosure. Most states now have statutes criminalizing the intentional exposure of others to the HIV virus.

- Angela Harris, St. Charles, Missouri, facing three counts of recklessly risking another person with HIV infection. Four additional people have come forward, including the mother of a 17-year-old boy with whom Harris had unprotected sex. Harris, 26, has known her status since she was 14 years old. *Susan Weich, St. Louis Post-Dispatch, April 13, 2006*
- Unidentified mother, Hamilton, Ontario, Canada, charged with criminal negligence causing bodily harm after refusing prenatal and postnatal care and ignoring advice that would have prevented her baby from acquiring HIV. At the time of the article, this was the only known case of someone being prosecuted for vertical transmission of the HIV virus. *The Toronto Sun, May 28, 2005*
- Anthony Whitfield, Olympia, Washington, convicted on 17 counts of criminal assault for having unprotected sex with 17 different women while knowing that he was HIV positive. Whitfield has been HIV positive since 1992. *Mark Fefer, The Seattle Weekly, December 1, 2004*
- Amazingly, although a majority of states now have laws criminalizing HIV exposure, *The Seattle Weekly* found only a dozen prosecutions throughout the United States through 2004. *Mark Fefer, The Seattle Weekly, December 1, 2004*

Do these current events change your attitude toward disclosure of medical information? Why or why not? In what way do they affect your attitudes about truthfulness and confidentiality?

PATIENT ACCESS TO MEDICAL RECORDS

An area of concern in patient confidentiality is patients' access to medical records. Over the past decade, many jurisdictions have enacted statutes allowing patients access to their medical records. Now HIPAA also mandates a specific patients' right of access to their own records. Some exceptions to this right exist, including psychotherapy notes, information compiled in anticipation of lawsuits, and other specific statutory exceptions. Patients also have the right to request a review of refusal to provide access with some exceptions including those mentioned above, records created in connection with correctional facilities, criminal proceedings, and research projects. Generally, parents have the right of access to their children's records. Facilities are required to have policies in place outlining the specific regulations, and imaging professionals should become familiar with the policies in their facility. In addition, the imaging department should have a policy in place that implements HIPAA with regard to patients' requests to view their radiographs. Imaging professionals should be familiar with that policy.

TORTS REGARDING CONFIDENTIALITY

Breach of Confidentiality

Confidentiality is the duty owed by health care providers to protect the privacy of patient information. This duty stems largely from the right to privacy, but courts have imposed liability based on statutes defining expected conduct, ethical duties owed to the

IMAGING SCENARIO

An imaging professional has a family member in the hospital and is staying on a cot in the patient's room. Early one morning she hears the nurses in the hallway giving report, which includes patients' conditions and treatment. She mentions this to the next nurse who comes into her family member's room. The nurse makes excuses about why the reports were given in a hallway rather than a private room. These include issues of safety for the patients and staffing shortages. In fact the nurse is quite put out that the imaging professional would bring this up, let alone question issues of staffing shortages. After this encounter the level of care for the imaging professional's family member seems to decline. The situation is exacerbated by the administration of the wrong IV medicine to the patient. At this point the imaging professional becomes very concerned about the care of all the patients on the floor.

Discussion questions
- What ethical and legal dilemmas has the imaging professional encountered?
- In what manner most meaningful to patient care should she handle this situation?

patient,[10] breach of the fiduciary duty to maintain confidentiality, and breach of contract or implied contract between patient and physician or health care facility.[11]

Regardless of the origin of the duty of confidentiality, imaging professionals clearly have an obligation to keep medical and personal information about patients in confidence. As health care providers, imaging professionals have access to a vast amount of information on patients. This duty of confidentiality extends to oral, written, and computer communication, as well as reproduction of records and employee conduct (Box 5-6). Breach of the duty to hold information in confidence may cause liability for the individual and the facility.

In certain circumstances, remedies are available through state and federal statutes to compensate patients for breach of confidentiality. Case law has confirmed that courts do award compensation for these breaches of confidence.[12]

The Code of Federal Regulation and many state laws provide a high level of confidentiality for patients receiving treatment for drug or alcohol abuse.[13] These requirements have generally caused providers to refuse to disclose even whether a certain individual is a patient. Many states have enacted legislation protecting confidential information regarding HIV or AIDS status, and courts have been willing to allow claims based on these statutes. Unless disclosure is mandated by patient consent, statute, a duty to warn third parties, or the special circumstances surrounding HIV and AIDS, imaging professionals have a clear duty to maintain confidentiality of medical and related information regarding patients.

Defamation

The tort of **defamation** is based on the right to maintain a good reputation.[13] As stated earlier, the opportunity for defamation may arise in the delivery of patient care and is therefore worthy of discussion.

Defamation is the utterance or publication of an unprivileged false statement that hurts another's reputation. If the publication is oral, the defamation is slander; if written,

DEFAMATION
Defamation is the making of a false statement to a third party that is harmful to another's reputation. In the medical imaging setting, defamation may occur if something false that is harmful to the reputation is said to another person about a patient, a patient's family member, a visitor, another employee, or a physician.

| BOX 5-6 | **PATIENT CONFIDENTIALITY GUIDELINES** |

Verbal communication

Patient information should not be discussed where others can overhear the conversation, such as in hallways, elevators, the cafeteria, the shuttle bus, or restaurants. Discussion of clinical information in public areas is unacceptable even if the patient's name is not used. Doing so can raise doubts with patients and visitors about our respect for their privacy.

Written information

Confidential papers, reports, and computer printouts should be kept in a secure place.

Confidential papers should be picked up as soon as possible from copiers, mail boxes, conference room tables, and other publicly accessible locations.

Confidential papers should be appropriately disposed of, for example, torn or shredded.

Computer information

Passwords should not be shared with anyone else.

Passwords should not be written down and left where others can find and use them.

Once a user is logged on, no one else should be allowed to use the computer under that user's password.

Users should log off when leaving a workstation.

Reproduction and faxing of patient information

Before faxing a document, employees should make sure of the following:

Sender information is correct.

The receiving fax is in a secure location.

A patient release of information form allows faxing of the information.

The fax cover sheet contains a confidentiality disclosure, including notice that the information is not to be disclosed to another party and, if received in error, should be destroyed and the sender notified.

Receipt of faxed information

Fax transmissions should be removed immediately and delivered to the correct recipient.

Faxed information should be treated as confidential.

Information received in error should be destroyed and the sender notified.

Sensitive information

The following information should be released only through the health information department of the facility:

Communication between patient and psychotherapist or social worker

Sexually transmitted disease test results or visit notes

HIV test results and related information

Substance abuse rehabilitation treatment records

Sexual assault treatment records

Employee conduct

Only the information needed for job performance should be accessed.

Data must not be accessed simply to satisfy a curiosity. Looking up a friend's birthday, address, or phone number is unacceptable.

Modified from Massachusetts General Hospital, Department of Radiology: *Patient confidentiality guide,* Boston, 2006, Author.

it is libel. The publisher must be at fault at least to the degree of negligence. Harm must have resulted from the publication of the false and defamatory statement. Because the statement must be false, the truth is a total defense to a charge of defamation. However, a jury trial may be necessary to determine the truth.

If the false statement concerns criminal activity; a loathsome disease such as AIDS or venereal disease; business, trade, or professional misdeeds; or unchastity, no specific injury need be proved. These situations are termed *slander per se* or *libel per se.* Because no injury must be proven in libel or slander per se, the only facts to be proved are that a false and defamatory statement or writing was made to another person and the teller or writer was at least negligent in telling it.[13]

SUMMARY

- Imaging professionals are expected to tell the truth in situations in which others have a reasonable expectation of the truth. The location of the communication, the roles the communicators have in relationship to one another, and the nature of the material to be communicated are determining factors in the expectation of truth. Contract relationships and special needs are factors that determine whether a person has a right to information.
- Of all the types of obligatory secrets—natural, promised, and professional— professional secrecy is the most important because of the damages incurred as a result of its violation. In certain instances, professional secrets may be shared. This occurs most often when the good to be gained by sharing the information outweighs the evil of violating confidentiality, when the law indicates that it must be shared, or when special relationships indicate a need for an exception.
- The imaging professional has a clear duty to maintain patient confidentiality. However, a small number of exceptions to this duty exist and require the professional to disclose confidential information. Unless a situation meets one of the exceptions to the duty of confidentiality, disclosure may create liability for the individual and the facility.
- HIPAA (Health Insurance Portability and Accountability Act of 1996) has established conformity across the United States as to disclosure of health care information and clarifies situations for disclosure without patient permission. HIPAA has also created or reinforced patient rights to access their own records.
- Guidelines as to when confidentiality can be breached include the following:
  - Requirement for patient authorization
  - Existence of a statutory duty to disclose
  - Duty to warn third parties
  - AIDS confidentiality and reporting
- Although HIPAA has clarified the law to some extent regarding disclosure, the law concerning AIDS confidentiality and reporting is not as clear cut as the other exceptions to confidentiality. All states mandate physician reporting to public health, but jurisdictions vary as to the duty to inform third parties who may be infected. While imaging professionals generally are not involved, the imaging professional who also acts as a medical assistant may become involved in dilemmas

regarding the duty to disclose and should discover the status of the law in his or her jurisdiction.

- HIPAA mandates a specific right of patients to access their medical records. Some exceptions exist, including psychotherapy notes, information compiled in anticipation of litigation, and other statutory exceptions. Imaging professionals should know the policy in their facility and department with regard to patients' requests to see their films.

- The torts involved in confidentiality include defamation and breach of confidentiality. Breach of confidentiality is a violation of the strict duty of confidentiality, and defamation occurs when a false statement is made to another that harms a person's reputation.

- Oral defamatory statements constitute slander, and written defamatory statements constitute libel. Defamatory statements regarding criminal activity; loathsome diseases; business, trade, or professional misdeeds; and unchastity constitute slander or libel per se; in these situations no specific injury need be proved.

REFERENCES

1. Garrett TM, Baillie HW, Garrett RM: *Healthcare ethics, principles and problems*, ed 2, Englewood Cliffs, NJ, 1993, Prentice Hall.
2. American Hospital Association: *Values in conflict: resolving ethical issues in hospital care. Report of the Special Committee on Biomedical Ethics*, Chicago, 1985, Author.
3. Furrow BR, Greaney TL, Johnson SH, et al: *Health law: cases, materials and problems*, ed 5, St Paul, Minn, 2004, West.
4. *Tarasoff v Regents of the University of California*, 551 P.2d 334 (Cal. 1976).
5. *Thapar v Zezulka*, 994 S.W. 2d 635 (Tex. 1999).
6. *Nasser v Parker*, 249 Va. 172, 455 S.E.2d 502 (1995).
7. White JG: Physicians' liability for breach of confidentiality: beyond the limitations of the privacy tort, *SC Law Rev* 49(5):1271, 1998.
8. American Medical Association Council on Scientific Affairs: *Universal screening of pregnant women for HIV infection*, Report 1-01, Chicago, 2001, Author.
9. Rinaldi RC: *HIV blood test counseling: AMA physician guidelines*, Chicago, 1988, American Medical Association.
10. *Humphers v First Interstate Bank of Oregon*, 696 P.2d 527, 1985.
11. *Doe v Roe*, 400 N.Y. Supp. 2d 668, 1977.
12. *Doe v Roe*, No. 0369 N.Y. App. Div. 4th Jud. Dept., May 28, 1993.
13. Code of Federal Regulation, Title 42, Part 2 (1985).
14. Schwartz V, Kelly K, Partlett D: *Prosser, Wade, and Schwartz: cases and materials on torts*, ed 10, Westbury, NY, 2000, Foundation Press.

REVIEW QUESTIONS

1 Define truthfulness.
2 Expectations of truth vary with which three conditions?
   a. _____
   b. _____
   c. _____
3 The right to the truth is determined by the _____ _____.
   of the patient in many nonmedical situations (such as in preparing for death).
4 Informed consent and the need to make treatment decisions are examples of conditions for the _____ _____ _____ _____.

5 _____ is concerned with the keeping of secrets.

6 List the three types of obligatory secrets:

    a. _____

    b. _____

    c. _____

7 The most binding obligatory secret is the _____.

8 Describe the most common exceptions to confidentiality.

9 According to the AHA Committee on Biomedical Ethics, duties to disclose patient information exist in which situations?

10 Which of the following are origins of the duty of confidentiality?

    a. Right to privacy

    b. Statutes

    c. Ethical obligations

    d. Breach of contract issues

    e. All of the above

11 **True or False**   The imaging professional must always tell the whole truth.

12 **True or False**   The imaging professional has an obligation to the patient, profession, and society to maintain confidentiality.

13 **True or False**   An imaging professional who finds himself or herself in the role of the patient should not expect the same degree of confidentiality.

14 **True or False**   If the risk of keeping a secret outweighs the harm to the patient, no ethical decision making is necessary.

15 **True or False**   A deontologist believes that stricter rules of right and wrong should be used in keeping information confidential.

16 **True or False**   The duty of patient confidentiality is clear, and courts allow compensation for breach of confidentiality.

17 **True or False**   Imaging professionals owe an absolute duty of patient confidentiality.

18 **True or False**   Truth is a total defense against allegations of defamation.

19 **True or False**   Defamatory comments regarding a person's AIDS status are slander per se, and damages would not have to be proved.

20 **True or False**   Confidentiality of drug and alcohol abuse treatment information is mandated by the federal government.

21 **True or False**   Virtually all requests by third parties for records come from new health care providers.

22 **True or False**   Imaging professionals do not have to worry about statutory reporting because this duty lies only with physicians.

23 **True or False**   The duty to warn third parties extends to the imaging professional.

24 **True or False**   Imaging professionals when working in clinics and fulfilling the role of medical assistant may have to deal with warning people at risk for contagious diseases in accordance with the privacy policies surrounding this information.

25 **True or False**   The existence of legislation mandating strict confidentiality regarding information about patients' AIDS, HIV, and ARC status means that disclosure is never appropriate.

26 HIPAA stands for:
   a. Health Insurance Private Account Association
   b. Health Insurance Profit Accountability Act
   c. Health Information Portability and Accountability Act
   d. Helping Inform Physicians About Alcohol Abuse
27 **True or False**   State law overrides HIPAA regulations.
28 **True or False**   Patients always have an absolute right to their records.
29 **True or False**   VA hospitals are exempt from HIPAA regulations.
30 **True or False**   Imaging professionals should feel free to show patients their films and answer questions about them.
31 **True or False**   Under HIPAA, patients have the right to sue.
32 HIPAA's purposes include the following:
   a. To give patients a right of access to their records
   b. To create a national framework for privacy regulations
   c. To attempt to restore trust in health care delivery of information
   d. All of the above
33 **True or False**   Under HIPAA, when records are requested, all medical records of that patient are provided.
34 **True or False**   Under HIPAA, all requests for information require patient authorization.
35 **True or False**   Under HIPAA, patients have the right to see their psychotherapy notes.
36 **True or False**   Health care plans may decide if they want to participate in the HIPAA regulations.

CRITICAL THINKING *Questions & Activities*

1 What is the difference between not telling the whole truth and telling a lie? Why might one of these be admissible?
2 Cite a situation in which the place of communication is inappropriate for an expectation of truth in medical imaging.
3 Discuss the differences and similarities between natural and promised secrets.
4 If you were HIV positive, do you think your patients or employer would have the right to know? Why or why not?
5 Should a parent have the right to know a child's physical condition if it involves treatment? Why or why not?
6 Define confidentiality.
7 Identify exceptions to the duty to confidentiality.
8 Consider the following situation: With the health care system changing and third-party payers becoming stricter about coverage, imaging professionals (like other people) are concerned with their own health care services. Do you think your third-party payer has a right to know your health history and present conditions if they involve a communicable disease or drug history? Should you be able to expect privileged communication between you and your physician? Justify your answers. A group discussion may follow in which each person lists the consequences of the decision and possible alternatives.

9 Discuss situations that may potentially involve defamatory statements about fellow employees or patients.

10 Discuss the devastation a negligent breach of confidence may cause, such as in the scenario involving the dentist, Mary Smith.

11 Does the facility you are affiliated with have a policy regarding HIV-infected workers? If it does not, should it? Is protection of the patient more important than the rights of HIV-infected staff members?

12 Discuss the situation of an HIV-infected imaging professional who intends to put a student at risk through unprotected sexual intercourse. Does another imaging professional's duty to warn fall under the law or is it only an ethical obligation?

13 Play out a scenario in which a patient wants to see her x-ray films, an imaging professional who believes patients should have a right to access shows her the films, and the patient starts demanding that the imaging professional answer questions regarding the outcome of the study, what it means, and possible treatments. Discuss a better way to handle the situation and play the scenario again.

6 DEATH AND DYING

Death is a friend of ours; and he that is not ready to entertain him is not at home.

FRANCIS BACON

Chapter Outline

Ethical Issues
Value of Life
Definitions of Death
The Patient
Sanctity of Human Life
Suicide
Imaging Professionals and Suicide
Euthanasia
Patients' Rights Regarding Euthanasia
Advance Directives and Surrogates
Quality of Life
Ethics Committees and Services for Patients with
     Terminal Illnesses
Family in Death and Dying

Legal Issues
Definitions of Death
Determination of Death
Directives
Physician-Assisted Suicide
Competence and Life-Sustaining Treatment
No-Code Orders
Living Wills
Durable Powers of Attorney for Health Care
Family Consent Laws
Uniform Health Care Decisions Act
Absence of Advance Directives
Patients in a Persistent Vegetative State
Patients Who Have Never Been Competent

Learning Objectives

After completing the chapter, the reader will be able to perform the following:

- Provide definitions of life and death.
- Differentiate between the patient's and the imaging professional's role in death and dying.
- Identify the physical and ethical differences between active and passive suicide.
- State a perceived need for euthanasia.
- Develop arguments for and against the right to die.
- Define the meaning of quality of life and explain what affects it.
- List reasons for ethics committees.
- Cite the basis for the patient's right to forgo life-sustaining treatment.
- Define and understand differences between a persistent vegetative state and a minimally conscious state.
- Define how death is determined.

- Define life-sustaining treatment and its exclusions.
- Explain the difference between living wills and durable powers of attorney.
- Identify the limitations of living wills.
- Define the advantages of durable powers of attorney.
- Compare the ways in which powers of attorney influence the decision-making process of ancillary people such as physicians, ministers, and specified family members and friends.
- Identify the differences between persons in a persistent vegetative state and those in a minimally conscious state.
- Explain the difference between competency and decisional capacity.
- Contrast the treatment of persons who have never been competent and competent persons who have become incompetent.

Key Terms

abortion
active euthanasia
active suicide
competence
development
euthanasia
life
passive euthanasia

passive suicide
quality of life
sanctity of human life
slippery slope
suicide
surrogate
terminal illness

Professional Profile

I recall my first experience with death and dying when I was a student radiologic technologist. The image is still quite clear although it happened more than 30 years ago. The department was closed, and I was called in from home around 2:30 AM. A second-year student and staff technologist had also been called in. I was a first-year student.

We wheeled the stretcher with a young man who appeared to be about my age from the emergency department to the radiology department. He had been in a motor vehicle accident, and the gearshift lever from his car was sticking out of his chest. We moved him onto the table and began taking films. His breathing became erratic, and the staff technologist called the emergency room staff. Soon the entire room was filled with people and equipment. The scene was frantic, with everyone working to try to keep this young man alive. Unfortunately, they were unsuccessful, and he died on the x-ray table.

After all the paperwork was completed and the appropriate procedures were followed, he had to be moved from the x-ray table to the morgue cart. Because staff was sparse at that time of night, the three radiology personnel who were present had to help the night supervisor with the actual transporting of the body. I will never forget the way that young man's body felt. It was cold and hard, almost like stone.

That night was the first time I experienced death. That night was the first time I really thought about death. That young man had been alive when we started the examination. He was warm, he had feelings, aspirations, hopes, dreams, and fears. Then he was cold and hard. I thought about what he had experienced. Was he afraid, was he angry, did he see his short life flashing before his eyes? Was it just his body that was dead and did his soul live on to go to heaven or hell as I was taught in grade school, or is this life all there is? This experience bothered me for a very long time. I would wake up in the middle of the night and think of the way this young man's body felt. I would dwell on whether he knew he was going to die, whether he was prepared, what exactly it meant to die.

I now realize that each person must form his or her own answers to these questions. I also believe that some guidance on the ethical and legal issues of death and dying for the imaging student is appropriate. I was not prepared to deal with these issues as a first-year student, and I wish that I had been.

Terese A. Young, J.D., RT(R) (retired), CNMT
(Emeritus)
Co-author,
Ethical and Legal Issues for Imaging Professionals

ETHICAL ISSUES

Imaging professionals often have contact with patients who have critical or terminal conditions. Most of the imaging modalities (except radiation therapy) do not involve lengthy contact with patients. Nevertheless, regardless of the length

IMAGING SCENARIO

The portable and trauma team imaging professionals are called to the morgue to perform a radiographic examination on a young man with a gunshot wound. The bullet entered the right temple and is lodged in the brain. The images corroborate forensic analysis that indicates suicide. Before the fatal wound the young man appeared to have been muscular, handsome, and healthy. The youngest imaging professional questions why such a young man who had his whole life to look forward to would choose such a tragic ending.

The next day another staff imaging professional notes that the young man had recently been diagnosed with an incurable and inoperable brain tumor. This information leads to a discussion about the choices people make when they know they will die, perhaps painfully. Did this man have the right to end his life? In what way did the suicide affect his family and friends? Did his situation excuse his suicide? In what ways were the family dealing with not being able to say their final good-byes?

The young trauma imaging specialist wonders what she would do in such a situation. Would she choose to die a slow, painful death or end her life quickly? Does she have the right to determine the quality of her life and choose suicide or euthanasia even if both are illegal or considered immoral by many? How would she respond to a healthy young patient faced with the prospect of an early and painful death? Was there an obligation to counsel about possible treatments and pain control modalities that was not met or could have been handled better?

Discussion question
- What impact do the questions posed in this scenario have on the professional's compassion and quality of care toward patients?

of the therapeutic relationship, the imaging professional will encounter death and dying.

To help the imaging professional deal with questions regarding patients' rights, refusal of treatment, and quality of life, this portion of Chapter 6 discusses ethical concerns surrounding death and dying. The ethical dilemmas of patients and imaging professionals are emphasized.

VALUE OF LIFE

LIFE
Life is the entire state of the living thing.

Before imaging professionals consider questions of death and dying, they should understand the ethical issues surrounding **life**. Life may be considered as an element of human autonomy through which a person experiences a sense of self. It is defined as the entire state of the living thing; it encompasses the value of the self and is a determining factor in a person's "preconscious" standard of judgment. Thought, analysis, and action come from this fundamental sense of the value of life.

Traditional religious and secular beliefs celebrate the uniqueness of life, but when life begins and the way it ends remain points of contention. The imaging professional should consider the following aspects of life when making determinations in ethical dilemmas[1]:
- Life is the foundation of all other values of a patient.
- Life is the foundation of a patient's rights.

- The preservation and maintenance of a good quality of life are the goals of the patient entering the health care environment.
- A patient is motivated to enter the health care environment when capabilities and potentialities are radically affected. If a patient can regain these capabilities and potentialities, quality of life is greatly improved.
- A patient, except in the most extreme circumstances, has no rational desire greater than the desire for life. Nevertheless, in extreme circumstances a desire for death may not be irrational.

DEFINITIONS OF DEATH

Most people and cultures agree that physical life is a cyclic event with a beginning and an end. The life cycle is generally considered a good to be held in awe and respected. Some believe that the goodness of life may be judged by the decisions a person makes regarding actions and responses to others and the environment. Others believe that decisions concerning the goodness of life should be the person's own determination. Many arguments and problems are inherent in this philosophy; they are discussed later in this chapter, as are legal definitions of death, persistent vegetative state, minimally conscious state, and coma.

THE PATIENT

A discussion of the ethical dilemmas faced by the imaging professional requires a consideration of the ethics of the patient, including questions concerning passive and active suicide. Empathy with the patient provides the imaging professional with insight into these questions.

SANCTITY OF HUMAN LIFE

The ethics of the taking of human life becomes a consideration in a number of patient care situations, and imaging professionals may have to address this issue during their interactions with patients. Respect for the **sanctity of human life** entails an obligation not to infringe on an individual's decisions regarding life and an obligation not to take human life.[2] Nevertheless, questions about the sanctity of life arise in situations of assisted suicide and when patients are suffering from life-threatening disease or illness.

SANCTITY OF HUMAN LIFE
Sanctity of human life is the ideal underpinning the obligation not to take human life.

SUICIDE

Suicide is the act of knowingly ending one's own life. It may be accomplished either actively or by omitting treatment, which is a passive form of suicide. The individual must also have the intention to die.

Several arguments may be made against suicide (Box 6-1). Some find it unacceptable for religious reasons—God has lent life to the individual, and therefore that life is

SUICIDE
Suicide is the act of knowingly ending one's life.

| BOX 6-1 | **ARGUMENTS AGAINST SUICIDE** |

Many religions forbid suicide.
Life is the greatest good.
Suicide causes harm to the community.
Suicide causes harm to friends and family.

not the individual's to end. Others believe that human life is the greatest of goods and consider it precious. However, what if the patient has tremendous pain and therapy has caused such nausea and weakness that the patient cannot move from bed? Is life "good" at this level of pain and loss of dignity? Harm to the community is another argument against suicide. If one suicide leads to another (as has been observed with teenage suicides), does this not harm the community? A further argument against suicide is the harm it inflicts on family and friends. Suicide denies them time with their loved ones to plan, share, make amends, and say good-bye.

All these arguments have some logic, and laws to control and discourage suicide are based on such arguments. If suicide were declared legal, would more untimely deaths be associated with emotional problems and not just physical problems? Would the broken heart be cured more often with a bullet than with therapy and understanding?

Passive Suicide

Ethically, patients have the right to refuse treatment even if it brings about death. Of course, not all refusal of treatment leads to death. However, would a situation in which a patient knows the refusal of treatment will bring about death much more rapidly be considered a form of **passive suicide**? Some may consider passive suicide ethical if the good of the act outweighs the bad of the suffering. The scenario at the bottom of the page explores some of these issues.

Active Suicide

Some people can accept the idea of passive suicide because refusing treatment is a person's right and refusal of treatment does not seem to be an act of violence toward the self. However, when the young man in the imaging scenario on p. 118 shot himself to end his life quickly rather than die a painful and slow death, would some consider this **active suicide** wrong? Those who oppose suicide do so for various reasons. Some believe that life is sacred and must be cherished. Others believe that only God or some supreme being gives life and only that being should decide when it should end.

Suicide proponents also have their rationale. Many believe suicide is an individual right, analogous to a woman's right to an abortion. If a woman has the right to choose what will happen to her body, shouldn't an individual have the right to choose life or death? Some also argue that it is not only the supreme being that gives us life, that technology also allows humanity to produce life, and if humanity can produce life, why shouldn't it be allowed to decide when it should end? The technology that has been developed to prolong life also is used as an argument against the "God brought life, God should take it away" theory.

PASSIVE SUICIDE
Passive suicide is the refusal of treatment by a person who knows that refusal will lead to death.

ACTIVE SUICIDE
Active suicide is the taking of one's own life through a conscious act.

IMAGING SCENARIO

Pancreatic cancer is diagnosed in two patients, and the computed tomography scan indicates that the cancer has invaded many other organs. One patient has elected to discontinue nourishment to hurry death; the other patient elects to continue all treatment to sustain his life as long as possible.

Discussion question
- How do personal values, as discussed in Chapter 1, influence the weighing of reasons for refusing treatment as compared with continuing it?

| BOX 6-2 | REASONS FOR THE IMAGING PROFESSIONAL'S DUTY NOT TO COOPERATE WITH SUICIDE |

Assisting in or supplying the means to suicide is generally illegal.
Health care providers are devoted to healing.
Assisting in suicide is incompatible with professional obligation.

IMAGING PROFESSIONALS AND SUICIDE

Many imaging professionals have encountered patients who have no hope of becoming well and whose pain can no longer be controlled with drugs. Their lives are full of pain and suffering, and their desire to end their lives may be reasonable. If these patients discontinue treatment, they will suffer but die sooner. They could also overdose and end their suffering quickly. Whether the suicide is active or passive, imaging professionals should be careful not to make judgments. What should be the response of an imaging professional asked to interact with a patient determined to commit suicide (Box 6-2)? In what way should an imaging professional respond when approached by a patient who wishes to end life either actively or passively? These may be rare situations for imaging specialists, but they must be considered because of imaging professionals' changing interactions with patients and their families. Imaging professionals must recognize that each case is different. They may be required to participate in procedures involving patients who have elected to end nourishment and hydration. The imaging professional must remember that it is the value system of the patient that is important in such situations, not the value system of the imaging professional.

EUTHANASIA

Suicide is taken one step further when another person becomes involved. **Euthanasia** is the act of painlessly putting to death a person suffering from an incurable and painful disease or condition. Physician participation in euthanasia, or assisted suicide, has stirred great controversy recently (Box 6-3). The legal issues surrounding physician-assisted suicide are discussed in the legal section of this chapter.

Euthanasia may be either passive or active. The difference between the two lies in the methods, not the consequences. **Passive euthanasia** may be committed through the withholding of nourishment or through a decision not to perform cardiopulmonary resuscitation (CPR) on a patient who has stopped breathing. It is considered legal in certain instances because no one delivers a method of death. "Nothing" is done and that "nothing" leads to death. **Active euthanasia** is the performance of a specific act on the request or behalf of the patient to end life.

Professionals in the medical imaging services may see patients with terminal diseases, patients in horrible pain, or those in a persistent vegetative state (PVS) (the medico-legal definition of PVS is discussed in the legal section of the chapter). These imaging professionals may struggle with whether they should perform procedures that will add to the patient's pain and loss of dignity and autonomy (e.g., barium enemas). They may imagine themselves in the patient's position and hope that someone who cares about them would help hasten their death. At the same time, they should consider the consequences for the person "helping" to carry out a suicide. Imaging professionals should

EUTHANASIA
Euthanasia is deliberately ending the life of another to end suffering.

PASSIVE EUTHANASIA
Passive euthanasia is the ending of another person's life by withdrawing treatment.

ACTIVE EUTHANASIA
Active euthanasia is the ending of another person's life by an aggressive method to end suffering.

BOX 6-3	**PHYSICIAN-ASSISTED SUICIDE**

The physician who has drawn the most attention to the controversy over physician-assisted suicide is Dr. Jack Kevorkian. Dr. Kevorkian is a pathologist by training, although he has not held a position on a hospital staff since 1982 and he lost his medical license in Michigan in 1991.

Beginning in 1990 and ending in 1998, Kevorkian assisted in over 100 suicides. In all but the last case he gave the patient the means to commit suicide, but the patient carried out the final act using a device designed so that the patient could pull the trigger. On November 22, 1998, CBS's *60 Minutes* aired a videotape showing Kevorkian giving a lethal injection to Thomas Youk, a terminally ill 52-year-old man with amyotrophic lateral sclerosis (ALS). During the taping, Kevorkian asked Youk to sign a consent form, after which Kevorkian gave him a lethal injection. Kevorkian was convicted of second-degree murder and delivery of a controlled substance.

A Michigan judge sentenced Kevorkian to 10 to 25 years in prison. Having been repeatedly denied parole, Kevorkian remains in prison at this writing. He will next be eligible for parole in June 2007. Kevorkian has said that while he still believes in assisted suicide where it is legal, he regrets flouting the law and should have worked toward legalization of assisted suicide. He also says that if released, he will no longer assist suicides.

Data from http://medicine.creighton.edu/idc135/2004/group4a/index.htm; www.pbs.org/wgbh/pages/frontline/kevorkian/chronology.html; Martindale M: Dying Kevorkian wouldn't pick suicide, *Detroit News*, June 13, 2006; and http://www.cnn.com/US/9812/09/kevorkian.02/index.html.

also remember that they should not base their decisions on their personal values. The patient's values and needs are the important issues in these decisions.

The legal ramifications of euthanasia, especially active euthanasia, are tied to the act of murder. Indeed, many people believe that they are the same, and for this reason euthanasia is generally illegal in the United States. In Holland, where euthanasia has become an accepted procedure, some health care professionals and ethicists wonder whether this acceptance will become a **slippery slope** leading to the overuse and misuse of euthanasia. For example, will the euthanasia of a patient suffering from acquired immunodeficiency syndrome (AIDS) lead to the deaths of unwanted types of individuals and ethnic cleansing? No policies are currently in place regarding who makes these decisions, and the ways in which controls should be established remain controversial.

The moral and legal questions regarding passive euthanasia are more complex. The passive withdrawal of nourishment from a patient in a PVS seems less awful than the active euthanasia of a patient who is conscious and aware. However, after health care professionals and family members start making judgments for handicapped neonates or patients who are incompetent, in a PVS, old, or senile, the implications for patient autonomy become serious. Who decides who is fit to live? Does a person have to have consciousness and decision-making ability to be worthy of life? The potential for **development** and quality of life must be considered. If a neonate has a chance to develop and live (not necessarily by traditional standards), should that chance be given? Should cost and distribution of resources issues play a role in such decisions?

The controversies surrounding the euthanasia of neonates are often related to the issues in the **abortion** debate. Questions regarding when the fetus has a right to life,

SLIPPERY SLOPE
A slippery slope is present when one act leads to another and then to another at an accelerating rate.

DEVELOPMENT
Development is the ability to grow and continue the life process.

ABORTION
Abortion is the expulsion or removal of a usually nonviable fetus (a fetus that cannot live outside the uterus at that time).

IMAGING SCENARIO

> An imaging professional's father is dying from an aggressive cancer with no hope for recovery. The father has an advance directive explaining that he does not want the use of life-sustaining equipment. He becomes nonresponsive, and a family conflict develops concerning withdrawal of nourishment and hydration. Part of the family believes this is in the best interest of the parent—to hasten his death and end his suffering—and the other family members view this as killing him. They ask the imaging professional about the pain and suffering, the issues of active and passive euthanasia, and whether not using life-sustaining machines is equal to starving the man to death.

> **Discussion questions**
> • How can the imaging professional respond? Is there a right or wrong answer?
> • How often are family members required to make these type of decisions?

self-determination, and dignity have yet to be resolved. When aborting a fetus that can wave its arms and legs and suck its thumb is legal, but the legality of letting an anencephalic neonate be an organ donor is still in question, do such perceptions confuse the issues surrounding the processes of life and death? Ultrasonographers required to participate in fetal ultrasound examinations that may lead to abortive procedures must learn to deal with these dilemmas based on professional standards and personal conscience.

Euthanasia of patients at the beginning of life raises serious ethical questions. So too does the active or passive euthanasia of elderly people. Elderly patients should be evaluated by imaging professionals as individuals with value, not as "old people" who have lived long lives and are somehow expendable. The intellectual capacity and strength of elderly people may be failing (although many elderly people retain a high degree of intellectual capability), but a human being does not have to be a perfect specimen to have a reason for living. The fear of pain and loss associated with death may be as great to an 85-year-old as it is to a 35-year-old. The age of the patient should never prevent the imaging professional from granting the best care possible.

PATIENTS' RIGHTS REGARDING EUTHANASIA

The ethical questions surrounding the possibility that patients have a right to active euthanasia are complex. Consider the patient in hospice care with pain control who has been diagnosed with invasive liver and pancreatic cancer by a CT scan and has undergone radiation therapy for pain. Does this patient have the right to self-determination and a "good death" through euthanasia if all of these procedures have not lessened the pain, or must the patient continue to be in pain?

The exercise of rights requires a self; proponents of patient-chosen euthanasia consider it an act of self-determination. Therefore the person seeking euthanasia must completely understand the nature and consequences of the request. The person must be competent and as informed as possible. Ideally the person should have experienced the five stages of coming to terms with death:

1. Denial
2. Anger

3. Bargaining
4. Depression
5. Acceptance

In a scenario of legalized euthanasia, only after going through these phases would the patient be considered ready to make the decision regarding the commission of euthanasia.

ADVANCE DIRECTIVES AND SURROGATES

Advance directives and **surrogates** (who act on behalf of patients and may make decisions and grant consent for them in quality-of-life judgments) are increasingly important elements in decisions regarding euthanasia. A written explanation of the patient's wishes in the form of a living will or advance directive hastens the processes leading to passive euthanasia. Active euthanasia is still generally illegal, however, and many roadblocks stand in the way of its becoming an accepted procedure. The idea of lethal injections evokes perceptions of "doctors of death" and "angels of mercy." This is not the life-giving image most health care providers wish for themselves. Even with an advance directive, a patient in a PVS or a burn patient in hideous pain would have great difficulty finding a health care professional willing to run the risks inherent in active euthanasia. This is why active euthanasia currently is generally performed by a loved one—someone willing to run the risk of murder charges and a prison cell.

Proponents of active euthanasia believe that society has more compassion for animals that are suffering and in pain than it does for suffering human beings. Those opposed to active euthanasia believe that improved methods of pain control can enhance the quality of a patient's life. A concern for patient rights and autonomy may require imaging professionals to consider these divergent interpretations of the ethics of euthanasia.

Imaging professionals are charged with working to provide for the good of the patient's health; many believe this entails an obligation to maintain life under any circumstance. However, the patient's autonomy and freedom to choose treatment options may come into conflict with this ethical and professional obligation. In some instances imaging professionals may need to help prepare patients for death and help themselves and their patients to see that death is not always an enemy.

QUALITY OF LIFE

Quality of life has different meanings for different people. Factors influencing quality of life may include the capability of performing normal biologic functions, the stability of the powers of intellect and creativity, and emotional contact with others. Some persons may demand a maximum of these factors to feel their lives are worth living, whereas others have minimal needs and find the simplest interactions to be the rewards of life (Figure 6-1).

Most people fall into the middle of the quality-of-life spectrum. They may not demand maximal health and happiness, but they do not want to live in agonizing pain and without hope. The living will is one way to ensure that people's wishes regarding treatment in relation to their quality of life are honored. Living wills identify specific treatments to be initiated or discontinued when patients become terminally ill, are in great pain, or find themselves in a life-threatening situation. If a living will is not present and the patient's wishes are unknown, quality-of-life decisions are difficult to make. In such situations, the minimal requirements for quality of life must be recognized.

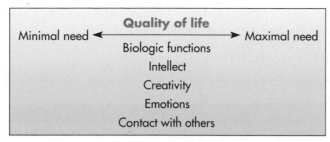

FIGURE 6-1   Factors involved in quality-of-life decisions.

Imaging professionals must not pass judgment on others facing these dilemmas; they can be decided only for the individual by the individual—not by others.

Quality-of-Life Problem-Solving Tools

The principles of beneficence and nonmaleficence and respect for autonomy are critical issues in a discussion of quality of life. Problem solving can be aided by the use of the following points (with modifications for imaging) from Jonsen, Siegler, and Winslade[3]:

- What are the prospects, with or without the imaging or radiation therapy procedure, for a return to a normal life? What is normal for this imaging patient?
- What physical, mental, and social deficits is the patient likely to experience if the radiation therapy is successful?
- Does the imaging professional have any biases that might influence his or her evaluation of the imaging patient's quality of life? Have life and work experiences tainted the professional?
- Does the patient's current or future condition indicate that life may not be what the patient would consider worth living? Has the patient stated this? How is this decision made?
- If the radiation therapy patient decides to discontinue or not begin treatment, does the patient have a plan? How could a therapy professional influence this plan?
- How will the patient deal with pain and be made comfortable? How would an imaging professional explain degree of pain if asked?

ETHICS COMMITTEES AND SERVICES FOR PATIENTS WITH TERMINAL ILLNESSES

Many hospitals have formed ethics committees to help health care professionals address the ethical problems surrounding termination of treatment and related issues. These committees have several missions. First, they educate the hospital, its employees, and its other constituencies. Second, they develop policies regarding problem areas, especially the problems of death and dying. Third, they act as advisory consultants to health care providers and families.

Ethics committees serve in an advisory capacity only. Ideally, their recommendations are exercised with practical wisdom in the patient's best interest.

In addition to ethics committees, other services exist in the health care community to provide aid to terminally ill patients. Among these are hospice care, home health care services, mental health services, social services, organizations for persons with specific terminal diseases, and pastoral and religious services. Often these services provide support to terminally ill patients and their families and help them deal with the many issues involved in the final portion of the life cycle.

FAMILY IN DEATH AND DYING

Medical imaging personnel often interact with patients' families during the dying process[4]:

> At a certain point in the dying process, the family members become secondary patients in need of information about the state of affairs and emotional support. Too often the families are neglected and left to fend for themselves. Yet, insofar as the health care professionals are dedicated to relieving suffering, the duty of compassion is in the role of all care givers. The duty to relieve suffering demands concern for the well and the living as well as for the ill and dying. Families, as well as those who are patients in a legal sense, have needs that should be respected.

Imaging professionals must interact with families in a manner that exhibits a caring and professional attitude. They must be approachable and ready to comfort grieving family members, no matter how difficult this duty may be. Professional empathy is crucial for the well-being of the patient and the patient's family.

LEGAL ISSUES

Many aspects concerning the patient's right to die remain unresolved. In fact, the only well-resolved issue is the recognition of the common law right of a patient to choose the form of treatment. As was stated in previous discussions of battery and informed consent, Justice Benjamin Cardozo established in the 1914 *Schloendorff* case that "every human being of adult years and sound mind has a right to determine what shall be done with his own body." This finding also underpinned the right to forgo treatment—because patients have a right to determine whether to consent to a particular treatment, they also have a right to refuse to consent to a particular treatment.[5]

The principle that competent patients have a right to forgo life-sustaining treatment was not articulated by any court until 1984.[6] According to a finding at that time, the competence of the patient is crucial to whether he or she has a right to forgo life-sustaining treatment; the method by which that right is exercised is also relevant. Unfortunately, courts have been reluctant to give a formal definition of competence. This section discusses legal and medical definitions of death and persistent vegetative state, minimally conscious state, competence, guidelines for its determination, and its significance for the right to die and the vehicles used to further that right.

As previously noted, laws vary by jurisdiction. Judicial decisions from one jurisdiction are not binding in others, although they may be considered by the deciding court. For these reasons it is important for imaging professionals to know the state of the law in their jurisdiction. The facility's legal counsel and risk management team should provide this information.

DEFINITIONS OF DEATH

For centuries, death has been evidenced by the contemporaneous cessation of heart and lung function. These functions were related to such a degree that the cessation of breathing would lead almost immediately to the cessation of heart function and the cessation of heart function would lead almost immediately to the cessation of breathing. In addition, the cessation of these functions was accompanied or immediately followed by cessation of all cognitive activity, all other brain function, and all responsiveness generally.

Because the disappearance of any heartbeat and the cessation of breathing were the simplest to identify, and because the advent of the stethoscope made the determination of heartbeat easier, the heart and lung test of death became not only the evidence of death but also the actual definition of death. The Uniform Determination of Death Act,[7] enacted in 1980, established two tests to determine death. The act states that an individual who has sustained either (1) irreversible cessation of circulatory and respiratory functions, or (2) irreversible cessation of all functions of the entire brain, including the brainstem, is dead. A determination of death must be made in accordance with accepted medical standards.[7]

The Uniform Determination of Death Act has been adopted, more or less in the form quoted above, in most states. There is now nearly a consensus among philosophers that the irreversible cessation of all brain function constitutes death, whether it be measured through tests of brain function itself or tests for cardiopulmonary activity.[8] Even the few dissenters who would return to the heart-lung criterion as the sole legal criterion agree that those who meet the whole brain death definition should be allowed to die.

New technologic developments, such as sophisticated ventilators and heart-lung machines, required this new definition of death. These machines allowed the heart to keep beating and the lungs to operate even in the absence of other indications of life. Before this technology the heart and lungs could not function without brainstem activity. After it was developed, the heart and lungs could continue to function even in the absence of a functioning brainstem.

The advent of successful organ transplantation techniques also rendered the heart-lung definition of death inadequate. Irreversible damage to the brainstem eventually leads to the cessation of function of the heart and lungs. However, this cessation takes some time, time in which potentially transplantable organs might not receive sufficient oxygen. Rather than delay the certain declaration of death and destroy the possibility of transplanting healthy organs, many suggested that death be declared early enough to make the organs available for transplantation. Ultimately, the heart-lung machine and organ transplantation techniques led to the acceptance of this alternative criterion for death—the traditional heart-lung criterion in most cases, and the newer "brain death" criterion in cases in which the use of life support systems or the potential for use of the decedent's organs for transplant made the traditional criteria impossible or inefficient.

DETERMINATION OF DEATH

The National Conference of Commissioners on Uniform State Laws, which promulgated the Uniform Determination of Death Act (UDDA) of 1980, also recommended some procedures for the declaration of death: the ventilator should be removed after death is declared; the physician (and not the family) should make the decision to declare death; the physician may choose to consult with others (although the physician may choose not to) before declaring death; and the declaration should not be made by someone with an interest in the subsequent use of the tissue of a patient.

Where no statute for brain death exists, courts have been willing to accept the brain death definition in the unusual cases in which it is an issue, although the courts would clearly prefer that the decision be made by legislative action. Because the declaration of death is a scientific medical matter, it is governed by medical standards, not legal ones. The UDDA states that this determination is to be made "in accordance with accepted medical standards."[7] Because those medical standards change over time and depend on the diagnostic tools available in different times and different places, it makes sense for good medical practice to determine what counts as good evidence that the definition of death has been met.

Currently a physician declaring death based on brain death criteria is constrained by good medical practice to confirm the absence of any response to stimulus and the absence of any spontaneous respiration and cardiac activity. The Ad Hoc Committee's instruction that life support systems not be removed before the declaration of death is made and that any physician involved in the subsequent transplantation of organs from a deceased person not be involved in the declaration of death remains good advice, although not required by law.

Generally, a physician declaring death has a certain leeway regarding the time death is declared. Although a delay in declaring death for financial gain (such as an extra day billed to the hospital) is inappropriate, delaying a declaration of death a few hours so that loved ones may see their family member "alive" once more may be very appropriate.

Persistent Vegetative State

In 1968, the Ad Hoc Committee for the Harvard Medical School to Examine the Definition of Brain Death proposed a new criterion to reflect the need for an alternative definition of death. This committee called the new criterion "irreversible coma," which includes the following characteristics: unreceptiveness and unresponsiveness, no movement or breathing, no reflexes, and a flat electroencephalogram. The Committee's use of the term *irreversible coma* has caused some problems, because the condition they were describing is not a coma at all, but irreversible lack of function of the entire brain.

The term *irreversible coma* was used to describe patients who are now generally referred to as in a persistent vegetative state (PVS), when all higher brain function is lost. PVS differs from brain death because the brainstem continues to function and the body is not dead. Basically, the connection is lost between the brain and the ability to carry out certain functions. Patients in a PVS may even seem to be awake but have no awareness of themselves or their environment. Imaging professionals should always treat these patients with respect and compassion.

Minimally Conscious State

Researchers have recognized that hierarchic levels of consciousness exist and that more precision is needed in the diagnosis of different levels of impaired consciousness. The distinction between PVS and minimally conscious state (MCS) is important because prognosis and treatment choices may be different for these two conditions.[10] These distinctions were brought to light in the case of Terri Schiavo, which is discussed in this chapter.

MCS is a condition of severely altered consciousness in which minimal but definite behavioral evidence of self-awareness or environmental awareness is demonstrated.[10] Scientists have developed criteria to diagnose MCS, which include functional interactive communication and functional object use.[10]

The natural history and long-term outcome of MCS have not yet been adequately investigated. No guidelines exist for the care of patients in MCS, and until sufficient data are available, the following consensus-based approaches to care are recommended. In all circumstances the patient should be treated with dignity and caregivers should realize the patient's potential for understanding and perception of pain. The distinction between PVS and MCS should be made by qualified professionals because the assessment will affect critical decisions, including changes in the level of care, disputed treatment decisions, and withdrawal of life-sustaining treatment.[10]

Life-Sustaining Treatments

CPR has traditionally been treated differently from other forms of life-sustaining treatment. CPR is the only form of life-sustaining treatment that is provided routinely without the consent of the patient, and it may be the only medical treatment of any kind that is generally initiated without an order of a physician. The following sections discuss orders that further a patient's wishes not to be resuscitated or undergo other life-sustaining treatments or procedures.

DIRECTIVES

Early cases that paved the way for recognition of directives include the 1976 Karen Ann Quinlan case[11] and the 1990 Nancy Cruzan case.[12] In response to the highly publicized Quinlan case, many states adopted statutes designed to give formal recognition to some form of written directives by patients; these directives are generally called *living wills*. The case concerned Karen Ann Quinlan's right to die. She collapsed at a party after ingesting alcohol and a tranquilizer and entered a PVS at the hospital. She was kept alive on a ventilator and with feeding tubes for years, against what Quinlan's family and friends felt was her will.[11] This section discusses the current state of the law regarding living wills and the treatments that can be withheld when a living will exists. Another well-publicized case helped further the development of the law regarding advance directives and living wills. The Nancy Cruzan case resulted in a Supreme Court split decision that refused to allow life-sustaining measures to be withdrawn from a woman in a PVS.

Although the outcome of the Cruzan case was controversial for proponents of the right to die, Justice Sandra Day O'Connor established in her opinion (which concurred in the result with the majority, but differed in the reasoning) some further guidelines and encouragement for use of durable powers of attorney. The durable power of attorney for health care decisions is an advance directive that is not limited to terminal conditions or specified treatments but instead appoints a person or persons to assume a substitute decision-maker role in the event the patient is unable to make decisions. The durable power of attorney as an advance directive tool, as well as situations in which no advance directive is in place, is discussed later in the chapter. The more recent, highly publicized case of Terri Schiavo highlights to an even greater degree what can happen when advance directives are not in place (Box 6-4). Think of the anguish all the family members endured in this case, the expense of the monumental legal battles that ensued, the wasted resources of judicial time and energy, when all of this could have been avoided had an advance directive, such as a power of attorney for medical purposes, been in place.

The role of imaging professionals regarding advance directives may appear small. However, nearly every day of imaging practice involves the provision of care for patients

BOX 6-4   **CASE STUDY: TERRI SCHIAVO**

In 1990, 26-year-old Terri Schiavo suffered cardiac arrest. Because her brain was deprived of oxygen, she lapsed into a persistent vegetative state and a feeding tube was inserted.

In 1998, Terri Schiavo's husband, Michael Schiavo, filed a petition to discontinue life support, and in 2000, the court ruled that feedings must be discontinued. In 2001, however, the court granted an appeal to Terri Schiavo's parents, Bob and Mary Schindler. Legal battles between Michael Schiavo and the Schindlers continued until 2005, attracting national media attention.

By March 2005, the legal case of Terri Schiavo had been appealed fourteen times, and motions, petitions, and hearings had all taken place in the Florida courts. There were also five suits in federal district court, but Florida legislation was overturned by the Supreme Court of Florida.

Ultimately, the U.S. Supreme Court refused to hear the case. Local and regional Florida courts also refused to hear the case, overturn earlier rulings, or order the reinsertion of the feeding tube. On March 18, 2005, Terri Schiavo's feeding tube was removed for the final time. She died at about 9 AM on March 31, 2005, at a hospice in Pinellas Park, Florida.

Modified from Holan AD, Jau don B: Timeline: Terri Schiavo's life, *The Tampa Tribune*, 2005.

TERMINAL ILLNESS
A terminal illness is a condition that leaves the patient irreversibly comatose or will lead to death within a year.

with **terminal illnesses**. An awareness of the state of the law enables imaging professionals to be more sensitive to patients, know the patients' legal rights, and ensure that both patients and professionals realize the options available to direct health care in the future.

PHYSICIAN-ASSISTED SUICIDE

As stated previously, physician participation in euthanasia, or assisted suicide, has stirred great controversy recently. The U.S. Supreme Court decided in June 1997 that states may ban assisted suicide but did not prohibit states from passing laws that would allow physician-assisted suicide. This Supreme Court case upheld the state laws in New York and Washington banning physician-assisted suicide. However, the Supreme Court also left the door open for states to allow physician-assisted suicide, if they so desire. The court found no constitutional right to physician-assisted suicide. The court also upheld New York's decision that a distinction exists between withholding medical treatment and actively assisting suicide.

The result of this Supreme Court decision is that each state may decide for itself whether the physicians in its state should be allowed to prescribe medication intended to end life if a terminally ill patient so wishes. Many states outlaw physician-assisted suicide. Oregon is the only state at present with a law allowing physician-assisted suicide. The debate will no doubt continue. Ethical and social issues are as important as the medical and legal ones.

Opponents of physician-assisted suicide say that the practice violates the sanctity of life; that a potential for abuse exists, especially against people lacking access to care and support; that burdened family members and health care providers may encourage the use of assisted suicide; that the ethics of medicine is strongly opposed to the taking of life; and that uncertainty in diagnosis and prognosis may lead to people being put to death who could actually recover.

Defenders of assisted suicide point out that decisions about time and circumstances of death are personal and competent persons should have a right to choose death; that justice requires treating all cases alike, and if competent terminally ill patients are allowed to hasten death by refusing treatment, assisted suicide should be allowed to accomplish that same goal; that physician-assisted suicide may be the only way to relieve suffering; that while society has an interest in preserving life, the prohibition on physician-assisted suicide excessively limits personal liberty; and that assisted death already occurs, although in secret, when such things as morphine drips, ostensibly used for pain relief, may actually be a form of assisted death or euthanasia.

The American Medical Association's position on physician-assisted suicide is stated in AMA Opinion 2.211[13]:

> Physician assisted suicide occurs when a physician facilitates a patient's death by providing the necessary means and/or information to enable the patient to perform the life-ending act (e.g., the physician provides sleeping pills and information about the lethal dose, while aware that the patient may commit suicide.)
>
> It is understandable, though tragic, that some patients in extreme duress, such as those suffering from a terminal, painful, debilitating illness, may come to decide that death is preferable to life. However, allowing physicians to participate in assisted suicide would cause more harm than good. Physician assisted suicide is fundamentally incompatible with the physician's role as healer, would be difficult or impossible to control, and would pose serious societal risks.
>
> Instead of participating in assisted suicide, physicians must aggressively respond to the needs of patients at the end of life. Patients should not be abandoned once it is determined that cure is impossible. Multidisciplinary interventions should be sought including specialty consultation, hospice care, pastoral support, family counseling, and other modalities. Patients near the end of life must continue to receive emotional support, comfort care, adequate pain control, respect for patient autonomy, and good communication.

COMPETENCE AND LIFE-SUSTAINING TREATMENT

Whether a patient has the right to forgo life-sustaining treatment, and the method by which that right can be exercised, depends fundamentally on whether that person is competent to make the decision. Courts have tried to use the traditional law of guardianship and conservatorship in dealing with the issue of **competence** regarding decisions about life-sustaining treatment. This assumes that a person is either legally competent or incompetent for all legal and medical purposes. More recently, some courts have rejected the all-or-nothing approach and have recognized the concept of "decisional capacity"—a term that focuses on the actual decision to be made—rather than "competency"—a term that focuses on the actual status of the patient. This concept accepts that a person may have the attributes to make some simple health care decisions and not to make other, more complex decisions. Similarly, a patient may be able to make certain decisions at some times but not at others.[8] In practice, these definitions do not suffice because strict adherence to them makes medical care for the incompetent impossibly burdensome by substantially increasing the caseload of the courts.[14]

COMPETENCE
Competence is the ability to make choices.

Courts have been reluctant to articulate a formula for determining competence. This is true even when the court has had to address specifically the competence of patients to forgo life-sustaining treatment.

To date, the most widely accepted test for determining patient competence comes from the 1980 President's Commission for the Study of Ethical Problems in Medicine and Biomedical and Behavioral Research. The Commission found that the capacity to make competent decisions requires "to a greater or lesser degree" each of the following[14]:

- Possession of a set of values and goals
- Ability to communicate and understand information
- Ability to reason and deliberate about one's choice

Unfortunately, these elements are somewhat ambiguous and difficult to apply. Although this test may assist courts in making judicial determinations of competence, it provides little practical help in the determination of whether a patient is capable of making the decision to forgo life-sustaining treatment.

Tools are available to help competent people make medical decisions before they become incompetent. One of these is the living will, which generally allows patients to state in advance (in addition to other treatment preferences) that in the event of terminal illness they wish to forgo life-sustaining treatment. Another tool is the durable power of attorney for health care decisions. This directive is broader than a living will and provides for a substitute decision maker to make health care decisions when the patient is not able. These tools are often combined into one document called a "Declaration Relating to Life-Sustaining Treatment and Durable Power of Attorney for Health Care Decisions,"[15] which states the person's desire, in the event of terminal illness, not to have life prolonged by life-sustaining procedures and also creates a substitute decision maker with regard to health care.

NO-CODE ORDERS

As discussed earlier, CPR has traditionally been treated differently from other forms of life-sustaining treatment. CPR is generally provided unless a formal "do not resuscitate" (DNR) order is entered on the patient's chart.

In the past, CPR was not discussed with patients. In the mid-1980s, health professionals feared the legal ramifications of not performing CPR, even when obviously futile or inconsistent with the wishes of the patient. This resulted in "slow codes" or "pencil DNRs," meaning that staff members would be instructed to provide resuscitation guaranteed not to be successful (for example, be slow in calling the code). Some institutions used a removable dot of a certain color on the patient's chart to indicate that a "slow code" should be called. These practices were intended to ensure that no record would be left that decisions were made not to resuscitate the patient.

The reaction to this process was the development of formal hospital policies that provided for open and honest decision making on DNR issues. Today, generally accepted principles of medical ethics require that hospitals maintain such policies, and many hospitals have delegated this responsibility to their ethics committees. Any hospital without such a policy could face legal liability if a patient is inappropriately resuscitated or not resuscitated because of the uncertain reaction of a nurse, physician, or health care worker within the institution. In fact, health care professionals have an absolute duty to respect the patient's wishes in the case of DNR orders. Nurses have been sued for failure to observe DNR orders[16] and have faced such claims as battery, negligent infliction of pain and suffering, and "wrongful life."[17] Imaging professionals must know the CPR status of each patient they are treating. This includes knowing where in the patient's medical record to find the information and consistently checking the CPR status.

Today, most hospitals have DNI ("do not intubate") policies. This is an important part of advance directive planning because intubation can be considered separately from resuscitation. A person may have trouble breathing or may not be getting enough oxygen before the heart actually stops beating or breathing stops. In such a case, if the condition continues, a full arrest will occur. If the patient is intubated, cardiac or respiratory arrest may be averted. It is important for health professionals to understand the policy of the facility, since refusal of resuscitation is not necessarily the same as refusal of intubation.[18] Discussions with a patient regarding advance directives should address this issue so the patient's wishes will be followed.

At the time of this publication, legislation requiring specific procedures is in place only in New York State. The statute is precise and complicated. Health care providers had feared that legislation would ensue in all states, creating a crazy quilt of medical procedures required by statutes, but no other state has followed suit.

LIVING WILLS

The 1976 Karen Quinlan case started a trend of statutes that formally recognize certain forms of written statements requesting that some types of medical care be discontinued.[8] These "living will statutes" differ significantly among the states. This situation prompted an attorneys' commission to draft the Uniform Health Care Decisions Act of 1993, which formulated a uniform statute that could be adopted by states.

Living will statutes, which still provide the governing law in most jurisdictions, differ in several respects. One significant variable in state statutes is a definition of who may execute a living will. In some states living wills may be executed by any person at any time, and in some states they may even be executed on behalf of minors. Other states require a waiting period or specify that a living will may not be executed during a terminal illness. In most states living wills are of indefinite duration, whereas in others they expire after a specified number of years. Some statutes address only patients who are "terminally ill," others include those in "irreversible coma" or in a "persistent vegetative state," and still others provide for different conditions to be present before the living will applies.[8] Some states require the same formality of execution as is required of a will, while others require different formalities.

Most statutes relieve physicians and health care providers of civil or criminal liability if they properly follow the requirements of the statute and implement the desires expressed in a legally executed living will. Many living will statutes do not apply to patients in a PVS, irreversible coma, or other medical condition that is not considered "terminally ill." Many living will statutes specifically exclude "the performance of any procedure to provide nutrition or hydration" from the definition of death-prolonging procedures and thus do not allow any statutory protection to those who remove nutrition or hydration from a patient.[8]

Many statutes require physicians who do not wish to carry out the requests of patients with living wills to transfer them to other health care providers who will. The statutes also provide that carrying out the provisions of a properly executed living will does not constitute suicide for insurance purpose. It is difficult to know whether the absence of litigation over the terms of living wills means that these documents are working or not working well at all.[8] Because of the variations in statute, the imaging professional and all health care providers must know what the law is with regard to living wills in their particular jurisdiction.

DURABLE POWERS OF ATTORNEY FOR HEALTH CARE DECISIONS

A durable power of attorney is a document executed by a competent person (the principal) to appoint another (an agent) to make health care decisions when the principal becomes incompetent. Any competent adult may be appointed as an agent under durable power of attorney statutes. An alternate agent may be appointed in case the appointed agent is unable or unwilling to act.

Durable powers of attorney may be limited in time, scope, or method of decision making at the discretion of the principal executing the document. For example, a principal may designate a person to make decisions regarding life-sustaining treatment, decisions that do not involve life-sustaining treatment, or any other subclass of decisions. An agent may be required to consult with designated others before making health care decisions or applying principles articulated in the document.

Agents are expected to apply the principle of substituted judgment when making health care decisions; that is, they are to make the decisions the principal would make if the principal were competent. However, the durable power of attorney document may specify other principles to be used by the agent to make decisions. Virtually no practical limits exist to the restrictions and conditions that may be placed on agents in durable powers of attorney for health care decisions.[8]

Durable power of attorney statutes became popular after the Cruzan decision in 1990. In her separate opinion, Justice Sandra Day O'Connor stated that she approved of durable powers of attorney and commented that the "practical wisdom" of such documents has been recognized by several states.[12] She also suggested that durable powers of attorney, which she described as "valuable additional safeguard[s] of the patient's interest in directing his medical care"[12] might have constitutionally protected status. Her opinion further indicated that courts may find that the U.S. Constitution requires states to follow the decisions of an appointed surrogate.[12]

The reasons that durable powers of attorney for health care decisions have become accepted so quickly by ethicists, physicians, medical institutions, and the law are easy to understand. These documents allow patients to decide who will make health care decisions for them and thus help safeguard autonomy.

Because durable powers of attorney do not require patients to anticipate what treatments are required in the event of incapacitation, they are much less likely than living wills to give rise to questions and concerns over whether patients have changed their minds. Because a durable power of attorney appoints a particular decision maker instead of defining a particular decision, it allows the decision maker to consult physicians and family members about proposed treatments. Although a durable power of attorney is not inconsistent with a living will (a principal may instruct an agent to follow the wishes expressed in the living will), it is generally a far broader document that may be applied to all health care decisions. As is the case with all state statutes, there are considerable variations from state to state and therefore imaging professionals need to be aware of the statutes that exist in their particular jurisdiction.

FAMILY CONSENT LAWS

Another concept involved in health care decisions by substitute decision makers has become law in many states. This is the concept that when no advance directive exists, physicians and health care facilities should look to family members to make health care decisions. Some states have adopted statutes to give formal recognition to a practice that is based in common sense and has been accepted for a long time.

These statutes vary from state to state, but generally they become effective only when a patient becomes incompetent; some require a certification of incompetence before the family is authorized to make health care decisions. The statutes authorize designated close family members to act on behalf of the patient, but never in the same hierarchy as is used to determine inheritance of the patient's estate. All these statutes require that a patient's designation (e.g., through a living will or durable power of attorney) be followed so that no conflict with the patient's wishes occurs. These statutes have been the subject of very little litigation. This is probably because all they do is bring formal recognition to an arrangement that is merely common sense and has been in use for a long time.

UNIFORM HEALTH CARE DECISIONS ACT

The Uniform Health Care Decisions Act (UHCDA) was developed to replace the Uniform Rights of The Terminally Ill Act, state durable powers acts, and parts of the Uniform Anatomical Gifts Act. It was approved by the National Council of Commissioners on Uniform State Laws in 1993 and by the American Bar Association House of Delegates in 1994.[8] This act, for those states that choose to adopt it, takes a comprehensive approach by placing into one statute the living will, called the "individual instruction"; the durable power of attorney, called the "power of attorney for health care"; a family consent law; and some provisions involving organ donation.[8] By 2004, some version of the uniform act had been adopted in Alabama, Alaska, California, Delaware, Hawaii, Maine, Mississippi, and New Mexico.

Under the UHCDA, the residual decision-making portion of the act is much like the family consent laws that were discussed previously. This section applies only if there is no applicable individual instruction or appointed agent. Although it specifies a familial hierarchy for decision making for a decisionally impaired incapacitated patient, it also allows the family to be superseded by an "orally designated surrogate," who may be appointed by the patient's informing the "supervising physician" that the surrogate is entitled to make health care decisions on his or her behalf. In the same manner the patient may disqualify the surrogate simply by telling the supervising physician. So, in essence, under the UHCDA, any health care decision will be made by the first available in the hierarchy[8]:

1. The patient, if competent
2. The patient, through an individual instruction
3. An agent appointed by the patient in a written power of attorney for health care, unless a court has given this authority explicitly to a guardian
4. A guardian appointed by the court
5. A surrogate appointed orally by the patient
6. A surrogate selected from the list of family members and others who can make health care decisions on behalf of the patient

The drafters of the UHCDA made it clear in their comments that one purpose of the statute was to ensure that these intimate health care decisions remain within the realm of the patient, the patient's family and close friends, and the health care providers, and that others not be allowed to disrupt that process. The court would rarely have a role in decision making under this statute and outsiders (including outside organizations) who do not think a patient is being adequately protected would have no standing to seek judicial intervention.[8] As stated previously, because of the variance in statutes among states, imaging professionals must know the status of the law in their jurisdiction.

ABSENCE OF ADVANCE DIRECTIVES

When no advance directive exists, no statute governs the choice of decision makers in the jurisdiction, and no family consent statutes exist to provide for decision making for incompetent patients, courts have attempted to protect the principle of autonomy by allowing others to make health care decisions on behalf of incompetent persons. The decision maker (i.e., a family member, a person appointed by the court, sometimes the court itself) must look at all potentially trustworthy sources of information and determine with sufficient reliability the decision the patient would make if competent.

Courts deciding such cases have used different tests to determine whether treatment may be withdrawn based on the strength and certainty of the articulation of the patient when competent and on the current condition of the patient. Before the Schiavo case the Karen Quinlan case was the most authoritative case on the subject, and in that case the court ordered that the "clear" and "unequivocal" desire of the patient to terminate treatment be carried out.[11] However, as the New Jersey Supreme Court stated in the *In re Conroy* case, if the desire of the patient is neither clear nor unequivocal, any apparent desire for the termination of treatment is honored only if the burdens of continued life clearly outweigh the benefits of treatment.[18] The Conroy decision went on to state that if the patient has never made any expression about whether life-sustaining treatment should be continued, such treatment must be continued unless doing so is inhumane.[18]

PATIENTS IN A PERSISTENT VEGETATIVE STATE

Only a short time after *In re Conroy* articulated the tests to determine whether life-sustaining treatment should be withdrawn, the inappropriateness of these tests for patients in a PVS became apparent in the case of Nancy Ellen Jobes. She was in a PVS in a nursing home as the result of surgery following a car accident. The Jobes court explained PVS by quoting the trial testimony of Dr. Fred Plum, who stated, "[Persistent] vegetative state describes a body which is functioning entirely in terms of its internal controls. It maintains temperature. It maintains heartbeat and pulmonary ventilation. It maintains digestive activity. It maintains reflex activity of muscles and nerves for low level conditioned responses. But there is no behavioral evidence of either self-awareness or awareness of the surroundings in a learned manner."[20]

A person in a PVS has no chance of return to a cognitive state, although the body of a patient with this condition may be maintained, sometimes without use of a ventilator, for years and perhaps decades. The Jobes court pointed out that the criteria used for evaluation of incompetent patients should not be used for patients in a PVS. Instead it said that if the particular patient clearly would have refused treatment under the circumstances, treatment should be withdrawn. If, however, the patient's wishes are not clear, "the right of a patient in an irreversibly vegetative state to determine whether to refuse life sustaining medical treatment may be exercised by the patient's family or close friend."[20] This liberal approach to patients in a PVS has been accepted in theory by many states.[8] As Justice John Paul Stevens pointed out in his Cruzan dissent, every court that has heard a request to terminate life-sustaining treatment for a patient in a PVS has ultimately approved the request—except the Cruzan court itself.[12] The district court in Florida, in affirming the trial court's decision to allow life-sustaining procedures to be withdrawn from Terri Schiavo,[21] used an approach set out in the previous Florida case of Estelle Browning.[22] (Estelle Browning had a living will but was being kept alive by a feeding tube, the termination of which was not covered by Florida's living will statute.) Based on the reasoning in the Browning case, the appeal court followed the clear and convincing standard of proof that allows the court to make decisions even in the face of inconsistent and conflicting evidence. The appeals court concluded that the trial court had clear and convincing evidence that Terri Schiavo, not after a few weeks in a coma but after 10 years in a PVS, with no hope of a medical cure, would wish to permit a natural death process to take its course. Other appeals and pleas, involving various issues and participation from various other entities, postponed the final removal of her feeding tube until March 18, 2005, and her death finally resulted on March 31, 2005.

PATIENTS WHO HAVE NEVER BEEN COMPETENT

If a patient has never been competent (e.g., if a patient has been profoundly mentally disabled since birth), the substituted judgment standard to determine the kind of life-sustaining treatment the patient would want is difficult to apply. Courts are divided on which standard to apply in such situations.[8] One court stated, "We recognize a general right in all persons to refuse medical treatment in appropriate circumstances. The recognition of that right must extend to the case of an incompetent, as well as a competent patient, because the value of human dignity extends to both."[20] It further asserted that the choice is not to be made by asking what a majority of competent people would choose, but rather by determining with as much accuracy as possible the wants and needs of the individual involved.[23]

Other courts have not been so concerned with the autonomy and dignity of persons who have been disabled since birth and think the "best interest" standard should be applied. The New York Court of Appeals, which has narrowly defined even a competent patient's right to forgo treatment, has declared that adults who have been incompetent since birth should be treated the same as children.[24] It has also established a default position requiring treatment in virtually all cases. As the court pointed out, a "parent or guardian has a right to consent to medical treatment on behalf of an infant. The parent, however, may not deprive a child of life sustaining treatment, however well intended."[24]

SUMMARY

- The value of life and its impact on the ethical decision-making abilities of the imaging professional influence choices concerning death and dying. Suicide, euthanasia, and problems surrounding quality of life are all issues that imaging professionals face in their work.

- Some may consider passive suicide ethical if the good of the act outweighs the bad (proportionality). Others may consider active suicide ethical in certain situations for the same reason. Nevertheless, this does not mean that the patient has the legal right to commit suicide; suicide and euthanasia are still illegal in most states.
- It is generally illegal for imaging professionals to participate in active euthanasia or a patient's active suicide even if the patient is terminally ill. In certain instances, however, imaging professionals may be involved in passive suicide or euthanasia by not performing procedures on a patient who has given orders not to be revived with heroic measures if his or her heart fails (no-code orders) or a patient for whom nothing else can be done medically.
- Quality-of-life issues are affected by what normal life means to the patient, how the patient's life will be affected if no treatment is given, what biases the imaging professional may have about quality of life, what options the patient who refuses treatment has, and how a terminally ill patient will be kept comfortable.
- The patient's right to forgo life-sustaining medical treatment stems from the common law right to choose the form of treatment. The reasoning behind the right to forgo life-sustaining treatment is that if patients have the right to determine whether they consent to a particular treatment, they also have the right to refuse to consent to a particular treatment.
- The principle that competent patients have a right to forgo life-sustaining treatment was explicitly articulated in a 1984 case. As suggested by this ruling, the competence of patients is fundamental to whether they have a right to forgo life-sustaining treatment and the method by which that right is exercised.
- Courts have been reluctant to define competence formally. In fact, definitive tests of competence are virtually impossible to articulate. The issue of the inability of a patient who has become incompetent to choose to forgo life-sustaining medical treatment was brought to the world's attention in 1976 through the Karen Ann Quinlan case. This case led to many living will statutes that give formal recognition to some form of written directives by patients.
- Although living wills serve a useful purpose, their use is limited to patients with terminal conditions. The treatment that may be withheld under a living will is limited to life-sustaining care, often specifically excluding nutrition and hydration.
- The well-publicized Cruzan case in 1990 helped further the development of the law regarding advance directives. Although the Missouri Supreme Court refused to allow the withdrawal of life-sustaining treatment, the opinion written by Justice O'Connor established some guidelines and encouragement for the use of durable powers of attorney. The Terri Schiavo case has underlined the importance of advance directives.
- A durable power of attorney for health care decisions is an advance directive that is not limited to terminal conditions or specified treatments but instead appoints a person or persons to assume a substitute decision-maker role if the patient becomes unable to make decisions. It is a much broader tool than a living will and in general allows health care decisions to reflect the wishes of the patient more accurately.
- Physician-assisted suicide is illegal in all states except Oregon.
- CPR has traditionally been treated differently from other forms of life-sustaining treatment. CPR is generally provided unless a formal "do not resuscitate" order is entered. Imaging professionals should know the status of their patients with

regard to DNR orders and know where to locate this information in the patient's record.

- Laws on death and dying vary tremendously among jurisdictions. Nearly every day of practice in imaging involves the provision of care for patients with terminal illnesses. An awareness of the state of the law enables imaging professionals to be more sensitive to these patients and their wishes and know the patient's legal rights and the imaging professional's responsibilities. It also enables them to ensure that both professionals and patients realize the options available to direct their health care in an often uncertain future.

REFERENCES

1. Husted GL, Husted JH: *Ethical decision making in nursing*, ed 2, St Louis, 1995, Mosby.
2. Garrett TM, Baillie HW, Garrett RM: *Healthcare ethics, principles and problems*, ed 2, Englewood Cliffs, NJ, 1993, Prentice Hall.
3. Jonsen AR, Siegler M, Winslade WJ: *Clinical ethics: a practical approach to ethical decisions in clinical medicine*, ed 5, New York, 2002, McGraw-Hill.
4. Beauchamp TL, Perlin S: *Ethical issues in death and dying*, Englewood Cliffs, NJ, 1978, Prentice Hall.
5. *Schloendorff v Society of NY Hospitals*, 105 N.E.92 (N.Y. 1914).
6. *Bartling v Superior Court*, 209 Cal. Rptr. 220 (Cal. App. 1984).
7. *Uniform Determination of Death Act*, 12 U.L.A. 340 (Supp. 1991).
8. Furrow BR, Greaney TL, Johnson SH, et al: *Health law: cases, materials and problems*, ed 5, St Paul, 2004, West.
9. Humber J: *Statutory criteria for determining human death*, 42 Mercer L.Rev. 1069 (1991).
10. Giancino JT, Ashwal S, Childs N, et al: The minimally conscious state, *Neurology* 58:349, 2002.
11. *In re Quinlan*, 355 A.2d 647(N.J. 1976).
12. *Cruzan v Director, Missouri Dept. of Health*, 497 U.S. 261, 190, 110 S.Ct.2841, 2857 (1990).
13. American Medical Association: *Policy compendium*, 2002-2003; *Decisions near the end of life*, 1991; *Physician-assisted suicide*, Dec 1993; updated June 1996.
14. *In re Cruzan*, 110 S. Ct. 2841 (1990).
15. Iowa State Bar Association: *Declaration relating to life sustaining procedures and durable power of attorney for health care decisions*, Des Moines, revised 2006, Author.
16. Tammelleo A: Malpractice insurance: for your protection, *RN* 60(10):73, 75-77, 1997.
17. *Anderson v St. Francis–St. George Hospital*, 614 N.E.2d 841 (1992).
18. *In re Conroy*, 486 A.2d 1209, 1232 (N.J. 1985).
19. National Hospice and Palliative Care Organization: *Questions and answers: artificial nutrition*, Alexandria, Va, 2005, Author. Available at www.webmd.com/content/Article/114/111424.htm.
20. *In re Jobes*, 529 A.2d 434, 438 (N.J. 1987).
21. *In re Guardianship of Theresa Marie Schiavo*, 780 So.2d 176 (2001).
22. *In re Guardianship of Browning*, 543 So.2d 258 (Fl. 1989).
23. *Superintendent of Belchertown State School v Saikewicz*, 370 N.E.2d 417, 427 (Mass. 1977).
24. *In re Storar*, 438 N.Y.S.2d 266, 240 N.E.2d 64 (N.Y. 1981).

REVIEW QUESTIONS

1 Life is the _____ _____ of the living thing.
2 Death is considered part of the _____ _____.
3 List three reasons why suicide may be considered wrong:
   a. _____
   b. _____
   c. _____

4 Define euthanasia.

5 In what ways do advance directives and living wills assist the health care provider?

6 Define persistent vegetative state.

7 List three factors involved in quality-of-life decisions:

　　a. _____

　　b. _____

　　c. _____

8 What is the difference between active suicide and active euthanasia? When may each situation present itself in medical imaging?

9 Discuss ways in which the law may interfere with and uphold patient rights.

10 In what way may an imaging professional cooperate with passive suicide or passive euthanasia?

11 When may an imaging professional ethically be involved in passive euthanasia?

12 True or False   Patients have the ethical right to refuse treatment.

13 True or False   Imaging professionals may assist in active suicide.

14 True or False   Active euthanasia is not against the law in the United States.

15 True or False   The right to forgo life-sustaining treatment is based on the principle of autonomy.

16 True or False   The principles of beneficence and nonmaleficence and respect for autonomy are important factors in quality-of-life issues.

17 True or False   The imaging professional's biases might affect his or her evaluation of the patient's quality of life.

18 True or False   Plans for comfort and palliative care are not concerns for quality of life of a terminally ill patient.

19 True or False   Imaging professionals may encounter personal issues of passive euthanasia.

20 True or False   The right to forgo life-sustaining treatment was first articulated by Justice Benjamin Cardozo in 1914.

21 True or False   Courts have articulated definite rules on ways to determine patient competence.

22 True or False   All the statutes in various states agree that any adult may execute a living will.

23 True or False   Living wills are limited in the conditions under which they are effective and the treatments they may authorize to be withheld.

24 True or False   Living wills always include authorization for the withholding of nutrition and hydration.

25 True or False   Living wills must be executed in the same manner as a last will and testament.

26 True or False   Health care workers should be concerned with criminal and civil liability for carrying out the wishes documented in a living will.

27 True or False   Justice Sandra Day O'Connor helped further the law regarding durable powers of attorney in the Cruzan case of 1990.

28 True or False   Durable powers of attorney for health care decisions have broader applications than do living wills.

29 True or False   The advantage of a durable power of attorney is that an attorney always makes the decisions and family members are not involved.

30 **True or False**   Durable powers of attorney for health care decisions appoint a particular decision maker instead of defining a particular decision.

31 **True or False**   Durable powers of attorney apply only to decisions regarding life-sustaining treatment.

32 **True or False**   When no advance directive exists and the wishes of the patient are not clear, life-sustaining treatment would probably be withdrawn.

33 **True or False**   The same rules apply for patients in a persistent vegetative state as for incompetent patients.

34 **True or False**   The same rules apply for persons who have never been competent as for competent patients who have become incompetent.

35 **True or False**   The terms "persistent vegetative state" and "minimally conscious" describe the same condition.

36 **True or False**   The terms "irreversible coma" and "persistent vegetative state" describe the same condition.

37 **True or False**   Physicians in all states have the right to help patients commit suicide if they think it is the right thing to do.

38 **True or False**   The Uniform Health Care Decisions Act combines the living will, durable powers of attorney, and organ donation laws and provides a method of making health care decisions for incompetent patients without advance directives.

39 **True or False**   Eight states have thus far adopted some version of the Uniform Health Care Decision Act.

40 **True or False**   The Uniform Determination of Death Act has helped to determine death by defining two tests: (1) irreversible cessation of circulatory and respiratory functions and (2) irreversible cessation of all functions of the entire brain, including the brainstem.

41 **True or False**   Using the tests in question 40, any health care professional can determine death.

CRITICAL THINKING *Questions & Activities*

1 What factors do you personally believe make life worth living? Defend your answers.

2 How many imaging professionals in your area have living wills? Talk to them and learn their reasons. Evaluate your own needs.

3 Make contact with chaplains and social services to review the types of services offered to patients with terminal illnesses.

4 Visit a hospice.

5 Do a case study on a patient who has received passive euthanasia.

6 Develop a list of criteria for establishing a plan for active euthanasia. The criteria and supporting factors should be recorded.

7 HEALTH CARE DISTRIBUTION

Health is more than just the absence of illness. Health is the presence of aliveness, energy, joy.

PETER McWILLIAMS, *PORTABLE LIFE 101*

Chapter Outline

Ethical Issues
Biomedical Ethical Challenge
Rights and Health Care
Scarcity and Distribution
Distribution Allocation Groups
Distribution Theories
Distribution Decision-Making Criteria
Traditional Care
Health Care Delivery Model and Managed Care
Patient-Focused Care
Quality and Cost Effectiveness
Imaging Professionals' Participation

Legal Issues
Access to Medical Care
Health Care Costs
Managed Care
History of Managed Care Organizations
Legislation and Regulation of Managed Care
Institute of Medicine and Risk Managed Care
Medicare and Medicaid
Patient-Focused Care
Impact on the Imaging Professional

Learning Objectives

After completing this chapter, the reader will be able to perform the following:

- Define the right to health care.
- List distribution allocation groups.
- Identify ethical theories of distribution of health care.
- List and use distribution allocation criteria.
- Define managed care and its implications for imaging professionals and imaging services.
- Define patient-focused care.
- Compare concepts of quality care and cost effectiveness.
- State the imaging professional's role in health care distribution.
- Define the problems that created the need for managed care.
- Identify the history and evolution of managed care.

- State the current state of the law with regard to managed care organizations.
- Define the concept and origins of modern managed care or risk managed care.
- Define the concept of patient-centered or patient-focused care models.
- State the legal implications of managed care, risk managed care, and patient-focused care.
- Identify legal safeguards provided by proactive approaches to cross-training and streamlining imaging services.
- List possible liability issues with regard to denial of authorization of testing and the possible roles of imaging professionals as patient advocates in managed care settings.
- Identify the liability issues these roles may create.

Key Terms

egalitarian theory
entitlement theory
fairness theory
health care
managed care
patient-focused care

practical wisdom
right
rights theory
triage
utilitarian theory

Professional Profile

When I graduated from a hospital-based radiography program many years ago, signing the application for the American Registry of Radiologic Technologists (ARRT) examination seemed like a mere formality. I was focused on taking the registry examination, so I gave little thought to signing the promise to adhere to the professional code of ethics. The imaging and radiation sciences professions have become much more complicated than I ever imagined when I became a radiographer. I could not envision the role that ethics would play in the delivery of imaging services over the life of my career.

My first encounter with an ethical dilemma occurred when I was a radiography student. A young couple brought their toddler son in for an abdominal radiograph. The father carried the child and very gently laid him on the table. The boy looked like a victim of child abuse, bruised and battered. Cancer was actually the culprit, and the radiograph was a follow-up to an intense radiation therapy regimen. The radiologist's interpretation of the radiograph suggested that more radiation therapy might be needed. The parents announced there would be no further medical intervention, and they carried their son out of the hospital, against medical advice. Many technologists were appalled and very critical of the parents. I remember thinking how much harder it would be to say "no more" than to cling to the tiniest shred of hope for your child.

I had another distressing experience just a few years later that I will never forget. I was summoned to do a stat portable chest examination on an older man. He was uncooperative, noncommunicative, and obviously very uncomfortable. I finally had to be very firm with him to get him to lie still and take a deep breath while I made the exposure. A few minutes later I returned to the unit with his radiograph, only to learn that he had expired. I felt angry that the doctor had ordered an imaging procedure for a patient so close to death, but mostly I was angry with myself for being gruff with a patient during what turned out to be his last moments on earth. It was a terrible feeling and a painful lesson.

The uncharted territory of new technology and advances in medicine changed ethical issues for me from words on paper into new processes for my daily work routines. Witnessing a patient's written consent suddenly meant more than pausing long enough to scribble my name on a form handed to me by a doctor while on my way to the break room. The waiting room sign-in sheet vanished. Gone are the view boxes in the main hallway where patients walked to the dressing rooms. Now fusion imaging technology and molecular imaging are blurring the lines between health care disciplines and creating areas of overlapping responsibility. Emerging areas of advanced practice are ushering in even higher levels of obligation and ethical responsibility.

Understanding the foundations of ethical decision making is the first step toward appropriate professional practice. Knowing the limits of your scope of practice, state laws, and institutional policies will keep you headed in the right direction. Let experience serve as your guide, and always listen to your inner voice. When in doubt, ask for clarification. As the delivery of imaging and radiation services becomes more sophisticated, addressing the ethical implications continues to expand as an important component of clinical practice.

Rebecca Ludwig, PhD, RT(R)(QM), FAEIRS
Interim Chairman & Associate Professor,
Director, Master of Imaging Sciences Program
Department of Imaging & Radiation Sciences
University of Arkansas for Medical Sciences
Little Rock, Arkansas

ETHICAL ISSUES

The ethics of health care distribution affects both imaging professionals and patients. The United States spends more on health care than any other nation. Despite increased spending on health care, the national health status has not always improved. Thus reform of the health care environment, services, patients' rights, and the imaging professional's changing role are topics that must be addressed. The ethical challenges inherent in health care are changing, and imaging professionals must be prepared to change. Changes require critical thinking, flexibility, and a continued desire to provide high-quality imaging services.

BIOMEDICAL ETHICAL CHALLENGE

In the 1940s, the patient's needs came first regardless of the cost. Health care's obligation was to serve and meet the needs. By the 1960s, cost was becoming a greater concern and diagnostic related groups (DRGs) were developed to control resource allocation. In the 1980s, the prospective payment system (PPS) further expedited a fairer and more equitable system of health care distribution.

In the 1990s, President Bill Clinton stated the following[1]:

> We must set and keep our sights on three goals: controlling rising health care costs, covering every American with at least a basic health benefit package, and maintaining consumer choice in coverage and care. Putting people first in health care calls for a fundamental reform of the system. It requires that we combine an appropriate and revised governmental role with reliance on the private sector to provide care and to compete to serve every person in this country. But that competition must take place under a restructured set of ground rules that foster competition to provide the best care at the best price, not to avoid covering the less healthy and to raise prices fastest for the sickest.

As we enter the 21st century, the ethical dilemma of fair and equitable health care distribution remains. Health maintenance organizations and preferred provider organizations, which are discussed later in the chapter, have had the opportunity to provide more care for more people. Whether they have fulfilled this goal is questionable.

As the public becomes more aware of new imaging technologies and their diagnostic importance, the medical imaging community has been affected profoundly by the health care distribution dilemma. Patients may respond to advertisements in the mass media by asking for these expensive new procedures. As such advertisements become more prevalent, questions regarding the ethics of health care industries marketing to target patients become more complex. Patients may feel entitled to the benefits of new technologies and may make demands on physicians and institutions to facilitate their needs. The reimbursement process, however, remains controversial. The patient, provider, and third-party payer must come to terms with the availability of services and the amount of reimbursement available for those services.

RIGHTS AND HEALTH CARE

RIGHT
A right is a claim or an entitlement.

HEALTH CARE
Health care is a practice, a commodity, an approach, or a collective responsibility to ensure the wellness of a population.

Before a right to health care can be discussed, the terms "right" and "health care" must be defined. A **right** in this context means a just claim or an entitlement. Americans tend to believe that all people deserve health care as a matter of course, but this may be a simplistic notion. Should all people, regardless of whether they pay for their health care, are homeless, or are financially irresponsible and cannot afford health care, be able to claim routine health care as a right?

The second term, **health care**, encompasses many elements. It may be perceived as a practice, a commodity, an approach, or a collective responsibility. *Health* may be described as a condition or frame of mind. All these definitions help inform a discussion of health care.

To answer the ethical question of whether a right to health care exists, medical professionals should ask whether health care is an element in autonomy and self-determination. Self-determination requires patients to participate in their own health care. Patients need knowledge, awareness, and continuing education regarding what they can do to maintain health to be full participants in their care. This is as important in the health care process as the provision of health care services. However, self-determination also requires patients to take responsibility for their health. Smokers who have chronic respiratory problems require many health care services, including chest studies, sinus radiographs, computed tomography (CT) scans, and other procedures. However, do such patients not bear some responsibility for their poor health? Should other patients suffer delayed access to imaging examinations because of the examinations required by patients who have not participated in their own health care? Should society pay the health care costs of those who do not take care of themselves?

SCARCITY AND DISTRIBUTION

Society is under many demands to provide health care for all citizens. The increasing costs of health care and the demands of a growing population place other stresses on an increasingly overburdened health care system. Nevertheless, many perceive a need for resources for the distribution of health care services to come from public as well as private sources because "society is under an obligation to the individual to promote the common good."[2]

Resources in health care are increasingly expensive and scarce. "A sound theory [of] distribution, then, must provide for priorities and a system of allocating resources that at least regularizes expectations in the light of what is politically and economically possible."[2] Society, patients, and providers must make difficult decisions to aid in this distribution.

DISTRIBUTION ALLOCATION GROUPS

Questions regarding health care resource allocation can be divided into three groups: macro-allocation, meso-allocation, and micro-allocation.[3] Macro-allocation questions ask how big the health care budget will be, who will pay for it, what end it serves, whether there is a right to this care, and what standards will be used to determine these factors. Meso-allocation questions ask how the health care budget will be divided, what health care needs will be addressed, how they will be prioritized, who will deliver these services, and what limits will best serve the efficient meso-allocation of health care. Micro-allocation questions ask who should get what share of the health care budget, whether the present distribution is equitable, how rationing of services is determined, and what factors should be used in the triage of patient needs (Figure 7-1).

DISTRIBUTION THEORIES

Prioritizing, or **triage**, is an ongoing decision-making process in health care. The determination of which patient is the most important, is in the most critical condition, has the greatest need, or has the best opportunity for a positive outcome is an evaluation process necessary for the distribution of limited resources. Triage, however, is much easier to practice at an administrative level than at eye level with a dying patient. Triage

TRIAGE
Triage is a system of prioritizing that encourages the delivery of treatment to those with the greatest opportunity for a positive outcome.

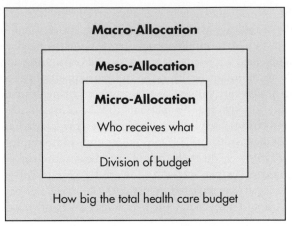

FIGURE 7-1 Resource allocation groups.

TABLE 7-1 **THEORIES OF DISTRIBUTION: PROS AND CONS IN IMAGING SERVICES**

Theory	Pros	Cons
Egalitarian	All persons have equal access to all imaging services	Patients' needs are different; scheduling and reimbursement would be different
Entitlement	All persons have needs	Patients must be involved in a contract to pay for services; theory more concerned with cost value of treatment instead of the intrinsic value of the service to the patient
Fairness	Balances dignity and equality of all persons with the inequality of their needs and circumstances	Identifying the differences (inequality of needs) can lead to subordinating the dignity of the individual to the convenience of the society
Utilitarian	Recommends providing the greatest good for the greatest number of people	Identifies patients as a group rather than as individuals

seems to be a practical method to bring justice and fairness to distribution, and society may see it as such, but it presents ethical conflicts.

The prioritization of patient needs influences imaging modalities. For example, breast imaging is often scheduled under pressure by patients and physicians after a lump has been found. Many breast imaging suites examine patients every 15 minutes all day long, and many of these patients have to wait for diagnostic examinations after discovery of an abnormality. Prioritizing these patients according to their needs is difficult. A number of theories have been advanced to aid the triage process (Table 7-1).

Egalitarian Theory

The **egalitarian theory** demands equal distribution of equal resources. This system believes every person is good and is equal. However, it does not address the fact that persons may not have equal needs. Moreover, whether this theory can be put into practice is uncertain. Carried to its logical conclusion, equal distribution of equal resources gives every imaging patient equal access to all imaging modalities. In what way would scheduling and reimbursement be handled under such a system?

Entitlement Theory

The **entitlement theory** sees the distribution of health care resources as a system of contracts. For this theory to work, a person must have a way to pay for the contract. The health care needs of the patient and the patient's ability to pay for required services do not fit into the value system to which some Americans are accustomed if those Americans believe they have a right to health care but are unwilling to pay for it. In addition, the theory seems to be grounded in the financial value of medical treatment rather than its intrinsic value.

Fairness Theory

The **fairness theory** tries to tailor health care distribution to balance the dignity and equality of all persons with the inequality of their needs and circumstances. The most important consideration in this theory is the ways in which advantaged and disadvantaged people receive care and who makes these decisions. Inequalities in health care distribution are frowned upon. "Identifying how these differences affect the person can easily lead to subordinating the dignity of the individual to the convenience of the society."[2]

Within the fairness theory, the equality of patients as individuals is weighed against differences in their needs and circumstances. This weighing leads to a number of difficult questions. Do pediatric patients who come from financially disadvantaged homes have a right to an imaging examination their parents cannot afford? Should imaging procedures on individuals with mental disabilities be limited because of these patients' limited intellectual and financial resources? The fairness theory answers yes to the first question and no to the second. All patients are equal under the law and equal in human dignity, and regardless of whether they are unequal in means and resources, they still have the right to health services. However, difficulties arise in the determination of the degree to which a patient is disadvantaged.

Utilitarian Theory

As noted in previous chapters, utilitarianism recommends the provision of the greatest good (in this case, health care services) for the greatest number. Under **utilitarian theory**, imaging departments look at patients as a group and not as individuals and seek to provide the most care for the most people. A utilitarianist would say that if a vascular laboratory can accommodate five uncomplicated procedures in one day, it should perform them instead of two long procedures. More patients are served in this way, and thus the greater good for the greater number is achieved. However, utilitarianism creates a number of problems. Individuals may have difficulty maintaining autonomy as the utilitarian theory is implemented.

Rights Theory of Justice

The **rights theory** of justice claims that individuals have a right to good health care because of their human dignity. In recognition of this dignity, society has an obligation to care for all people. This theory raises questions of rights and autonomy and the ways in which they are implemented.

Practical Wisdom and Distribution

The **practical wisdom** theory of distribution states the following[2]:

> Justice or distribution is accomplished through application of practical wisdom (right reason) to meet the demands of human dignity in the social circumstances of the time. Justice thus involves respecting human dignity and satisfying human needs and recognizing human contributions within the system and in ways that are characteristic of the system.

In other words, to serve the patient, imaging professionals must use practical wisdom to assess individual needs, ability to pay, scarce resources, and resource distribution. How are rights balanced with scarce resources? Who makes these decisions?

DISTRIBUTION DECISION-MAKING CRITERIA

According to Armstrong and Whitlock, there are six criteria—need, equality, contribution, ability to pay, effort, and merit—that will aid the health care professional in ethical problem solving when a fair distribution of scarce resources is required.[4] These criteria, modified for imaging, are explained as follows:

1. Need. Need seems to be an obvious and useful criterion; however, this is complicated by whose perception of need is used to make the distribution decision. The imaging patient may determine that a much more expensive procedure is needed than the physician has ordered. Thus need is not always the best criterion to use in allocation dilemmas.
2. Equity. The concept of equity rarely serves well as an effective criterion for allocating health care resources. Each imaging patient may require a different type and number of imaging examinations depending on his or her health. It would make no sense to expect each patient to have an equal type and number of examinations.
3. Contribution. The consideration of contribution requires a determination of what an individual might be expected to give to society at a future date. Does the imaging patient have the ability to contribute something useful? Should younger imaging patients be given priority over the elderly? Is there an ethical means of evaluating these future contributions?
4. Ability to pay. Decisions based on ability to pay are of limited benefit in making allocation decisions based on the individual situation. Imaging professionals recognize the values of compassion and giving, and denial of health services based on the imaging patient's inability to pay is counter to the fundamental belief in generosity and charity. However, the ability to pay may be considered a compelling criterion for consideration when decisions involve elective treatment and the imaging patient was able to choose his or her health plan. At this point the third-party payer may determine the allocation of resources.
5. Patient effort. The imaging patient's effort may be a useful criterion for patients who fail to heed medical advice or do not make an effort to help themselves.

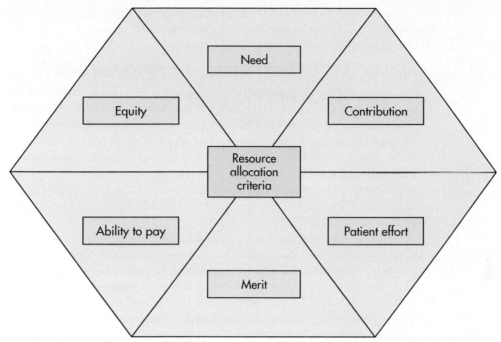

FIGURE 7-2 Resource allocation criteria.

It would be reasonable to consider the value of repeating imaging procedures on a person who continues high-risk behaviors after being warned by a physician to discontinue them. Patient effort may be a controversial criterion because of the complexity of withholding and limiting resources.

6. Merit. The best criterion on which an imaging professional could base an ethical allocation determination might be merit. Merit is the potential to benefit from the additional investment of limited health care resources. The criterion of merit requires that decisions be based on data or evidence. Do the data support the successful outcome of a vascular imaging procedure? Conflicting data and sources may complicate a merit-based decision.

The preceding criteria are useful in dealing with ethical dilemmas in allocating imaging resources. They raise important questions when choices are necessary, and they provide the imaging professional with an awareness of what imaging administrators face when solving distribution dilemmas (Figure 7-2).

TRADITIONAL CARE

Traditional care allows patients to choose their own physicians and facilities for health care services; however, a patient must be able to pay for those services. Each individual must have traditional insurance or be able to pay for the services. The more choices allowed to the consumer, the greater the cost of insurance. Traditional care provides high-quality health care for those with traditional insurance coverage and those who can pay for these services, but uninsured persons and those unable to pay find it difficult to obtain high-quality services.

Inequity of service, escalating health care costs, and demands from society have caused the U.S. health care system to become more sensitive to market forces. These factors have led to the development of managed care.

HEALTH CARE DELIVERY MODEL AND MANAGED CARE

Imaging professionals must understand the health care delivery model of managed care so that they may address the challenges that reforms in health care distribution have presented to imaging services. **Managed care** is an all-encompassing term that includes any type of system to coordinate the care and treatment of patients. Managed care is designed to provide better access, improved outcomes, more efficient use of resources, and controlled costs for the patient.[5] More simply, managed care is any type of delivery and reimbursement system that monitors or controls the type, quality, use, and costs of health care.[6] The aim of managed care is to reduce unnecessary or inappropriate care and reduce costs (Box 7-1).[7]

Whether managed care has accomplished the intended objectives is still to be determined. Not everyone has access to health care services, and whether the quality of care has increased or has at least been maintained at its previous level is unclear. Persons who were outside the system are still outside. Moreover, quality of care seems to be far down the list of objectives for most corporations; it is judged more by patients' perceptions of quality than by quality standards developed by the professional medical community.[7]

Managed care is having an impact on the ethical dilemmas faced by imaging professionals. It complicates the imaging professional's problem solving by adding questions concerning the needs of patients (both inside and outside the system), the medical community, and managed care corporations. Nevertheless, managed care will remain an integral part of the health care distribution system for some time to come[7]:

> Managed care takes many forms and is under so many different corporate structures that it is impossible to say it is categorically good or bad. The fact is that managed care is predominant in nearly every section of the country, and we must be able to adjust to the new way of providing patient care to our patients, making sure that we practice diagnostic imaging within the bounds of ethics.

PATIENT-FOCUSED CARE

Managed care is not the only model affecting health care and the imaging services. **Patient-focused care** also plays a significant role in the imaging professional's changing environment. Health care organizations and imaging services traditionally were designed to meet the fiscal needs of the organization. Now, following the lead of business and industry, they are currently developing and investing in services that address the demands and needs of the patient.[8]

The primary objectives of patient-focused care are to move hospital care services closer to the patient's bedside and decentralize hospital services, including radiology services. Patient-focused care also seeks to implement teams of multiskilled cross-trained health care professionals (including imaging professionals) to provide patient care.

The requirements of multiskilling and cross-training for imaging professionals lead to ethical considerations that have an impact on imaging practice. Cross-training may require imaging professionals to perform functions that were previously performed by other health care professionals such as nurses and medical technologists. Critics of patient-focused care

MANAGED CARE
Managed care is any type of delivery and reimbursement system that monitors or controls types, quality, use, and costs of health care.

PATIENT-FOCUSED CARE
Patient-focused care is a health care distribution model that calls for decentralization of patient care services and cross-training of health care professionals.

| BOX 7-1 | **WHAT IS MANAGED CARE AND HOW DID IT EVOLVE?** |

Managed care is a fusion of the two functions that historically were regarded as separate, the financing of medical care and the delivery of medical services.

1880s to 1960s

Managed care is not a new concept. Prepaid plans existed as early as the early 1800s, when employers paid physicians a few cents per employee to take care of the needs of all their factory employees. In the 1920s and 1930s, doctors and hospitals took care of patients through prepaid plans with payment by employers. Providers were not happy with this system, and hence the traditional fee-for-service or indemnity plans (like Blue Cross and Blue Shield) emerged. These dominated the health care market until the 1970s, when the increasing cost of health care prompted more incentives for managed care and the government decided to help reform the health care system through legislation.

1970 to 1990

The HMO Act of 1973 provided federal money to spur the growth of HMOs. However, America was not ready for managed care at that time and few employees signed up for this option. As the cost of health care continued to grow, in the mid to late 1980s, employers expressed concerns that their health care costs were preventing them from being competitive in the international market. Big business started listening when managed care offered some solutions in the form of new types of HMOs that gave employers more choices and physicians a larger measure of autonomy, while still achieving the goals of lower costs, use of practice guidelines, and coordination of care among providers.

Several different HMO versions emerged, and they began to be recognized under the umbrella of managed care organizations. As managed care became more common, the cycle of trying to appease consumers and providers and being unable to control costs accelerated.

State legislation attempted to rein in the managed care organizations. However, the Employee Retirement and Security Act (ERISA), although intended to protect employee pension plans, also affected health care and prohibited states from regulating managed care organizations. Managed care organizations had virtually no or very limited liability when they made medical decisions to deny care.

Early 2000s

In the early 2000s, the U.S. Supreme Court decided three different cases that opened the door for consumers to sue managed care organizations when they make erroneous medical decisions. State tort laws as well as state regulation of managed care organizations now apply. Unfortunately, this ability to litigate against managed care organizations also contributes to higher health care costs.

Emergence of Risk Managed Care

In response to the problem of state and federal insurance mandates and the resultant continuing trend of cost increases, a supportable solution emerged from the Institute of Medicine (IOM) and its reports on medical errors. The solution is based to a large extent on evidence-based risk managed care. This concept uses guideline-driven protocols, monitoring of provider standards, and financial incentives for provider compliance. Risk managed care is often referred to in terms of quality and patient safety. The IOM sees risk managed care as an improvement over managed care because medical decision making is aboveboard and subject to increased scrutiny and scientific validation.

Modified from Mclean TR, Richards EP: Health care's "thirty year war": the origins and dissolution of managed care, *NUU Annual Survey of American Law* 60:283, 2004.

believe this cross-training and decentralization may lead to the loss of professional identity.[9] Critics also question the amount of training a professional requires to perform a variety of functions. The training issue leads to a consideration of the degree of competence an imaging professional must possess in other disciplines and the impact this competence or lack of it may have on the quality of patient care in the imaging services.

QUALITY AND COST EFFECTIVENESS

The new methods of health care distribution provide ethical challenges for imaging professionals. Maintaining quality, providing access to more individuals, and cutting costs are problems for all imaging professionals. During this time of challenge and change they need to aspire to increase the quality of imaging services to maintain their professional status. The provision of more and better care with fewer resources requires sacrifice and planning on the part of imaging facilities. As medical imaging becomes more competitive and is forced to change, proactive facilities will thrive. They will be more cost effective, efficient, concerned with service, and driven by market factors. They will be survivors.[5]

Cost effectiveness may result from improved efficiency, empowerment of employees, and sensible delegation of duties. Efficiency may be improved by flattening schedules through elimination of peaks and filling in of low-use time. Cross-training employees to function in many capacities improves the use of personnel. Wise application of automation also may improve efficiency.

Institutions may compete in cost effectiveness by improving their awareness of the efficiency of their services. This determination provides the basis for ensuring that patients receive the most cost-effective and highest quality imaging services.

Imaging professionals and departments can help streamline performance by recognizing that they are in the service business. The focus of this business is the delivery of responsive, prompt, caring, and high-quality service.

Imaging professionals and departments can improve their performance by being aware of market considerations. The health care industry in general and medical imaging facilities in particular are under growing pressure to change. This pressure is driven by ever-increasing health care costs that must be borne by government, industry, and society. These cost considerations present a challenge to provide more cost-effective health care services without sacrificing the quality society has come to expect. Providing more cost-effective medical imaging in the face of evolving technologies that require more expensive facilities and equipment and more competent personnel is not easy. Imaging professionals will need to make the best use of their time, increase their productivity, and become multiskilled. They must be able to deal with change and be flexible in their assignments to enable their imaging department to become more competitive, cost effective, and market driven. Facilities that become more cost effective will survive; those that cannot make this transition will not.[5]

IMAGING PROFESSIONALS' PARTICIPATION

Health care providers cannot be all things to all people or meet the needs of everyone. Choices regarding the distribution of health care must be made, implemented, and evaluated.

Individuals and society have priorities for health care and must make health care decisions based on them. Priorities are both intrinsic and extrinsic—the priorities people

IMAGING SCENARIO

A high school student from a small rural town comes to her hometown physician with complaints of dizziness and headaches. He sends her to the nearest hospital for magnetic resonance imaging (MRI). The radiologist reads the MRI as a cyst in her brain. Her local physician is very concerned and presents the family with the worst case scenario. Her parents are self-employed and pay for all medical bills out of pocket because of extremely high insurance rates. The patient is sent to the university hospital where she has multiple tests, including a myelogram and another MRI. The myelogram leaves her with a terrible headache for several days. After the tests are completed and read, the specialist at the university hospital explains that the cyst in her brain is actually a portion of one of her ventricles. The radiologist who read the initial MRI read it incorrectly. The patient has an inflamed nerve in her neck, which caused the headaches and dizziness. Her family has incurred a debt of several thousand dollars because of the inaccurate reading of the MRI. After some inquiry it is determined that the radiologist who mis-read the MRI had had only a 2-week course in reading MRI images. The family confronts the radiologist about the inaccuracy and explains the anxiety, pain, and cost incurred. He is very difficult and states that he has no financial obligation in this situation.

Discussion questions
- Were there issues other than money?
- How did health care allocation and distribution of services enter into this ethical dilemma?
- Who was responsible for the anxiety, pain, and cost incurred?

IMAGING SCENARIO

An overweight woman in her eighties arrives for radiographs of her knees. She has great difficulty and pain when walking. She talks with the imaging professional about how she hopes for new knees because she still leads an active life and hasn't been able to exercise much because of the pain. The imaging professional notices how much boney destruction and arthritis are present in both knees. Later the professional learns from the patient that she was denied the surgery because of her age and weight. The patient is very depressed and asks the imaging professional what she thinks.

Discussion questions
- How would the six criteria for allocation decisions affect the imaging professional's thought process concerning the woman's right to surgery?
- What should she say to the patient?
- What would you do if this were your relative?

personally hold may not be the same as the priorities they recognize for society. Imaging professionals must remain continually aware of the problems and opportunities of health care service distribution. It is hoped that, as imaging professionals develop a heightened awareness of the ethical challenges posed by changes in health care distribution, they too will be survivors.

LEGAL ISSUES

Research into the state of health care in America shows that the system is in turmoil, although it is a different turmoil than when the first edition of this book was published in 1999. The problems are virtually the same: barriers that limit the access of many Americans to health care and the high and rapidly rising cost of health care. These problems brought about changes in health care in the late 1990s and early 2000s that had an impact on health care professionals, including imaging professionals. Now even more changes are occurring as the face of medicine is changing significantly. This section provides an overview of changes in the practice of medicine and the legal impact of these changes on imaging professionals.

ACCESS TO MEDICAL CARE

The problem of access to medical care has grown worse over the past decade. Between 2001 and 2002, the number of Americans not covered by health insurance grew from 41.2 million to 44.6 million. An estimated 15.2% of the population lacked health insurance for all of 2002, up from 14.6% in 2001. In 2005, almost 7 million more people in the United States were uninsured than in 2000. This is true even though Medicaid coverage has expanded dramatically and although the State Children's Health Insurance Program, created in 1997, now covers more than 5 million American children.[10,11]

Many lack drug coverage, and the ever-growing loss of retiree benefits has a huge impact on the ability to obtain needed pharmaceuticals. Approximately 30 million Americans who are insured for hospital or physician services do not have drug coverage, while many others have limited coverage.[10]

A survey performed by the Kaiser Family Foundation and the Harvard School of Health in 2005 showed that 62% of those struggling to pay medical bills have health insurance, underscoring how increasing premiums, deductibles, and gaps in coverage are affecting families. The survey showed that 28% of adults were unable to pay for some form of medical care in the preceding year. That is nearly double the 15% who reported such a problem in 1976.[12]

HEALTH CARE COSTS

By any measure, Americans spend a great deal on health care; in 2002, $1.6 trillion was spent on health care, $5440 for every man, woman, and child. Factors contributing to the increased costs include demographic changes (the population is getting older and requiring more health care); administrative costs (private insurance systems cost money to administrate); malpractice insurance (physicians feel the need to practice defensive medicine, premiums are disproportionately high for certain specialties and geographic areas); labor costs; and technology (the constant need to update equipment as more advanced systems are introduced).

The rapid increases in health care costs have had some disturbing consequences. The rise in premiums for employment-related insurance is driving employers to pass an ever-increasing share of the expense of health insurance on to employees, either by requiring them to bear an increased share of the premium through cost sharing or by cutting back on benefits. Managed care organizations came into existence to offer a more cost-effective way to provide health care.[10] In the continuum of health care delivery, managed care served this goal to some extent (Box 7-1). Whether managed care is still accomplishing that goal and at what cost is a matter of varying opinion (Boxes 7-2, 7-3, and 7-4).

MANAGED CARE

A managed care organization is a reimbursement framework combined with a health care delivery system, an approach to the delivery of health care services that at one time contrasted with fee-for-service medicine. Many physicians and patients have voiced their opposition to managed care over the years. Among employers, opposition lies mostly with concerns over liability for health care decisions made by the plans (Box 7-2).

Physicians' opposition is twofold. The first problem involves the restriction of physicians' practice patterns by requiring preapproval, sometimes denying diagnostic tests, monitoring drugs prescribed, and limiting the circumstances under which patients may be referred to specialists, as well as the specialists to whom patients may be referred. The second problem is the financial relationship of physicians with managed care entities (Box 7-3).

Patients' opposition is generally based on the restrictions imposed on physician and hospital choices. Patients fear that they will become seriously ill and the plan will not come through with the best doctor or hospital (Box 7-4).

Today virtually all private health insurance means managed care. Perhaps the most understandable definition of "managed care" is that it represents a fusion of two functions that once were regarded as largely separate: the financing of medical care and the delivery of medical services. As of 1997, between 80% and 98% of private health insurers appeared to fall into the broad category of managed care.[10]

BOX 7-2	EMPLOYERS' OPINIONS ABOUT HEALTH MAINTENANCE ORGANIZATIONS

Two thirds of Americans receive their health insurance through their employers. However, few employees are offered a choice about their health insurance coverage. In fact, five out of six employers offer only one coverage option. In addition to having fewer choices, employees are being forced to pay at least part of their health care premiums. Only one third of Americans had their health care premiums paid by their employers in 1995, compared with 62% in 1984.

Although employers generally believe that managed care has resulted in better patient care, they voice concerns about proposals that would allow patients to hold health plans liable for patient care decisions. According to a Harris poll in February 2000, 38% of employers would be likely to stop providing coverage for some or all of their employees if they became legally liable for coverage decisions.

Modified from Shalgian C: Perspectives on managed care: a call for change, *Bull Am Coll Surg* 85(4):14, 2000.

| BOX 7-3 | PHYSICIANS' OPPOSITION TO MANAGED CARE |

While a majority of employers believe that managed care has improved the quality of care for patients, many physicians have developed a dislike for managed care. A study conducted by the MEDSTAT Group and J.D. Power and Associates found that nearly seven out of ten physicians consider themselves to be "anti-managed care." The dissatisfaction with managed care is found among physicians both in private practice and in academic medicine. In a *New England Journal of Medicine* study, 80% of medical students, residents, faculty members, and medical school deans believed that patients have better access to service under a fee-for-service plan. The same study pointed out that 70.6% believed that the doctor-patient relationship is better for patients in the fee-for-service plans.

A growing segment of the physician community believes that dramatic changes are needed in the nation's health care system. A survey conducted by Strategic Health Perspectives in January 2000 found that 83% of physicians believe that fundamental changes are needed or that the nation's health care system needs to be completely rebuilt. This figure is up from 67% who expressed the same concerns in 1984.

These opinions are shared by both specialists and primary care physicians. According to a study conducted by Henry J. Kaiser Family Foundation in July 1999, 75% of specialists had a negative overall impression of managed care's impact on the medical service available to patients. Among primary care physicians, 66% agreed. The study went on to ask whether, if a member of their own family were sick, they would worry that the health plan would be more concerned about saving money than about determining the best treatment. Among the physicians, 46% percent would be very worried and 39% would be somewhat worried about the incentive for plans to save money.

Physicians have voiced much opposition to managed care. This opposition is twofold. The first problem involves the restriction of physicians' practice patterns by requiring preapproval and sometimes denial of diagnostic tests, monitoring the drugs prescribed, and limiting the circumstances under which patients may be referred to specialists, as well as the specialists to whom patients may be referred. The second problem is the financial relationship of physicians with the managed care entities.

Modified from Shalgian C: Perspectives on managed care: a call for change, *Bull Am Coll Surg* 85(4):14, 2000.

Managed care has virtually replaced traditional fee-for-service medicine. Some may try to differentiate the two by stating that an HMO is more "managed" than a fee-for-service plan, but the utilization review associated with the latter may have even stricter controls on individual treatment decisions. A more logical way to look at various types of health plans (and the way most courts now look at plans when determining liability of managed care organizations) includes three factors[10]:

1. The degree of risk sharing between the providers and the primary bearer of risk (whether an insurer or self-insured employer)
2. The degree to which administrative oversight constrains clinical decisions
3. The degree to which enrollees in a plan are required to receive their care from a specified roster of providers

| BOX 7-4 | **PATIENTS' OPPOSITION TO MANAGED CARE** |

In a 1998 study conducted by the Kaiser Family Foundation, individuals were asked, if they were sick, how concerned would they be that their health plan may be more worried about saving money than about the patient's best interest. The study showed that 33% would be very worried, while 26% would be somewhat worried. Interestingly, in a similar study conducted the year before only 18% of patients were very worried about this problem. Like physicians, it seems patients are becoming increasingly distrustful about the potential for financial incentives under managed care interfering with treatment and coverage decisions.

The study also showed that Americans would support a law that would allow patients to sue a health plan for malpractice, like they can now sue a doctor. The study revealed that 73% of the respondents would support such a law, up 9% from the year before.

According to a 2000 poll by the Kaiser Family Foundation, 72% of the American public support legislation to require HMOs, other managed care plans, and health insurance companies to provide people with more information about their health plan, make it easier to see medical specialists, allow appeals to independent reviewers when someone is denied coverage for a particular medical treatment and give people the right to sue their health plan.

From Shalgian C: Perspectives on managed care: a call for change, *Bull Am Coll Surg* 85(4):14, 2000.

The following definition of managed care organizations is commonly used in health law, policy literature, and many state regulatory statutes.

- Health maintenance organizations (HMOs) usually limit members to an exclusive network of providers, permitting their members to go to out-of-network providers only in extraordinary circumstances, such as medical emergencies. They have also historically emphasized preventive care and usually use incentives such as capitation payments to direct the behavior of their professionals and providers.
- Point of service plans (POSs) resemble HMOs but allow their members to obtain services outside the network at an additional cost and often subject to gatekeeper controls.
- Preferred provider organizations (PPOs) are organized systems of health care providers who agree to provide services on a discounted (usually fee-for-service) basis to subscribers. PPO subscribers are not limited to plan providers but face financial disincentives, such as larger deductibles or larger copayments, if they elect nonpreferred providers. PPOs usually pay their providers on a fee-for-service basis and often use utilization review controls for certain kinds of services, such as hospital admissions.
- Provider-sponsored organizations (PSOs), also called integrated delivery systems (IDSs), physician-hospital organizations (PHOs), and provider-sponsored networks (PSNs), are networks organized by health care providers themselves. They contract directly with employers or other purchasers of health benefits to provide their own services on a capitated basis.[10]

Hybrids of all these types of managed care organizations exist, including plans that for an additional premium allow individuals to choose a physician or allow the physician to spend more time with the patient. The possibilities are endless when it comes to the creation of managed care plans.

HISTORY OF MANAGED CARE ORGANIZATIONS

Early Prepaid Plans

Many think that prepaid health care is a new concept, but prepaid health care actually began in the early 19th century, when some individual physicians entered into contracts with employers to treat employees for payment of a few cents per employee. These physicians cared for all factory employees, regardless of the amount of care per patient and the cost of that care. Such arrangements represented the first prepaid health care in the United States.[13]

The model was expanded in the 1920s and 1930s to include a few hospitals. In exchange for a prepaid fee from an employer, the hospital would treat all employees at no additional charge, regardless of the level of care or time required. Most providers were uncomfortable with this idea of payment in advance, and mainstream providers focused instead on the development of what is now called traditional indemnity insurance, or fee for service, through the creation of Blue Cross, Blue Shield, and other commercial health insurance companies. Under this type of insurance, the more care the patient received, the more payment to the provider, and the less care, the less payment. Under this system providers had no risk and the roles of provider and insurer were clearly divided.[13]

Indemnity or "Fee-For-Service" Plans

Indemnity plans, or "fee for service," flourished during the first half of the 20th century. By the 1960s and 1970s, however, economists and policymakers pointed to three major problems with this traditional employer-sponsored private insurance system: rising costs, variation in care, and uncoordinated care.[13]

Rising costs were attributed to the fact that everything the provider did meant more payment, which encouraged more testing, hospitalization, and use of other services. A cycle emerged in which providers offered more care, consumers appreciated the additional treatment, insurance paid for it, and employers were charged a higher premium.[13]

Variation of care came to light in the 1970s. In a Dartmouth College study of the specific type of care patients received, people in a small town who went to their local doctors with similar sets of symptoms would be treated in a particular way, while those who traveled to a doctor or hospital in a neighboring town might receive very different treatment. Clearly, when the type of treatment provided depends on the region in which a patient lives or the hospital the patient visits, this is not the most efficient way to practice medicine.[13]

Lack of coordination of care was a problem with the private health insurance, or "fee-for-service" model. Patients could visit any specialist, and the insurance company would pay the bill. Since no single health care provider was coordinating or managing the care, patients were basically navigating the health care system on their own. This sometimes resulted in doctor shopping, and when numerous doctors prescribed various medications without knowing what medications had been prescribed by other doctors, adverse reactions were a consequence.[13]

Later Managed Care

In the 1970s, managed care companies, both those already existing and many more that arose, announced that their model was the solution to the problems associated with fee-for-service plans. Costs would be contained by providing an incentive in the form of a capitated fee to providers who would receive the same amount no matter how much care they provided. Geographic variation would be addressed when physicians were directly employed by the networks, reducing physician autonomy. A managed care company could look at the research on a particular disease and determine the most efficient and effective course of treatment, create practice guidelines or protocols, and instruct its physicians on how to practice. Prepaid plans also said they could coordinate the management of patient care through a gatekeeper system. The primary care physician would not only deliver primary care, but also oversee, coordinate, and manage the care received by the enrollee, the most significant role being the determination of when a patient should be referred to a specialist and to what specialist the patient should be referred.[13]

Although the systems worked, there was much opposition from physicians and patients, some of which continues today. Patients were reluctant to join HMOs and lose their ability to choose their physicians. Physician providers objected to the loss of autonomy and the efforts of managed care to instruct their practices. They sometimes felt that they were providing less care, which meant a lower quality of care for patients.[13]

System in Crisis

Managed care emerged as a national issue during Richard Nixon's presidency in the early 1970s. As a result of Nixon's desire to reform the health care system, Congress passed the HMO Act of 1973, which set aside federal money to help spur the growth of HMOs around the country and required large employers to offer their employees an HMO option. Americans were not ready for HMOs in 1973, and despite the option, few signed up for HMO coverage. While HMO enrollment remained low, health care costs continued to rise, from 6.2% of the U.S. gross national domestic product in 1962, to 7.3% in 1972, to 10% in 1980, and to 12.5% in 1990. In the mid to late 1980s, employers' health care costs rose to such an extent that they expressed concern that they were becoming uncompetitive internationally. Big business started listening to the solutions offered by managed care advocates.[13]

Evolution of Modern Managed Care

In the late 1980s and early 1990s, new forms of HMOs emerged. For-profit and not-for-profit commercial insurers recognized that Americans did not join HMOs because they wanted the freedom to choose health care providers and that physicians wanted autonomy to practice as they saw fit. Therefore the commercial insurers decided to offer consumers some freedom of choice and to provide doctors with some measure of autonomy while still achieving the goals of lower costs, practice guidelines, and coordinated care.[13]

The insurers created a new type of HMO, called an independent-practice association (IPA). Unlike an HMO in which patients had to obtain care from clinics owned by the plan and physicians were directly employed by the plan, enrollees could choose a doctor from a booklet listing hundreds of physicians who had signed contracts with the plan to treat its patients. The next step in the evolution was the point of service plan (POS). In addition to the benefits of the IPA (a large choice of enrolled physicians), POS enrollees could have the option to choose a nonlisted physician if willing to pay a higher percentage of their own health care bill. Insurers claimed these two new plans would provide the freedom of choice employees wanted and autonomy physicians demanded, while still offering cost savings, practice guidelines, and a gatekeeper physician. Employers bought into these newer, looser forms of managed care. However, costs were still rising, consumers were still unhappy with reductions in their freedom of choice, and physicians continued to be displeased about the compromise of their autonomy.[13]

LEGISLATION AND REGULATION OF MANAGED CARE

As managed care became more common, the problems of appeasing consumers and providers and the inability of the managed care organization to control costs accelerated. In an attempt to somehow control how managed care plans treat consumers, almost every state has enacted some form of a patient protection act. Some include a provision that managed care organizations must pay for emergency room visits if a "prudent person" would have viewed the situation as an emergency. Others eliminate the gatekeeper role to allow patients direct access to specialists, establish review boards to examine denial of treatment, and give consumers the right to sue managed care organizations for wrongful denial of care.[13]

ERISA Versus State Law

Since so many states had enacted their own patient protection acts, it may seem surprising that Congress would feel it necessary to consider and debate a national patient bill of rights act in 2001. The reason derives from the Employee Retirement and Security Act (ERISA) enacted in 1974. The purpose of ERISA was to put an end to the pension scandals of the 1950s and 1960s in which employers virtually robbed employees of the pensions they had been promised. The methods included inadequate capitalization of pension plans, tricky vesting rules through which employers were able to lay off employees just before they became vested in the plan (e.g., vesting might take effect at 30 years, and employees were laid off at 29 years and 6 months).[14]

ERISA affects health care because it included a preemption clause stating that individual states are preempted, meaning prohibited, from regulating employee benefit programs including HMOs, unless they are part of the traditional state regulation of insurance. Whether state law or ERISA mandates managed care in a particular circumstance is important for several reasons. The most important is what happens when a patient sues an HMO for wrongfully denying care, which results in harm. If ERISA preempts the state law, ERISA eliminates the powers the state law gives its citizens to sue. The bottom line is that when ERISA rules, any lawsuit must be filed in federal court and the maximum the plaintiff can recover is the actual cost of the treatment that was denied. If ERISA does not preempt the state law, the damages available to plaintiffs generally include actual damages, damages for past and future pain and suffering, and even punitive damages. This can be a huge difference, often several times what would be awarded in federal court. The courts took many years and many interpretations to establish a concrete meaning of the preemption clause.[14]

Although money can be saved by reducing the charges for services and by reducing unnecessarily expensive services or unneeded services, it is often difficult to determine what can be cut without harm and what is a necessary service. Physicians struggled with decisions about what tests and procedures could be eliminated under managed care. As the courts recognized ERISA preemption of state tort lawsuits and of state regulation of medical decision making by managed care organizations, ERISA-qualified managed care organizations became more ruthless in their cost cutting and less concerned about quality of care.[14]

In response to the situation created by ERISA preemption, physicians, patients, their lawyers, and state regulators pushed the courts to rethink this preemption. Physicians had taken the brunt of the fallout from the ERISA preemption. Even into the late 1990s, with the courts holding that ERISA plans could not be sued for interfering with medical decision making, treating physicians enjoyed no preemption and were the sole available targets in lawsuits. So, while physicians were forced to deliver lower quality care or risk losing their jobs or contracts with the insurer, they could not use the insurer's policies as a defense when sued for medical malpractice.[14]

Ultimately, the U.S. Supreme Court responded to concerns about ERISA preemption with three decisions that greatly limit the ability of managed care organizations to control the care delivered to their patients.[14-17] With some exceptions these cases carved out medical decision making from ERISA preemptions. Plans that continue to directly control medical decision making are subject to lawsuits and to state regulation of their decisions.[14]

INSTITUTE OF MEDICINE AND RISK MANAGED CARE

While state regulation of managed care organizations solves some problems, it will probably result in an increase of health care costs, since the mandated review options available in virtually all states generally result in reversal of the denial of care. The reviewer has no incentive to deny the care and every reason to approve it, rather like the traditional fee-for-service models before managed care.[14]

A supportable solution to the problem of state and federal insurance mandates and rising health care costs has come from the Institute of Medicine (IOM) and its reports on medical errors. Although these reports are somewhat controversial, painting a grim picture of needless patient suffering and death, they do identify a key problem—the lack of good information on the best treatment options for common medical conditions. Major research programs have been established to develop standard protocols for treatment of many medical conditions, including such diseases as asthma and diabetes. The rationale is to improve quality of care, but reducing costs is also an objective.[14]

The IOM envisions that the treatment protocols will replace managed care with a system of "risk managed care." The key features of evidence-based risk managed care include use of guideline-driven protocols, monitoring of provider standards, and financial incentives for provider compliance with guidelines. The IOM sees risk managed care as an improvement over managed care because medical decision making will be aboveboard and subject to increased scrutiny and scientific validation.[14]

MEDICARE AND MEDICAID

The discussion has thus far been on managed care. However, many Americans are covered by Medicare and Medicaid.

Medicare, provided by the federal government and administered through the Centers for Medicare & Medicaid Services (CMS), is the nation's largest health insurance program, covering nearly 40 million Americans.[10] Medicare is for people 65 years of age and older, some disabled people under 65 years of age, and people with certain other disease processes. It has two parts, Part A (which has no cost to most patients after age 65 or if they qualify for disability under Medicare) and Part B (which most people pay for monthly). Part A generally pays for care in the hospital, critical access facility, skilled nursing facility, or hospice, as well as some home health care. Part B generally requires payment by the enrollee and partially covers doctors' services, outpatient hospital care, and some other medical services that Part A does not cover, such as the services of physical and occupational therapists and some home health care when these services are medically necessary.

Medicaid is a joint and voluntary program between the federal government and the states. Its mission is to provide health insurance coverage to the nation's poor, the disabled, and the impoverished elderly. The federal government sets minimum eligibility standards and coverage requirements for Medicaid. Because Medicaid is an entitlement program, states choosing to participate must provide specified care to everyone who is eligible under guidelines developed by the federal government. Each state administers its own Medicaid programs.

Both Medicare and Medicaid face major financial issues as costs associated with these programs continue to rise. During more lucrative years, some states expanded eligibility criteria for Medicaid as a way to provide health coverage for the working poor and others without access to health insurance. As a result, more individuals become eligible during economic downturns, increasing demands for funding and services. In addition, as the population ages, the number of people in need of long-term care also increases.

Programs have been put in place to try and deal with some of the costs of care not covered by either program, particularly pharmaceutical coverage. These programs have recently been enacted and will likely take some time to evolve to where they need to be.

Medicare has made attempts to lower costs of services by using the managed care networks. This has met with mixed success and is changing rapidly, so it is not addressed here except to raise awareness of the issues.

PATIENT-FOCUSED CARE

As discussed earlier in this chapter, patient-focused care is a concept being implemented in an attempt to limit costs while providing better quality care. Patient-focused, or patient-centered, care attempts to centralize patient services using the unit-based model seen with nursing care.

In the patient-centered care model, patients have a team of health care workers assigned to them. This can include a specific nurse, radiographer, laboratory technologist, respiratory therapist, social worker, and other allied health professionals. Under this model the specific team assigned to the patient provides all patient care. Legal issues regarding the radiographer may arise with the patient-centered care model. As discussed in Chapter 2, specific standards of care exist for many of the subspecialties of radiography, ultrasound, nuclear medicine, and radiation therapy, and the standard of care for each specialty applies to any imaging professional performing that task, whether specifically trained or not. Standards of care exist for other health care professions as well. For example, imaging professionals performing electrocardiography or phlebotomy would be held to the standards of persons trained in that field. Consideration must be given to risk exposure when imaging professionals attempt this type of care in the radiology setting. There may be alternative ways to use this model, however, such as having one imaging professional coordinate the scheduling and performance of all imaging procedures for a particular group of patients.

IMPACT ON THE IMAGING PROFESSIONAL

Trends toward managed care, risk managed care, and patient-focused care have grave implications for imaging professionals and should be given some thought. Under managed care, costs are reduced through decreased use of testing, preauthorization requirements, and contracting with facilities that have streamlined their delivery systems to offer lower prices. If fewer tests are ordered, fewer imaging professionals are needed to perform those tests. If preauthorization cannot be obtained and the managed care organization will not pay for the procedure, fewer examinations will be performed. Therefore, if health care delivery systems are streamlined, imaging professionals may lose their jobs.

Risk managed care involves ever-increasing requirements for quality and safety. Evidence-based clinical care guidelines associated with risk managed care continue to evolve and must be taken seriously. These guidelines provide a standard of care that, if not followed, can result in legal liability. As discussed in Chapter 2, imaging professionals must be aware of the guidelines in their department, facility, and state. The risk management department is an important source of information, as is keeping current in professional organizations.

In patient-focused care, allied health professionals, including imaging professionals, are part of a team that offers complete care to a particular group of patients. Under this system, imaging professionals may become involved in providing other patient services when their imaging services are not needed. They may also find themselves reporting to nursing personnel in their assigned unit. Standards of care must always be considered with regard to any care an imaging professional is asked to provide. The standard of care for a person trained to perform any task will apply to an imaging professional providing that service, whether the imaging professional is specifically trained to do so or not.

Imaging professionals must cope with the challenges of managed care, risk managed care, and patient-focused care. To survive professionally and protect themselves legally, they must strive to be proactive. Cross-training and certification in other areas is one way to be proactive, as are voluntary self-examination, improvement of efficiency, and continuing education in appropriate areas.

Cross-training may have legal implications for imaging professionals. Cross-training in another area and achieving certification are proactive ways in which imaging professionals may deal with the changes caused by managed care and protect themselves legally. If imaging professionals do not cross-train, they may find themselves in an ethical and legal dilemma if they are required or expected to perform procedures for which they are not trained and with which they do not feel comfortable. Imaging professionals in private practice may want to train as medical assistants or nurse assistants before they are forced to do so by the downsizing that comes with managed care, the use of stricter guideline-driven protocols that comes with risk managed care, and the other tasks they may be asked to do under the patient-centered care model.

Imaging professionals have the obligation and opportunity to scrutinize their own cost efficiency. If they can identify wasteful practices or wasted time, they can streamline

IMAGING SCENARIO

You are a staff radiologic technologist in a small rural hospital. The department performs diagnostic radiology, computed tomography (CT), ultrasonography, and nuclear medicine. When the CT area is busy, your supervisor often asks you to go and help. You do not mind this and have actually learned a great deal about CT from observing. Thus far your assistance has been limited to transporting patients, developing films, and generally assisting the technologist. The CT technologist has never asked you to perform any patient studies.

One day the CT technologist calls in sick with the flu, and the part-time technologist who generally fills in is also ill. Your supervisor approaches you and insists that you "fill in" in CT. The emergency room has a patient from a motor vehicle accident for whom they have just ordered an abdominal CT to rule out a fractured spleen. Your supervisor explains that the hospital administration will be very upset if this patient has to be transported to another facility because the radiology department could not provide services.

You do your best to follow the protocols and perform the CT, and the images look satisfactory to you. The radiologist interprets the study as normal, and the patient is sent back to the emergency room and eventually admitted for observation. During the night, the patient bleeds internally and is rushed to surgery, where a fractured spleen is discovered. Later, the hospital receives a request for the medical records from the patient's uncle, an attorney.

Discussion questions
- To what standard of care would your performance in obtaining the abdominal CT scan be held?
- Even if the CT was performed perfectly, would the fact that you are not certified in computerized tomography have an impact on the legal outcome?
- Are state and national licensure issues evident here?
- Would this mishap affect facility accreditation?

their own practices before it is done by administrators who do not understand the imaging department. This allows control of the cuts to stay in the hands of knowledgeable imaging professionals who can make these reductions where they will have the smallest impact on patient care. Voluntary self-assessment and improvement of cost efficiency allow imaging professionals to maintain more control over their own risk management.

Managed care may pose other risks for imaging professionals. For example, denial of recommended treatment by the HMO or PPO may have legal consequences. Under managed care, more testing is performed on an outpatient basis. The interpreting physician reviews all ordered studies and recommends any additional procedures to be performed. Often, however, the physician must first obtain authorization from the managed care organization or the facility will not be paid. Although liability for imaging professionals is unlikely, they may be drawn into litigation as witnesses if indicated treatment is denied.

What obligations do imaging professionals have if an interpreting physician recommends another study but the authorization for that study is denied? Must they

IMAGING SCENARIO

A 28-year-old female outpatient with abdominal pain is examined in the radiology department. The treating physician's office has not seen the patient but has phoned in orders for an abdominal ultrasonographic examination. The examination is performed and is unremarkable. The ultrasound technologist, however, through communication with and observation of the patient, realizes that her pain is actually in the pelvis on the left side. The technologist also notes that the pain has increased in severity since the patient's arrival. These observations are passed on to the interpreting physician, who then recommends a pelvic ultrasonographic examination. The treating physician's office calls back to inform the technologist that authorization for the examination is denied, and the patient is to come into the office the next day.

Discussion questions
- Does this imaging professional have an obligation to act as an advocate for that patient?
- Could this imaging professional be subject to liability if the patient goes home and has an ectopic pregnancy that ruptures during the night?

communicate the seriousness of the recommendation to the ordering physician so that he or she can decide whether to fight the denial? Although unlikely, the potential exists for patients to leave the imaging department with an undiagnosed fracture, ruptured appendix, fractured spleen, or other life-threatening condition when authorization for recommended additional diagnostic testing is denied. Because of their unique relationship with patients, particularly outpatients, imaging professionals may be the only health care professionals who communicate with and observe patients sufficiently to recognize and inform the interpreting physician of the severity of the patient's symptoms.

Does the imaging professional then have an obligation to become a patient advocate? Is liability possible if an imaging professional sends a patient with serious symptoms home because a managed care organization has not authorized further testing? Although no case law exists on the subject, the standard of care of the imaging professional would most likely create some kind of obligation to at least communicate concern to the interpreting or ordering physician.

SUMMARY

- Many people in modern society assume that they have the right to health care. This right has evolved from an obligation to provide medical care by health care institutions and professionals to a rationed system of distribution. However, most also agree that with this right comes the responsibility for ensuring individual health care by taking part in wellness programs.
- Distribution of health care and imaging services is affected by distribution allocation groups. Ethical decision making at national, state, community,

institutional, and department levels is served by a determination of the group in which the distribution dilemma might be categorized:
  - Macro-allocation (how big the health care budget is)
  - Meso-allocation (how the budget is divided)
  - Micro-allocation (who gets what portion of the budget)
- A sound theory of distribution must be developed, accepted, and employed to facilitate patients' and society's growing awareness of health care issues. The theories of health care distribution include triage, the egalitarian theory, the entitlement theory, the fairness theory, the utilitarian theory, and the rights theory of justice.
- Six criteria aid the imaging professional in decisions regarding distribution of scarce resources: need, equity, contribution, ability to pay, patient effort, and merit. Merit may be the best criterion, from an ethical standpoint, on which allocation decisions should be made.
- Justice in health care distribution should involve "practical wisdom." Imaging professionals must keep in mind individual needs, scarce resources, and resource distribution when making health care distribution decisions.
- Traditional care provides consumers with freedom of choice for health care services as long as they have the ability to pay for these services, either with health insurance or on their own.
- *Managed care* refers to any type of delivery and reimbursement system that monitors or controls the type, quality, use, and costs of health care. Its aim is to reduce costs, increase access to health care services, and improve patient care. Whether these aims and objectives have been accomplished remains to be seen. Ethical problem solving for imaging professionals has been further complicated by managed care.
- Quality and cost effectiveness entail the provision of better quality health care with fewer resources. Ways to facilitate this objective include empowering employees, delegating tasks, cross-training employees, and applying automation wisely. Institutions and individuals must provide high-quality customer service to ensure that patients receive cost-effective and high-quality imaging services.
- Imaging professionals make daily decisions about the distribution of health care services. To survive in this changing environment, imaging professionals must develop a heightened awareness of ethical decision-making procedures in health care distribution dilemmas.
- Virtually all care today is managed care, a fusion of two formerly separate functions, the financing of medical care and the delivery of medical services. "Managed care" encompasses many organized forms of care, including the following:
  - Health maintenance organizations (HMOs)—a network of providers
  - Point of service plans (POSs)—availability of care outside the network at an additional cost to the patient
  - Provider-sponsored organizations (PSOs), integrated delivery systems (IDAs), physician hospital organizations (PHOs), and provider-sponsored networks (PSNs)—all these are networks of providers that contract directly with employers for service on a capitated basis
- Prepaid health care is not a new concept. It has been around since the early 1800s but has undergone many changes since its inception.

- The Employee Retirement and Security Act (ERISA), enacted in 1974 for the purpose of dealing with pension scams, also covered health plans and preempted or prevented state tort lawsuits and state regulation of managed care organizations until the early 2000s, when three U.S. Supreme Court cases allowed consumers to sue managed care organizations for making erroneous medical decisions and imposed state regulation on managed care organizations.
- Before the Supreme Court cases, a managed care organization governed by ERISA could be sued only in federal, not state, court. This meant that a plaintiff's recovery for the erroneous denial of medical care causing harm to the plaintiff was limited to only the actual cost of the denied care. A state court could also award such damages as economic loss (such as loss of wages, actual and future), pain and suffering (past and future), and infliction of emotional distress. The amount recovered in state court could easily be several times more than in federal court.
- As a result of the liability to which managed care organizations now became exposed, a system of risk managed care emerged, based in large part on medical error reports by the Institute of Medicine, which identified the lack of good information on the treatment of many common medical conditions.
- The risk managed care concept is evidence based and involves the use of guideline-driven protocols, the monitoring of provider standards, and a financial incentive for provider compliance. Issues of quality and patient safety are connected with this concept.
- Patient-focused or patient-centered care is a concept that involves a team approach to patient care. This team might include a specific nurse, radiographer, laboratory technologist, respiratory therapist, social worker, and other allied health professionals who are responsible for care of a patient or group of patients.
- Managed care, risk managed care, and patient-focused care can have grave legal consequences for imaging professionals, who should view them with an eye toward risk management.
- To survive professionally and protect themselves legally, imaging professionals should strive to be proactive. Proactive approaches include cross-training and certification in other areas, voluntary self-examination, improvement of efficiency, and education and continuing education in appropriate areas.

REFERENCES

1. Clinton WJ: The health care platform, *Adv Admin Radiol* 3:28, 1993.
2. Garrett TM, Baillie HW, Garrett RM: *Healthcare ethics, principles and problems*, ed 2, Englewood Cliffs, NJ, 1993, Prentice Hall.
3. Fisher A: *The effects of health care allocation*, electronic document, Catholic Resource Network, Trinity Communications, Manassas, Va.
4. Armstrong CR, Whitlock R: The cost of care: two troublesome cases in health care ethics, *Physician Executive* 24(6):32, 1998.
5. Barnes JE: Batten down the hatches, *Adv Admin Radiol* 3:38, 1993.
6. Congressional Budget Office: *Effects of managed care: an update*, Washington, DC, March 1994, US Government Printing Office.
7. Folland S, Goodman AC, Stano M: *The economics of health and health care*, New York, 1993, Macmillan.
8. Strasen L: Redesigning hospitals around patients and technology, *Nurs Econ* 9(4):233, 1991.

9. Pack DA: Patient-focused care and the future of radiography, *Radiol Technol* 65(6):375, 1994.
10. Furrow B, Creasey TL, Johnson SH, et al: *Health law: cases, materials and problems*, ed 5, St Paul, Minn, 2004, West.
11. U.S. Census Bureau: *Numbers of Americans with and without health insurance rise*, Census Bureau Reports, Washington, DC, 2003, Author.
12. Appleby J: Even the insured can buckle under health care costs, *USA Today*, Aug 31, 2005.
13. Spearer M: *A system on the fringe: roots of the prepay system*, Columbia University Interactive, 2006, http://cero.columbia.edu/1134/web/main/1134_m_s_top.html.
14. Mclean TR, Richards EP: Health care's "thirty year war": the origins and dissolution of managed care, *NUU Annual Survey of American Law* 60:283, 2004.
15. *Pegram v Herdrich*, 530 U.S. 211 (2000).
16. *Rush Prudential HMO, Inc. v Moran*, 536 U.S. 355 (2002).
17. *Kentucky Ass'n of Health Plans, Inc. v Miller*, 123 S. Ct. 1471 (2003).

REVIEW QUESTIONS

1 Describe four ways in which health care may be defined:
 a. _____
 b. _____
 c. _____
 d. _____

2 List two ways present-day health care differs from health care in the 1940s:
 a. _____
 b. _____

3 Resources in health care are increasingly _____ and _____.

4 List three allocation groups:
 a. _____
 b. _____
 c. _____

5 List and describe the four distribution theories:
 a. _____
 b. _____
 c. _____
 d. _____

6 The six criteria helpful in ethical decision making regarding distribution are:
 a. _____
 b. _____
 c. _____
 d. _____
 e. _____
 f. _____

7 Critics of patient-focused care believe that cross-training and decentralization may lead to the loss of _____ _____.

8 List four ways in which cost effectiveness can be improved:
 a. _____
 b. _____
 c. _____
 d. _____

9 True or False   An entitlement may be the same thing as a right.

10 True or False   The egalitarian theory uses a system of contracts.

11 True or False   Macro-allocation is how the health care budget is divided.

12 True or False   Meso-allocation is the entire health care budget.

13 True or False   The criterion of distribution of contribution is the most ethical criterion.

14 True or False   Ability to pay should be the most important criterion in health care.

15 True or False   Merit, from an ethical standpoint, is the best criterion for distribution.

16 True or False   Managed care controls the type, quality, and costs of health care.

17 True or False   Cross-training does not require the imaging professional to function in areas other than imaging.

18 True or False   Cost effectiveness and the maintenance of high-quality imaging services are the essence of customer service.

19 True or False   Imaging professionals need not worry about liability when they are told to perform procedures for which they are not properly trained.

20 True or False   The standard of care for an imaging professional in a particular area of imaging is that of a professional trained and certified in that particular area of expertise.

21 True or False   Under managed care, the imaging professional can do nothing to control risk.

22 True or False   The managed care organization may be responsible for outcomes if it denies authorization for treatment or testing.

23 True or False   Managed care has fused together two functions that were once separate: the financing of health care and the delivery of medical services.

24 The term "managed care" encompasses:
a. Fee-for-service indemnity insurance
b. Blue Cross and Blue Shield
c. Managers of nursing homes
d. HMOs, POSs, PSOs, IDAs, PHOs, and PSNs

25 True or False   ERISA was formulated to regulate managed care.

26 True or False   Before the early 2000s, ERISA prohibited lawsuits filed in state court against managed care organizations with regard to medical decisions that denied care, causing harm to patients.

27 True or False   It made no difference in outcome whether lawsuits regarding denial of care were filed in state or federal court.

28 True or False   Treating physicians may be found liable if they do not appeal the denial of treatment or testing they believe is essential.

29 True or False   Imaging professionals may be involved in litigation as witnesses when additional testing in the radiology services is recommended and authorization is denied.

30 True or False   Imaging professionals may have a responsibility to become patient advocates if they become aware of the severity of an outpatient's illness and testing is denied.

CRITICAL THINKING *Questions & Activities*

1 Discuss an individual's right to health care and compare it with the person's responsibility for personal health.

2 Compare and contrast the theories of distribution and select the one you feel is most appropriate.

3 Develop a plan for providing more care with fewer resources in radiology services.

4 Explain the imaging professional's role in health care distribution.

5 Explain how justice involves respecting human dignity and satisfying human needs.

6 Identify your present state of wellness and initiate a plan to improve it.

7 Interview a health care provider who has come from another country, such as Canada, that has a different type of health care system.

8 Evaluate the cost effectiveness of your imaging area, and develop an improvement plan.

9 Discuss any personal experiences with the health care or managed care system that indicate a need for improvement.

10 Select two teams to debate the managed care issue. Each team should create fact sheets to include areas of cost effectiveness, needs, distribution, and quality. Providing more care with fewer resources and maintaining quality should be the key factors of concern. Videotape or audiotape the presentation.

11 Discuss subspecialty areas available in your state for cross-training and certification.

12 Review the imaging scenarios presented in this chapter. Discuss options available to imaging professionals for dealing with such dilemmas.

8 STUDENT AND EMPLOYEE RIGHTS AND RESPONSIBILITIES

Respect for the fragility and importance of an individual life is still the first mark of the educated man.

NORMAN COUSINS

Chapter Outline

Ethical Issues
Ethical Theories
Models
Autonomy and Informed Decisions
Truthfulness and Confidentiality
Justice
Values
Legal Issues
Contract Law
Due Process

Substantive Due Process
Procedural Due Process
JRCERT Due Process Requirements
Whistleblowing
Malpractice Liability Insurance
Employee Rights
Exceptions

Learning Objectives

After completing this chapter, the reader will be able to perform the following:

- Compare and contrast the relationship between the imaging student's and the imaging profession-al's rights, responsibilities, and ethics, including the following considerations:
  - Ethical theories, and models
  - Autonomy
  - Informed consent
  - Truthfulness and confidentiality
  - Justice
  - Values
- Identify the legal doctrines affecting the relationship between the student and the education program and the imaging employee and employer.
- State the origin of due process.
- Define substantive and procedural due process.

- Explain why accrediting organizations may also impose due process requirements on educational programs.
- List the obligations of educational programs regarding restriction of student rights.
- Identify the procedural due process protections available when substantive rights are restricted.
- Define whistleblowing.
- State the serious nature of whistleblowing and what to consider before doing so.
- Explain the option of carrying personal malpractice insurance.
- Identify and discuss the doctrine of employment at will.

Key Terms

due process
employment at will
procedural due process
substantive due process
whistleblowing

Professional Profile

At the height of my career as program director for nearly 15 years, I was faced with an ethical dilemma that challenged me on all levels—as an administrator, educator, technologist, and individual.

It began when I was forced to make the unfortunate determination to fail a group of three students. The decision stemmed from a relatively common incident that eventually snowballed into the ultimate test of my fortitude. I caught a group of three students cheating on a class project. The plagiarism was so glaring that after consulting with two colleagues I decided to fail the students on this project on the grounds of cheating. Unfortunately the students' grades going into the project could not withstand a zero on the project and would ultimately cause them to earn an F for the course. Without a passing grade earned for the course, the students would be unable to progress the following semester to their internship. Although it was not an easy decision, the situation escalated until the dean, who did not have an educational background but rather a management background, and the director of the school stepped in and overturned my decision.

I was appalled and found myself face to face with a textbook example of a moral dilemma. One of the goals I emphasized to the students, advisory board, and staff in my program was that nuclear medicine and the imaging and radiological sciences were trying to reach professional status and move out of being labeled as vocational or technical job skills. We strived to provide our students with a well-rounded education to sharpen and hone students' oral and written skills, ethical and legal knowledge, and patient care skills, as well as technical abilities. How can you do that if you are allowing students who cheat to enter your profession and dilute the integrity of your field? When a colleague commented on the glaring contradiction the school displayed between teaching medical ethics and actually practicing it, I could not resign myself to teaching nuclear medicine technology including medical ethics when it seemed the school did not uphold the very basics of ethics in the classroom.

In the end, I made the decision to leave the program I built and the career I loved so much. Above all, other faculty and I felt that we were nuclear medicine technologists and we were responsible for training people to become our peers. Prior to being an educator, I stood for my profession and was very proud of what I felt were very high ethics in nuclear medicine. In regard to cheating on something as simple as a project or an exam, I worried about the trust factor that is involved with dosages or patient care ethics.

Ethics are important in any profession, but I think more important in the health field and even more important in a field striving to reach professional status. When you start lowering the bar and letting things slide, you dilute the integrity of your field. Sometimes you just have to stand up for what you believe in.

Carole South-Winter, MEd, CNMT, RT
Executive Director
Reclaiming Youth International
Chair of the Board
Association of Educators in Radiologic and Imaging Sciences
Lennox, South Dakota

ETHICAL ISSUES

Ethical issues often come into play in discussions of the rights of imaging students and imaging professionals. As prospective imaging students select and apply to the educational programs of their choice, and then progress through their professional careers, a variety of ethical dilemmas may present themselves.

Programs that teach imaging skills provide a variety of educational experiences. Each of the various modality programs offers unique opportunities for developing skills in

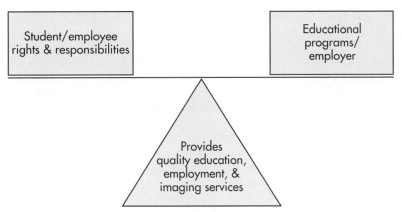

FIGURE 8-1 Balance of rights and obligations.

technology, socialization, and human relations. As students develop each new skill, complete their educational program, and become employees, the opportunities for interaction and dilemmas regarding student and employee rights and responsibilities grow.

Both imaging programs and students have concerns about student rights. Imaging employers and professionals have continuing concerns about the issue of rights. In each imaging setting both parties involved have ethical obligations to each other; these obligations may extend to the relationships among students, imaging professionals, and others in the medical imaging environment. The correct balance of the rights, responsibilities, and obligations between students and educational programs, as well as the rights, responsibilities, and obligations between imaging professionals and their employers, provides high-quality educational programs, high-quality employment opportunities, and high-quality imaging services (Figure 8-1). This chapter discusses these issues and provides examples of ethical dilemmas concerning rights and responsibilities that students and imaging professionals may encounter during education and employment.

ETHICAL THEORIES

The three ethical theories discussed in Chapter 1—consequentialism, deontology, and virtue ethics—serve as guidelines for ethical problem solving both for educational programs and imaging students and for imaging employers and imaging professionals. The choice of theory determines the basis on which each participant interacts within the educational and imaging environment (Table 8-1).

Consequentialism

Consequentialism evaluates an activity according to whether it can provide the greatest good for the greatest number. An application review committee at an imaging program may use this theory by selecting a large number of students with high grade point averages and significant clinical experience because this facilitates rapid comprehension of educational materials, which allows the students selected to include a greater variety of modality experiences in their education. Student applicants with great desire to learn but lower grade point averages might consider this theory a roadblock to their goals of

TABLE 8-1 **ETHICAL THEORIES IN RELATIONSHIP TO STUDENT RIGHTS**

Theory	Example
Consequentialism: the greatest good for the greatest number	Imaging students with the highest grade point averages may be selected to facilitate more educational opportunities for the group as compared to selection of students with lower grades who might require more teacher attention and progress more slowly through modalities, or imaging professionals who learn more quickly may be selected for advancement situations before an equally proficient professional who learns at a slower rate
Deontology: formal rules of right and wrong	Formal rules may serve as a foundation of educational programs and policies or imaging department policies and procedures regarding disciplinary processes and opportunities for students and employees
Virtue ethics: holistic approach to problem solving using practical wisdom	Students and employees may use intellect and practical reasoning when asserting their rights as students or employees in a method useful to themselves and in the educational or employment environment

becoming imaging professionals. The same concept is relevant in the imaging professional's development as he or she strives to learn new modalities. The professional with the ability to learn at a faster rate may be selected to move up the career ladder before the slower learner. Thus the greatest good of a busy department may be served before the needs and desires of an individual employee. Each imaging student or employee has the right to question these choices and has the responsibility of displaying his or her desire to learn and facilitate the needs of the imaging program and department.

Deontology

Deontology uses formal rules of right and wrong for reasoning and problem solving and judges an action on its merits alone, not on any possible consequences it may have. These formal rules may serve as the foundation of educational programs and student guidelines outlining student rights. A formal structure may be used to guarantee equal disciplinary processes and opportunities for students. A similar structure may be used to establish the employee handbook. Each imaging student and employee has the responsibility to recognize the need for formal rules and structure within the imaging department and educational program. Students and employees need to read the handbooks and signify that they understand and will abide by the rules and regulations.

Virtue Ethics

Virtue ethics, a holistic approach to problem solving using practical wisdom, may play a significant role in the educational and professional experience. Imaging students may determine that by integrating intellect and practical reasoning, they may assert their rights and demonstrate their responsibilities as students in a method useful to themselves and the educational program. When they become imaging employees, they may use this as a foundation for problem solving in their professional practice.

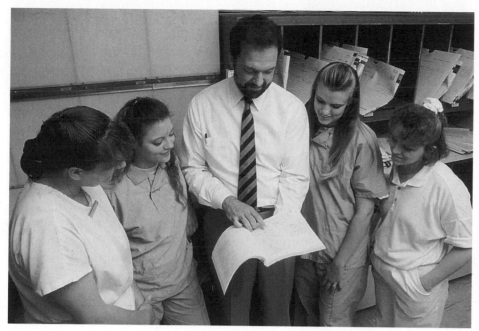

FIGURE 8-2 Students' rights involve problem solving.

MODELS

Although ethical theories provide a foundation for solving problems concerning students' and employees' rights and responsibilities, the model of care employed also helps define the ethical structure within which decisions are made (Figure 8-2). The model chosen—engineering, priestly, collegial, contractual, or covenantal—determines the ways in which interactions take place between students and educational programs or employers and employees. (See Chapter 1 for a more thorough discussion of these models.)

Students and imaging professionals who feel as though they have lost their identity within the educational and imaging process may be working within the engineering model. An instructor or physician who displays a godlike or fatherly attitude toward students or employees may be employing the priestly, or paternal, model. A cooperative effort between students and teaching programs or imaging professionals and patients is evidence of the collegial model. When students enter an educational program, they enter into a businesslike arrangement that defines the relationship between the student and the program. Rights and responsibilities may be defined within this arrangement. Imaging professionals enter into an employment agreement with an institution or organization in a similar fashion. These are examples of the contractual model. After the contract, including aspects affecting student or employee rights, has been agreed to by both parties, an understanding based on traditional values and goals develops between the student and the program or the employer and employee (see also contract law later in the chapter). This understanding is a crucial element of the covenantal model, which is based on trust and shared experiences within the educational program or the imaging environment. The model most often employed in imaging education and the imaging department is a combination of the contractual and covenantal models. A good example of this combined approach within the radiologic sciences is the learning contract in clinical education.[1] An example of this in the imaging employment area is a contract signed by an imaging professional for tuition reimbursement.

As a result of the explosion in technology and the ever-increasing knowledge base required for clinical practice, programs are having difficulty providing students with all they need to know to function competently in a continually changing work environment. To facilitate the adequate education of students and prepare them for employment in the evolving health care system, educational programs have developed learning contracts, which are formalized and mutual agreements between instructors and students that guide learning experiences.[2] Because they are contracts between programs and students, they require trust. Students enter the program trusting that they will be appropriately prepared to provide high-quality imaging services, and instructors trust that students are adequately motivated to uphold their responsibilities to study and perform their duties. When used properly, learning contracts may be valuable methods to provide needed experiences for students.[3]

Needed Imaging Experience = Students + Programs + Learning Contracts

The rapid evolution of technology not only affects educational programs but may also affect the imaging department and the imaging professional. New equipment and new technology often require continued education for the imaging professional. When professionals are asked to increase their knowledge base and responsibility level within the imaging area, they are often reimbursed in some method. This requires trust by both parties. Each has an obligation and responsibility to uphold the agreement and to maintain high-quality imaging services.

Needed New Technology = Imaging Professional + Employer + Reimbursement Method

AUTONOMY AND INFORMED DECISIONS

The exercise and protection of student and employee rights involve autonomy and informed decisions. The individuality of each student and imaging professional is an integral aspect of the educational and employment experience. Each student and employee has the right to be respected and treated with dignity and consideration. Students have the right to expect high-quality education by high-quality instructors. Because student abilities and experiences differ, educational programs must be creative in classroom and clinical methodology. Imaging employees have the right to expect fair and equitable treatment from their employers, but they may also have differing abilities and experiences. Employers must fairly evaluate their imaging employees and provide growth opportunities for them.

Programs that respect student autonomy provide realistic and current employment opportunities for graduates. However, some programs that have noted poor results in their cost-benefit analyses face an ethical dilemma regarding employment. To maintain current faculty numbers, such programs may have to keep enrollment numbers at a maximum even if job opportunities are limited and graduates may face a very difficult job search.

IMAGING SCENARIO

In a hospital that has just experienced staff radiographer layoffs, a senior radiography student is assigned to the surgical rotation with a staff technologist. The staff technologist is sent home early because of a low procedure count, and shortly thereafter a disaster code is called. Several accident patients are arriving, and some of them are going to surgery. The student is sent to surgery while the staff radiographers are busy with trauma patients in the department.

During the surgical procedure the C-arm fluoroscopy equipment malfunctions and the student cannot correct the problem. By the time the staff radiographer arrives to fix the C-arm equipment, the patient has died.

The surgeon is furious with the student and shares his anger with the other surgeons. The student is embarrassed and devastated.

Discussion questions
- What is the ethical dilemma?
- Whose problem is this?
- Are there remedies to this situation?
- How could the student have better dealt with this situation?

BOX 8-1	**QUESTIONS RAISED DURING COST-BENEFIT ANALYSIS IN THE IMAGING DEPARTMENT**

Is student labor being exploited?
Is the widespread use of student imaging professionals ethical?
Are clinical assignments to include students and imaging employees being made fairly, ethically, and with an eye to keeping costs down?
Are education expenses for the program justified by the labor potential of the students?

The cost effectiveness of clinical education is often a concern for administrators.[4] One of the primary concerns of administrators is whether the value of labor contributed by students offsets the cost of educating them. Indeed, the use of student labor in clinical settings is an ethical concern for educational programs and imaging students contemplating their rights in the educational environment. If students believe they are being used in place of staff radiographers for cost savings to a department, they may question their clinical assignments. Moreover, educators may have difficult ethical decisions to make concerning student rotations if they feel pressured by administrators to provide more student contact hours in the clinical setting. The rights of the students may be endangered if issues of cost savings by staff reduction are contemplated (Box 8-1). Imaging students are responsible for maintaining the safety of their patients and recognizing imaging procedures in which they are competent.

When issues of staffing and cost savings clash with student competency and clinical assignments, the student and the educator should be mindful of the accreditation requirements for student supervision set forth by the Joint Review Committee on Education in Radiologic Technology (JRCERT). JRCERT defines direct supervision as student

BOX 8-2	**REQUIREMENTS FOR INFORMED DECISIONS**

Information
Attention
Review

supervision by a qualified practitioner who reviews the procedure in relation to the student's achievement, evaluates the condition of the patient in relation to the student's knowledge, is present during the conduct of the procedure, and reviews and approves the procedure or image. Students must be directly supervised until competency is achieved. This supervision ensures patient safety and proper educational practices. JRCERT also states that all repeat radiographs by students will be supervised by a qualified practitioner.[5]

The cost effectiveness of maintaining an imaging department is an ongoing battle for both administrators and educators. Imaging professionals may feel as if they are not regarded as individuals when they are not involved in decision making and planning. Often departments can become so hectic that imaging professionals are shifted about and schedules changed with little notice. They may regard this as less than professional treatment by their employers. It is most important to remember that the driving force and responsibility for both the employer and the employee should be the needs of the imaging patients.

An emphasis on informed decisions encourages student autonomy by providing the prospective student with important information about the educational program and its policies and procedures. This exchange of information enables the student applicant to make informed decisions concerning participation in the program. After students have chosen and entered their programs, they are typically given a vast amount of information about their future didactic and clinical educational experiences. It is their responsibility to read, digest, and question this information until they have an operative knowledge that will facilitate their educational process. Educators should review this information periodically to ensure that students are provided with current and updated information that will help them obtain the skills and knowledge necessary to become qualified imaging professionals (Box 8-2).

The exchange of information is one of the most important communication tools in the imaging department. When the administrator keeps the employees informed, they recognize their importance in departmental decision making. Imaging professionals should be aware of the location of all informational materials pertinent to their activities in the department. Staying informed is also an important responsibility of the imaging professional. The process is a two-way street. Professional literature and organizations are excellent tools in making informed decisions.

TRUTHFULNESS AND CONFIDENTIALITY

Students and imaging professionals have a right to the truth during the informed decision process when they have a contractual agreement with the educational program or their employer. They also have a right to expect confidentiality during their education or employment. Truthfulness and maintenance of student and employee confidentiality are crucial elements in the relationships among students, instructors, imaging employers, and employees. Students put their trust in their instructors, who have the power to affect their future. They must be able to believe that when they ask even ethically difficult questions, they can expect the truth. A student who shares a personal confidence with an instructor should have the reasonable expectation that this confidence will be kept. However, this expectation of truthfulness and confidentiality may give rise to ethical dilemmas if the student expects to obtain truthful information that involves the confidentiality of another, or if the student makes a statement in confidence that may cause harm to another if it is kept secret. For example, a student may reveal a drug problem to an instructor with the intention of finding assistance and treatment. After a short period the instructor becomes aware that the student often works under the influence of drugs in the clinical area. The instructor faces a dilemma regarding conflicting ethical obligations. If the instructor explains the problem to the program director, the confidence of the student will be betrayed. However, if the greater good is served, the violation of student confidentiality may be acceptable. In this case, from a legal perspective, quality of care and patient safety dictate a breach of the confidentiality between student and instructor. This situation should be covered in the policies and procedures of the educational program and the student handbook, and therefore the student should be aware of the consequences of such actions. Such questions involve a balancing of student rights and responsibilities with the rights and responsibilities of the educational program to maintain an appropriate environment for imaging education and services.

A similar situation may occur when an imaging professional shares a drug dependency problem with an administrative imaging professional. The drug-dependent professional has placed trust and confidence in someone who is being asked for assistance. As in the educational situation, the balance of the employee's rights and responsibilities and the rights and responsibilities of the imaging organization to maintain high-quality imaging services and patient care has ethical and legal implications.

JUSTICE

A positive environment for imaging education and employment must also encourage justice and fairness (Box 8-3). Justice in imaging educational programs and imaging employment is enhanced through appropriate application of ethical theories and models and the creation of an educational and imaging environment in which student and employee autonomy, informed decisions, truthfulness, and confidentiality are valued.

Students and imaging professionals expect to be treated fairly. Fairness, however, is difficult to define. One student's or employee's perception of fairness may not be the same as that of another. The following examples illustrate the dilemmas resulting from differing conceptions of fairness.

A class of vascular imaging students is preparing for clinical evaluation. Each student has done a 2-month rotation in the vascular laboratory and has had differing clinical experiences according to the procedures available. One of the students asks for

---

BOX 8-3	**COMPONENTS OF A POSITIVE LEARNING ENVIRONMENT**

Truthfulness
Maintenance of student and employee confidentiality
Justice
Fairness

an extension because the laboratory was slow during the student's 2-month rotation. The instructor denies the extension by explaining that the students were instructed to simulate procedures to practice when no actual clinical procedures were available in the laboratory. The student believes the situation is unfair because simulations are not the same as clinical experience. Is the student being treated fairly? Is the student being responsible for his or her own competency? What if all students demanded the same type and number of experiences before being considered competent? Such questions raise the issue of whether justice has the same meaning for all persons and whether a formula for fairness can be defined.

A formula for fairness may also be important in the imaging employment situation. When new modalities are implemented in a large and busy imaging department, several imaging professionals may view the arrival of the new technologies as an opportunity for advancement. They may all feel entitled to career ladder advancement. The administrative professional may have difficulty in making this decision without alienating certain employees. Justice for one may not seem justice to all. Personal and professional responsibility may not always share the same pathway.

VALUES

A value is a worthwhile or desirable standard or quality.[5] Students, educational programs, employers, and employees have particular values and standards that must become aligned for students to have a valuable educational experience and imaging professionals to have a valuable professional experience. Student values motivate action and guide educational choices. Employee values motivate action and guide professional choices. Educational program values and standards are determined by organizational goals and mission. These organizational goals and mission are also the foundation of the imaging department's goals and mission. The values and standards of imaging programs are further determined by the JRCERT Standards for an Accredited Educational Program in the Radiologic Sciences. The importance of these values and standards is applicable to the interactions between the imaging and radiation sciences professional and the employer. These standards address a variety of issues important to students and employees as listed and modified here:

- Program mission and goals/institutional mission and goals
- Program integrity/institutional integrity
- Organization and administration
- Curriculum and academic practices/standard operating procedures and practices
- Learning resources/mentoring and resource availability
- Student services/employee services
- Human resources
- Student rights/employee rights
- Educational opportunities/continued education opportunities
- Students' physical safety/employee safety
- Program fiscal responsibility/institutional responsibility
- Physical resources
- Program effectiveness and outcomes/institutional ranking and credentials

All these issues are important aspects of the interactions between students and educational programs. The employee-employer relationship is affected by these issues. They are discussed further in the legal portion of this chapter.

Another set of standards important to imaging students and the imaging professional is the American Registry of Radiologic Technologists (ARRT) Standards of Ethics (see Appendix A). These standards are divided into two parts. The first part, the Standards of Ethics, serves as a guide by which registered technologists and applicants for the registry may evaluate their professional conduct as it relates to patients, health care consumers, employers, colleagues, and other members of the health care team. The second part, the Rules of Ethics, defines specific standards of minimally acceptable professional conduct for all currently registered technologists and applicants. They are enforceable rules intended to promote the protection, safety, and comfort of patients. Registered technologists engaging in any misconduct or the inappropriate activities listed in the Rules of Ethics are subject to sanction (Box 8-4).[6]

BOX 8-4   **SOURCES OF ORGANIZATIONAL STANDARDS FOR IMAGING PROFESSIONALS AND DEPARTMENTS**

Personal and institutional values
Standards of the Joint Review Committee on Education in Radiologic Technology
Ethical standards of the American Registry of Radiologic Technologists and
   American Society of Radiologic Technologists

IMAGING SCENARIO

An imaging student is assigned to a rotation with an imaging professional who seems to be having some emotional problems. The imaging professional has recently been divorced and has received a diagnosis of chronic depression. During this rotation the imaging professional tells the student in confidence about many of his issues. The student is becoming very concerned about the imaging professional's judgment, emotional welfare, and imaging skills. The student covers for the imaging professional after a series of mishaps. A difficult physician encounter in the surgical suite finally pushes the imaging professional over the edge. He walks out of the operating room leaving the student alone to complete the C-arm examination of a very critically injured patient. The examination goes badly because of the delay, and the patient suffers a stroke. The imaging administrator is contacted by an irate surgeon, the imaging professional has a complete meltdown and ends up in the mental health unit, and the student is called in to answer many questions by the program director and the administrator.

Discussion questions
- What issues of student and employee rights complicated this situation?
- Who was at fault and why?
- How could the student have handled this differently? Was there a confidentiality issue?
- Whose rights suffered, and whose were most important?
- Was there liability involved in this?
- Should the administrator and educator have been more aware of the situation?

Students and imaging professionals have the responsibility to understand and abide by the ARRT Standards of Ethics. When they apply for the registry and maintain their registry status, they should be aware of the applicable standards, including those concerning moral turpitude and conviction of a crime. These standards remain in place despite the ethical concerns of educators, students, imaging administrators, and imaging professionals regarding issues of confidentiality arising from the requirements of the certification body.

LEGAL ISSUES

Students entering educational programs for the imaging professions are taking a large and significant step into a new world that offers opportunities but also brings legal and ethical dilemmas. An awareness of legal rights for both students and employees may aid students in their interactions with the educational program and later as imaging professionals employed in the health care field.

This first part of this section provides an overview of legal concepts that may have an impact on student rights. These concepts are defined in contract law and due process as provided for in the U.S. Constitution and state constitutions. Specific due process procedures with regard to student complaints and grievance procedures are also addressed in the JRCERT standards and will be discussed.

A basic overview of employment law is included because it is an important consideration for students, as well as imaging professionals as employees. Among employment issues are the option of personal malpractice insurance and whistleblowing.

CONTRACT LAW

When entering an educational program, the student enters into a contract with that program. Students should read such contracts carefully and be aware of both their own obligations and responsibilities and those of the educational program.

In general, contract law is based on the premise that parties can agree to almost any transaction as long as both parties know to what they are agreeing.[7] However, exceptions to this premise exist. One exception occurs when the bargaining power of the parties is greatly mismatched and the contract is grossly unfair to the party with less bargaining power.[7] In such a situation a court will not enforce a contract "which no man in his senses, not under delusion, would make on the one hand, and which no fair and honest man would accept on the other."[8]

This contract law applies to student contracts with educational programs and also to student handbooks, guidebooks, and departmental policies and procedures that establish the relationship between students and institutions. Unless a contract or the contents of a handbook or guidebook are grossly unfair to the student or program, the contract is valid and both parties must honor its provisions.

The validity of the contract between the student and the educational program, however, does not mean that disciplinary action can be taken arbitrarily or unreasonably. Every individual has certain guaranteed rights, and among them is the right to due process in a disciplinary action against a student of a school or educational program. These constitutional guarantees exist in public and private institutions, schools, and colleges.

DUE PROCESS

An important legal concept in education law is due process. **Due process**, as it pertains to schools, outlines specific procedures that must be followed when disciplinary action is taken against a student.[9] These guidelines must be followed to ensure fundamental fairness and reasonableness.

The Fifth and Fourteenth Amendments to the U.S. Constitution are the origin of due process rights in America. The amendment states that "no state shall deprive a person of his life, liberty, or property without due process of law."[10] This guaranteed right protects individuals from any legislative, executive, or administrative action that, in the court's opinion, is found to be arbitrary. If the court makes such a finding, the action is invalid. The policy and procedures manual for the program and student handbook should also ensure these due process rights.

In 1975, the U.S. Supreme Court extended due process rights to education, reasoning that the state, in creating the public school system, had created an entitlement it could not remove without due process.[9] *Goss v Lopez* involved the suspension of several high school students for as long as 19 days without a hearing.[11] The court held that the damage to a student's educational opportunities and reputation caused by a 10-day or longer suspension was severe enough to require due process before imposition. The court further held that, except where a student's presence in the school presents a clear and present danger, notice and hearing should precede suspension and expulsion. Public and private institutions, schools, and colleges are subject to fundamentally fair due process procedures with regard to a student's guaranteed rights.[11]

Due process, as defined by the courts, has two elements—substantive due process and procedural due process.[12] The substantive element defines and regulates the rights of citizens and defines the circumstances under which those rights may be restricted.[12] The procedural element provides an opportunity for citizens to refute attempts by government to deprive them of their rights provided by the substantive element (substantive rights).[12]

SUBSTANTIVE DUE PROCESS

Dr. Michael Ward, while chairman of JRCERT, related substantive due process to radiologic science educational programs. **Substantive due process** requires a school to show that denial of any of the student's rights to life, liberty, or property is a valid, objective, and reasonable means of accomplishing a legitimate objective. In addition, any infringement on these rights must have a valid relationship to the improvement of the educational system.[13]

Dr. Ward used an example to further understanding. Radiology programs commonly forbid students from wearing long, dangling earrings in their contact with patients. The fact that the director of education does not approve of long earrings is not a reasonable and valid reason for this infringement on student rights. However, if one of the school's objectives is to provide a safe and healthy environment for students in the clinical setting, and one of the means of accomplishing this is to deny students the right to wear dangling earrings because patients might accidentally pull them off, the chances of the school's meeting the requirements of substantive due process are much better. Things have come a long way since Dr. Ward's original statements in his 1994 paper. Radiologic technology schools must by now have adopted due process procedures to ensure students' rights in

DUE PROCESS
Due process as it pertains to schools outlines specific procedures that must be followed when disciplinary action is taken against a student.

SUBSTANTIVE DUE PROCESS
Substantive due process is the notion that the rights of citizens and the circumstances under which those rights may be restricted must be clearly defined and regulated.

this area. Dr. Ward's rationale, however, certainly helps us understand the concepts of procedural due process, substantive due process, and the JRCERT due process standards.

PROCEDURAL DUE PROCESS

After an investigation has established that a substantive right is being denied or infringed upon, procedural due process comes into play. **Procedural due process**, unlike some legal rules, is not a fixed concept but must be determined by the circumstances at hand.[14] The U.S. Supreme Court invoked a balancing formula to determine the exact procedural safeguards needed in a particular context.[14] According to Dr. Ward, in the context of denying students' rights in a radiologic sciences educational program, authorities must provide at least the following[14]:

- A written statement regarding the reasons for the proposed action
- Formal notice of a hearing where the student may answer the charges
- A hearing at which both sides may present their case and any rebuttal evidence

The procedure is not fixed, as stated previously. However, the process must be commensurate with the length of the suspension or the detriment that may be imposed on the student.

According to Dr. Ward, the administration of discipline should guarantee procedural fairness to an accused student. The educational institution has an obligation to clarify standards of behavior it considers essential to its educational mission and community life. Schools should avoid imposing limitations on students that have no direct relevance to their education.[13]

Dr. Ward further stated that disciplinary proceedings should be instituted only for violations of standards of conduct formulated with significant student and faculty participation and published in advance through student handbooks or a generally available body of institutional regulations. If the misconduct results in serious penalties and accused students question the fairness of the disciplinary action, they should be granted on request the privilege of a hearing before a committee. The only legal concern regarding the composition of the hearing committee is that no conflict of interest or bias exists. Impartiality is the essence of fair judicial treatment.[14]

Dr. Ward pointed out the specific elements of procedural due process regarding hearings involving students. They include the following[14]:

- Accused students must receive notice of the time and place of the hearing, as well as the charges and specific grounds against them.
- Students must have an opportunity to be heard and must know the evidence against them.
- The allegations against a student must be presumed untrue until they are found to be true by direct, competent evidence of misconduct. This presumption that the allegations are untrue allows accused students to remain silent during disciplinary proceedings without such silence being held against them.
- Students' status should not be altered pending action on any charges, nor their right to attend classes or be present on the campus or in the clinic, except for reasons related to their own or others' physical or emotional safety.

According to Ward, other fundamental rights of the accused include the issuance of written findings of fact and the right to an appeal. These findings of fact should ensure that the hearing committee makes a decision based only on clear and convincing evidence presented at the hearing.

Legally, schools do not have to provide an appeal process. However, JRCERT's *Essentials and Guidelines of an Accredited Program for the Radiographer* provides that an appeal process should be defined and available to students.[15] Legally, judicial review is available to students to determine whether the hearing body violated their rights.

Appeals procedures help ensure that the student's interests are balanced against the school's sometimes contrary interests. Fairness and reasonableness should be the basis of the outcome of any such procedures.

The guidelines set out previously should be included in the policies and procedures of the program, handbook, and contract. These specify the guidelines to be followed by both parties. They also create an opportunity for the parties to sign off on these procedures, signaling their acceptance.

JRCERT DUE PROCESS STANDARDS

The current JRCERT standards address due process in the radiologic education field. Standard 2, "Program Integrity," states that "the program demonstrates integrity in representation to communities of interest and the public, in pursuit of educational excellence, and in treatment of and respect for students, faculty, and staff." Specifically, objective 2.4 states that the program must have due process standards that are readily accessible, fair, and equitably applied.[16]

Generally, student handbooks set out the due process standards for each facility. These include criteria both for program dismissal on academic grounds, with information on subsequent eligibility to remain in the program, and for program dismissal on clinical grounds (or clinical suspension). If suspension occurs, due process requires a review of that suspension by an impartial group such as a student affairs council, consisting of members of the faculty of the institution, at least one of whom should be from the radiologic science faculty. Generally, policies also define a time frame for this review, such as 1 week.

Program dismissal on academic grounds generally relates to grades and course requirements. Policies should define how academic disputes should be addressed. These policies should include a first-level challenge as well as an alternate route for resolution and a final alternative consisting of an appeal to an unbiased party or panel. Under most policies this might include first bringing the academic challenge to the instructor. If the challenge cannot be resolved at that point, it can then be presented to the program director. If the issue still remains unresolved, it can then be presented to an impartial panel including perhaps the university dean and a representative from both the nursing school faculty and the allied health professional school.

Policies on program dismissal on clinical grounds may include failure to maintain an acceptable grade point average but will also include clinical misconduct criteria. While this conduct is defined somewhat differently by each institution, it generally encompasses violation of the acceptable standards of professional conduct, the clinical setting's standards of conduct, or any act that places patients or clinical personnel at risk. These should be enumerated in the student or employee handbook, but they generally include intoxication, substance abuse, sexual misconduct, acts classified as felonies, refusal to provide proper patient care, and misrepresentation or misuse of institution or patient information or equipment.

Policies should define how disputes based on clinical grounds should be addressed. Due process requires a basic strategy to deal with such disputes. Policies for the resolution of a grievance that is related to facility policies and is nonacademic in nature may vary somewhat by institution but should proceed similarly to the following. The first avenue would be an attempt to resolve the grievance between the student and the other person involved. If the grievance cannot be resolved at this level or the individual involved is unavailable, a written grievance could be made to the program director. At that point the program director would investigate and respond to the student. There should typically be a time limitation for this response, such as 2 weeks. If the grievance could not be resolved at this point, the student could file a written request to meet with the dean and representatives of the school of nursing and the allied health professions. If this does not result in resolution, the student could ask in writing for an appointment with the vice president for academic affairs or the appropriate representative in the particular institution. If the grievance remains unresolved at this point, the student could file a petition with the vice president for academic affairs to form a nonpartial committee consisting of administrators, faculty members, and students to review the grievance. Upon review of the grievance, a written decision would be composed and would be the final and binding end to the student's nonacademic grievance. A time limit such as 2 weeks for the written decision would be appropriate.

WHISTLEBLOWING

Imaging professionals have generally chosen their profession because they want to take care of and help patients. Part of that profession is being an advocate for patients and doing what the professional may feel is needed to draw attention to unsafe or poor quality practices. Certainly the first avenue of that advocacy is within the organization, exhausting all levels of internal communication. If that strategy is unsuccessful, however, other paths can be pursued through national, state, regulatory, and sometimes legal agencies. For the imaging professionals and all health care providers to be able to do this without fear of retaliation from employers, a network of whistleblower laws has been enacted over the years. The following discussion includes what the laws really mean in terms of protection when the professional reports inappropriate or unsafe conditions.

In the United States legal protections for whistleblowers vary, often depending on the subject matter of the **whistleblowing** and the state in which it arises. A patchwork of laws grant protection to whistleblowers. These have their basis in the First Amendment, which states that "Congress shall make no law .... abridging the freedom of speech ... or of the right... to petition the Government for a redress of grievances."[17]

The Civil Service Reform Act of 1978 applies to labor organizations that represent employees in most agencies of the executive branch of the federal government. Under this act, the Office of Labor-Management Standards, a division of the Department of Labor, published a final rule on June 2, 2006, effective October 2006, that requires labor organizations in the federal sector to inform members of their democratic rights, including, among other things, the right to exercise free speech without fear of retaliation.[18]

Congress amended the Civil Service Reform Act of 1978 with the Whistleblower Protection Act of 1989. This act substantially strengthened the protection for whistleblowers in the federal government. It charges the Office of Special Counsel (OSC) with protecting the employee-whistleblower, allows the employee to pursue the case under the Merit Systems Protection Board if the OSC fails to act, and allows the whistleblower to obtain attorney fees and costs associated with litigation.[19]

Other whistleblower protection provisions are included in the Occupational Safety and Health Act. An employee may file a complaint with the Occupational Safety and Health

Administration (OSHA) if he or she is the subject of discrimination by the employer because the employee is involved in protected safety or health concerns, including (among other things) the reporting of environmental concerns and violations of Nuclear Regulatory Commission rules and regulations. There are time limits, however, for the reporting of complaints, sometimes as soon as within 30 days of the alleged discrimination.[20]

In addition to the above and other federal acts that may offer protection to employees for blowing the whistle on unsafe practices, many states have enacted statutes or have adopted common law remedies or public policy exceptions. These statutes, common law remedies, and public policy exceptions generally shield whistleblowers from retaliatory discharge for reporting alleged violations of any law, regulation, ordinance, or public policy. As discussed earlier, laws vary tremendously depending on the subject of the whistleblowing and often the state in which the violation occurs. Strict time limits exist for reporting complaints, again depending on the subject and the state.

As can be surmised from the previous discussion, a true patchwork of laws make up whistleblower protection. Because it is difficult for an employee to sort out what law, regulation, or principle will provide protection and therefore what time frame must be followed, advice from legal counsel or a professional organization should be sought before the whistle is blown.

Although whistleblower laws exist to protect employees from retaliation when reporting concerns, whistleblowers need to understand that their battle will probably be difficult. Such was certainly the case with Barry Adams, a registered nurse who had unsuccessfully exhausted all the internal channels of communication regarding unsafe patient care and dangerously low staffing levels before going public. Adams was threatened with the loss of his job, and in spite of previous reviews that were excellent, he was eventually fired. He sued and won his case. The hospital appealed and lost again.[21]

As Adams discovered, blowing the whistle can be a life-altering experience—either for better or for worse. The whistleblower who stops an unethical practice in his or her organization and is rewarded for the behavior can feel a deep sense of accomplishment. However, the whistleblower who attempts to stop an unethical practice and is punished may have to live through many harrowing experiences, including, as Barry Adams experienced, loss of job and difficult court proceedings.[21]

What Employees Should Consider Before Blowing the Whistle

Competition in health care seems to push managed care organizations into trying to do more with less to cut costs and may well affect quality and patient safety. While laws exist to protect whistleblowers from retaliation, it is a serious step and employees must be realistic when considering blowing the whistle (Box 8-5). One author has suggested some necessary conditions that should be established before blowing the whistle[21]:

- The reason the whistleblower is blowing the whistle should be because he or she sees a grave injustice or wrongdoing occurring in his or her organization that has not been resolved despite use of all appropriate channels within the organization.
- The whistleblower morally justifies his or her course of action by appeals to ethical theories, principles, or other components of ethics, as well as relevant facts.
- The whistleblower thoroughly investigates the situation and is confident that the facts are as she or he understands them.
- The whistleblower understands that her or his primary loyalty is to patients unless other compelling moral reasons override this loyalty.

BOX 8-5	CHECKLIST FOR THE WHISTLEBLOWER, OR THINGS EVERY WHISTLEBLOWER SHOULD KNOW

If you identify an illegal or unethical practice, reserve judgment until you have adequate documentation to establish there is wrongdoing.

Do not expect those who are engaged in unethical or illegal behavior to welcome any questions or concerns you have about the practice.

Seek the counsel of someone you trust outside the situation to provide an objective perspective.

Before acting, if at all possible consult with your professional organization or legal counsel.

You are not protected in a whistleblower situation from retaliation until you blow the whistle.

Blowing the whistle means reporting your concerns to your employer, a national or state agency responsible for regulation of the institution for which you work, or in the case of criminal activity, law enforcement agencies. You may also report concerns in accredited facilities to a national accrediting group such as the Joint Commission on the Accreditation of Healthcare Organizations and receive protection for retaliatory action.

All whistleblowing should be done in writing to employers as a formal complaint when notifying state or national agencies of concerns. Concerns expressed in writing provide a record of the date and circumstances under which you brought an issue to the attention of an employer or a regulatory agency. The written word provides credibility that a word-of-mouth complaint does not.

Document all interactions related to the whistleblowing situation and keep copies for your personal file of every piece of written documentation related to the situation. Such documentation could include memos that describe the interactions or a personal log of the interactions for future reference.

Keep all documentation and interactions objective.

Remain calm and do not lose your temper. When those you are documenting become aware of your activities (and they will), they might attempt to provoke you.

Remember, blowing the whistle is a very serious matter. The results can be negative for everyone involved, so do not frivolously blow the whistle. Make sure you have correct facts before taking action.

Modified from Texas Nurses Association, 2006. Available at www.texasnurses.org/wkplaceadv/whistleblower.htm.

- The whistleblower ascertains that blowing the whistle most likely will cause more good than harm to patients; that is, patients will not be retaliated against because of the whistleblowing.
- The whistleblower understands the seriousness of his or her actions and is ready to assume responsibility for them.

MALPRACTICE LIABILITY INSURANCE

An issue involving legal protection for imaging professionals revolves around the issue of professional liability insurance. Imaging professionals often ask whether they should carry their own professional liability (malpractice) insurance. The answer is maybe. Generally, an imaging professional's employer (i.e., hospital, clinic, radiologist, etc.) carries liability insurance that will both defend the radiographer in the event of a suit and indemnify (pay for) any expenses and damages assessed to the imaging professional in the event of a negative outcome. It is important for imaging professionals to be certain that they are covered by their insurer's liability policy for both defense and indemnification.

Instances certainly exist when a radiographer should carry private liability insurance. Circumstances in which private insurance would definitely be wise include employment by a business rather than traditional employment, such as portable or mobile imaging modalities (MRI, CT, nuclear medicine, ultrasound, x-ray), moonlighting at a facility other than the primary employment, or sharing employment among two or more entities. The rule for the imaging professional is to be sure of having coverage by his or her employer, whoever that might be, and if employer coverage is at all questionable, to self-insure.

The other side of this issue is that personal liability insurance is relatively inexpensive (less than $200 per year at the time of this writing). In addition, imaging professionals should be aware that the institution's insurance probably will not provide coverage for any activity the insurer considers out of the scope of employment, privacy violations, defamation claims including slander and libel, or assault and battery. Although a personal policy may cover some of these acts, the imaging professional should find out exactly what is covered before purchasing personal liability insurance.

Another argument some attorneys make for carrying private insurance is that the interests of the hospital and the imaging professional may not be the same. When depending on the institution's insurance, the imaging professional is also bound by whatever defense the institution and its defense attorney decide to follow. If private insurance exists, the imaging professional may be entitled to legal representation of his or her own (depending on the wording of the policy).

Professionals may also want to familiarize themselves with the trends in their state or region. In many states radiologic technologists and other health care professionals are seldom named as parties in a medical liability suit, with the named parties being the hospitals and physicians. In other parts of the country, health care professionals are frequently named parties. The institution's risk management department or legal counsel would be a good source for such information.

EMPLOYEE RIGHTS

A set of rules different from student rules governs the employment relationship. Health care workers, including imaging professionals, working in private health care facilities without employment contracts are generally subject to a legal doctrine called **employment at will**. This is the employment relationship most imaging professionals have with their employers.

Employment at will allows employers and employees to terminate their relationship for no cause, subject to the restrictions of antidiscrimination and other statutes. This doctrine varies considerably among the states, but some generalizations may be made.[16]

EXCEPTIONS

Employees at will may have a claim for wrongful discharge if their situation falls within one of the exceptions to at-will employment in the jurisdiction. However, none of these exceptions has developed a position that health care workers should have special exceptions from the at-will doctrine.[16]

EMPLOYMENT AT WILL
Employment at will is a policy that allows employers and employees to terminate their relationship for no cause, subject to the restrictions of antidiscrimination and other statutes. The concept of an implied contract provides an exception to the policy, as does the public policy exception.

IMAGING SCENARIO

An imaging professional who has recently moved to town is hired to perform general diagnostic procedures. As is generally the case, no employment contract exists. The imaging professional is very critical of the way things are done at the facility that has hired her. She repeatedly refers to the facility in which she previously worked, insisting things should be done as they were there. On several occasions, she ignores the policies and procedures of her current employer and performs procedures according to the policies and procedures of her previous employer.

The employee is counseled and written up for these infractions according to the personnel policies in the employee handbook. When her conduct does not change, she is terminated. She thinks this grossly unfair and seeks legal advice, stating that she was merely trying to improve the quality of patient care and do things the way they should be done.

Discussion

Employment at will. This employee is probably an employee at will because she did not enter into an employment contract.

Exceptions to employment at will. The imaging professional argues that the employee handbook should be construed as an implied contract and she therefore falls under an exception to employment at will. However, even if the employee handbook can be construed as an implied contract, it contains provisions for the discharge of employees under certain situations. As long as the facility followed those procedures, including counseling and written reprimands, discharge is allowed.

The employee also argues that she was merely trying to improve the quality of patient care and her way was the better way to do things. Such an exception would have to fall under the public policy exception to employment at will. Courts have recognized these exceptions in very limited circumstances; these circumstances generally do not include a health care worker trying to improve patient care. See whistleblowing for a more detailed discussion.

Implied contract is the most common exception to the at-will doctrine. This doctrine allows an employee handbook or personnel manual to be perceived as an enforceable contract. In such situations the court reviews the handbook or manual to determine whether it represents a contract and whether that contract prohibits discharge of the employee.[16]

The second most common exception to the at-will doctrine is the public policy exception, which allows for a claim of wrongful discharge if the plaintiff is discharged for conduct protected by specific state mandates.[16] This exception is quite narrow, generally requiring identification of a specific statute or state law that has been violated. Examples of the public policy exception include discharge that is in retaliation for the filing of a worker's compensation claim or because an employee served on jury duty against the employer's wishes. In the past, courts were generally unwilling to recognize a public policy exception for health care workers who claimed they were discharged for criticizing or taking steps to improve the quality of patient care or for actions the employee claimed were based on personal moral principles.[16] More states are now recognizing such an exception, however, and various statutes also allow protection for employees from retaliation in certain situations (see whistleblowing).

As briefly stated previously, employment at will is subject to restrictions imposed by antidiscrimination statutes. These statutes are discussed in Chapter 9.

SUMMARY

- Student rights and responsibilities are partially determined by the imaging student's and program's choices of ethical theories and models. Employee rights and responsibilities are also determined by selection of ethical theories and models. Each theory and model provides problem-solving techniques and helps guide interactions between students and educational programs and imaging employees and employers.
- Autonomy and informed decisions are important elements in considerations of student and employee rights and responsibilities. An informed decision process allows students access to information concerning application requirements for the program and other information necessary for appropriate imaging education. This process helps maintain student autonomy. An informed decision process allows imaging employees information in selecting career advancement opportunities and necessary continued education. Knowledge is important to the maintenance of the "self" of the student and the imaging employee.
- Mutual truthfulness and confidentiality enable students and educational programs to trust one another. The same concept enables employees and employers to trust one another in the imaging environment. Students and imaging professionals have a right to expect confidentiality regarding their personal communications and records as long as this does not cause harm to another. They each have the responsibility to be truthful and maintain confidential information.
- Justice or fairness is sometimes difficult to determine in an imaging program or an imaging department. Actions that seem fair to one student or employee may seem unfair to another. In such situations, ethical problem solving using appropriate theories and models becomes important to imaging students and imaging professionals.
- Values and standards are desirable qualities that imaging students and employees should use in setting goals for themselves in their personal and professional lives. The JRCERT and ARRT standards provide ethical guidelines for educational programs, students, and imaging professionals.
- The legal rights of students and employees in imaging and radiation sciences are generally based on contract law and due process. Unless the contract is grossly unfair to the student or employee, it is valid and the student and the educational program have obligations to fulfill its provisions. The same obligation exists for the imaging professional and the imaging employer.
- All American citizens have a right to due process that originated in the Fifth and Fourteenth Amendments to the U.S. Constitution. In 1975 the U.S. Supreme Court held that this right extends to students. Due process has two elements—substantive due process and procedural due process.

- Substantive due process requires radiologic science education programs to avoid placing restrictions on students that have no direct relevance to their education. After an investigation has established that restrictions on a student's substantive rights have been made, procedural due process requires procedural safeguards. These include a written statement regarding the reasons for the proposed action, formal notice of a hearing in which the student may answer the charges, and a hearing at which both sides may present their case and rebuttal evidence.
- The educational institution has an obligation to clarify the standards of behavior it considers essential to the educational program. Disciplinary proceedings should be initiated only for violations of standards that have been formulated and published in advance in student handbooks or generally available institutional regulations. If the misconduct may result in serious penalties and accused students question the fairness of the action, they should be entitled to a hearing before an unbiased committee.
- The procedural process of such a hearing must include the following:
  - The accused student receives notice of the time and place of the hearing and the specific charges.
  - Accused students must have an opportunity to be heard and know the evidence against them.
  - Students must be presumed innocent and their silence must not be used against them.
  - Student status should not be altered unless a threat to the student's or others' safety is evident.
- Written findings must be issued, and the student should be granted the right to an appeal. Judicial review is always available to students to determine whether the hearing body violated their rights.
- JRCERT has adopted due process standards that must be followed for an educational program to be accredited.
- Personal professional liability insurance may be appropriate for imaging professionals in some circumstances.
- Blowing the whistle means reporting concerns about unsafe conditions or poor quality care to the employer, the national or state agency responsible for regulation of the institution, or, in the case of criminal activity, law enforcement agencies.
- In the United States, legal protections for whistleblowers vary, often depending on the subject matter of the whistleblowing and the state in which it arises. A patchwork of laws grant protection to whistleblowers.
- The rules regarding fair employment are different from the rules regarding education.
- Employment at will is the legal doctrine that covers imaging professionals in private health care facilities without employment contracts. Employment at will means that employers and employees may terminate the employment relationship at any time for any reason. Exceptions to this doctrine include antidiscrimination statutes, the implied contract exception, and the public policy exception.
- Antidiscrimination statutes are discussed in Chapter 9. The implied contract exception allows an employee handbook or personnel manual to be considered a contract for employment. In any dispute, the court reviews the document in question to determine whether it represents a contract and whether that contract prohibits discharge. The public policy exception allows claims of wrongful discharge for conduct allowed by specific state statutes or mandates.

REFERENCES

1. Renner JJ, Stritter F, Wong H: Learning contracts in clinical education, *Radiol Technol* 64(6):358, 1993.
2. Knowles M: *Self-directed learning: a guide for learners and teachers,* Chicago, 1975, Follett.
3. Knowles M: *Using learning contracts,* San Francisco, 1986, Jossey-Bass.
4. Ballinger PW, Diesen MS: The cost effectiveness of clinical education, *Radiol Technol* 66(1):41, 1994.
5. Joint Review Committee on Education in Radiologic Technology: *Standards for an Accredited Educational Program in Radiological Sciences,* Adopted January 1996, Revised 2001, Chicago, Author.
6. Rokeach M: *Beliefs, attitudes, and values,* San Francisco, 1968, Jossey-Bass.
7. American Registry of Radiologic Technologists: *Annual report to registered technologists,* St Paul, Minn, 1997, Author.
8. Dawson J, Harvey W, Henderson S: *Cases and comments on contracts,* Mineola, NY, 1990, Foundation Press.
9. *Hume v United States,* 132 U.S. 406 (1889).
10. *Goss v Lopez,* 419 U.S. 565 (1975).
11. *The Constitution of the United States of America,* Amendment 14, Section 1, 1868.
12. Mawdsley RD: *Legal problems of religious and private schools,* ed 3, Topeka, Kan, 1995, National Organization on Legal Problems of Education.
13. Rotunda R, Novak J: *Treatise on constitutional law,* ed 2, St Paul, Minn, 1992, West.
14. Ward M: Due process of law and student rights, *Radiol Technol* 65(3):187, 1994.
15. *Mathews v Eldridge,* 424 U.S. 319 (1976).
16. Joint Review Committee on Education in Radiologic Technology: *Essentials and guidelines of an accredited program for the radiographer,* Chicago, 1990, Author.
17. *The First Amendment to the U.S. Constitution,* Dec. 15, 1791.
18. U.S. Department of Labor, Employment Standards Administration, Office of Labor-Management Standards, Jan. 25, 2005. Available at www.dol.gov/esa.
19. Whistleblower protection act, 5 u.s.c. §§ 1201, *et seq.*
20. Office of the Federal Register: Title 29. In *Code of federal regulations,* Washington, DC, US Government Printing Office.
21. Fletcher JJ, Sorrell J, Silva MC: Whistleblowing as a failure of organizational ethics, *Online Journal of Issues in Nursing,* Dec. 31, 1998. Available at http://www.nursingworld.org/ojin/topic8/topic8_3.htm.

REVIEW QUESTIONS

1 Both _____ and _____ have concerns about student and imaging professional rights.
2 _____ provide guidelines for interactions between students and educational programs.
3 The ethical model used to facilitate the learning contract is a combination of the _____ and _____ models.
4 Autonomy includes which of the following?
   a. The self
   b. Informed consent
   c. Respect
   d. All of the above
5 The provision of a trusting environment for imaging students and employees requires _____ and _____.
6 Another term for fairness is _____.
7 Define standards.
8 List two organizations that provide standards for imaging students.
9 Give an example of the use of each model of care within the clinical setting.

10 What are three requirements for informed decisions?

    a. _____

    b. _____

    c. _____

11 What are four components of a positive learning or employment environment?

    a. _____

    b. _____

    c. _____

    d. _____

12 What is the origin of due process law?

13 List and define the two elements of due process law.

14 When a school takes disciplinary action against a student, what actions do procedural due process require?

    a. _____

    b. _____

    c. _____

15 **True or False**   Accrediting bodies such as JRCERT also impose due process requirements.

16 Define and describe the legal employment doctrine that applies to most health care workers.

17 List the exceptions to employment at will.

18 **True or False**   The cost effectiveness of imaging programs may provide educators and students with ethical dilemmas.

19 **True or False**   Contract law prohibits parties from making unfair contracts.

20 **True or False**   Contracts between students and educational programs may include student handbooks and guidebooks.

21 **True or False**   A contract is valid even if it is grossly unfair to one of the parties.

22 **True or False**   If a student's contract is valid, educational institutions can take any disciplinary actions they desire.

23 **True or False**   Substantive due process defines the rights of citizens and the circumstances under which they may be restricted.

24 **True or False**   Procedural due process applies regardless of whether substantive rights are affected.

25 **True or False**   Educational programs may restrict student rights in any way they like.

26 **True or False**   Educational programs have an obligation to clarify behavioral standards essential to the educational program.

27 **True or False**   Standards of conduct cannot be published in student handbooks or institutional regulations.

28 **True or False**   Hearings may be held by committees composed entirely of educators and the program director.

29 **True or False**   If students do not speak at hearings to defend themselves, their silence may be used against them.

30 **True or False**   A student is entitled to a written finding of facts from a hearing.

31 **True or False**   Factors other than those presented at the hearing may be used in the decision-making process of the hearing.

32 **True or False**   If the hearing committee finds the student guilty of misconduct, the student has no other options but to accept the penalty.

33 **True or False**   The same rules govern employment and educational programs.
34 **True or False**   Imaging professionals never need to carry personal professional liability insurance.
35 **True or False**   Employers cannot discharge employees except if they find misconduct.
36 **True or False**   Whistleblowing consists of bringing concerns to employers; national, state, or regulatory agencies; and sometimes law enforcement agencies.
37 **True or False**   Cost incentives associated with managed care sometimes compromise patient safety and quality of care.
38 **True or False**   Your employer will welcome your efforts to blow the whistle on unsafe and poor patient quality practices.
39 Whistleblower protection against retaliation has its basis in which of the following laws?
   a. Federal laws
   b. State laws
   c. First Amendment to the U.S. Constitution
   d. Common law
   e. All of the above
40 **True or False**   You will be protected from retaliation no matter when you report retaliation by your employer.
41 **True or False**   You should feel free to make a complaint about unsafe practices without investigation or documentation.
42 **True or False**   Because there are laws to protect against employer retaliation for whistleblowing, there will be no consequences to the whistleblower.
43 **True or False**   The greater good must be considered in issues of truthfulness and confidentiality.

CRITICAL THINKING *Questions & Activities*

1 How does motivation guide student choices?
2 Which ethical theory do you believe protects student rights to the greatest degree? Why do you believe this?
3 Provide a scenario regarding the lack of student autonomy caused by a poorly informed decision-making process. Discuss your reasoning.
4 Describe a situation in which the truth may be a detriment to student rights. Defend your answer.
5 Define fairness. Is fairness the same for all students? Provide examples to support your answer.
6 What role did your values play as you explored your educational opportunities? Did your personal values ever come into conflict with the educational program's standards? Why do you think this occurred? What alternatives could have been implemented to rectify the situation?
7 How do you feel about the issue of sanctions being imposed on technologists who make statements in confidence to educators? How would you feel if you were the person involved in the process? How would you react if you believed your confidentiality was being infringed?

9 DIVERSITY

I find the great thing in this world is not so much where we stand,
as in what direction we are moving.

OLIVER WENDELL HOLMES, SR.

Chapter Outline

Ethical Issues
Diversity Defined
Diversity and Ethics
Diversity and Values
Legal Issues
Institute of Medicine Report
Cultural and Linguistic Competency

Mandates Regarding Discrimination and Cultural
    Diversity
What Does Cultural and Linguistic Competency
    Mean to the Radiologic Technologist?
Antidiscrimination Statutes in Employment Situations
Antidiscrimination Statutes in Patient Treatment
    Situations

Learning Objectives

After completing this chapter, the reader will be able to perform the following:

- Define diversity and describe interaction patterns.
- Define the implications of a study in diversity.
- Compare the ways in which diversity and ethical problem solving relate to each other.
- List ways that values affect issues of diversity.
- State and discuss the 2004 Institute of Medicine reports and resulting mandates.
- Identify the current state of cultural diversity in the health care professions.
- Define linguistic and cultural competencies.

- List the mandatory culturally and linguistically appropriate service standards for most health care providers.
- Identify and discuss the law regarding discriminatory patient treatment.
- State and discuss the origins of discrimination law.
- Identify the two types of sexual harassment.
- Define sexually harassing behavior.
- Identify the prima facie case of employment discrimination and hostile work environment, including sexual harassment.

Key Terms

cultural competence
diversity
hostile work environment sexual harassment
-isms
linguistic competence

multiculturalism
prima facie case of employment discrimination
quid pro quo sexual harassment
sexual harassment

Professional Profile

A sonographer in a busy hospital radiology department performed survey obstetric sonograms before the performance of amniocentesis procedures. She localized a preliminary site and requested that the radiologist come in and verify the amniocentesis site. The sonographer read several of the reports regarding the amniocentesis localization procedures and noticed that the radiologist dictated that the site was selected by the sonographer and included her name in the report.

During the amniocentesis procedure, the radiologist came into the room but would offer no advice to the obstetrician regarding the accuracy of the selected site. The rate of multiple sticks during amniocentesis procedures, as well as the morbidity and mortality rates, were above the national norms at this institution.

The sonographer was faced with a legal, moral, and ethical dilemma. The technical supervisor did not want to get involved. The sonographer realized that contact with the higher levels of the hospital's administration, including legal counsel, could bring serious consequences, including dismissal. The ethical implications regarding the welfare of the patients, however, compelled the sonographer to arrange a meeting with the chief administrator and the hospital lawyer. After the meeting, the radiologist was told to cease these practices or risk losing his contract to provide services to the hospital. An in-service educational program was held for all obstetricians on staff to review amniocentesis procedures.

This physician was trying to transfer legal liability to the sonographer. Many court cases within the medical field have upheld the legal doctrine of respondeat superior, or the "captain of the ship" doctrine. The presence of the radiologist in the room during the procedure established his supervisory role. The lack of any guidance or response during the procedure does not diminish or transfer the legal responsibility. Including the name of the sonographer in the report does not transfer legal liability. Indeed, because the sonographer is an employee of the hospital, the physician in effect was trying to transfer liability to the hospital. The sonographer must stay within the limits of the institution's job description and national scopes of practice.

Beth Anderhub, MEd, RDMS
Director, Ultrasound Program
St. Louis Community College, St. Louis, Missouri

ETHICAL ISSUES

Imaging students must prepare themselves for a variety of experiences, interactions, and problem solving in their careers. Every patient and situation is unique. This uniqueness may lead to dilemmas that require imaging professionals to employ ethical problem-solving skills.

Imaging professionals, as well as other health care professionals, should be able to identify and accept differences among people. These differences include much more than skin color or native language. Imaging professionals must be knowledgeable about patient attitudes and perceptions regarding imaging procedures. Their mission is not to change patients so that they are all similar but to better understand the differences of their patients as they go about their work.[1]

Imaging professionals should develop their interpersonal qualities at all educational levels. Educational programs should emphasize an appreciation and respect for diversity. According to the proceedings from the American Society of Radiologic Technologists (ASRT) National Education Consensus,[2] issues of diversity will have an increasing impact on the imaging profession in this century. The ASRT House of Delegates has adopted a position statement consistent with the goals of cultural competency.[3]

Imaging professionals are challenged to provide imaging services to individuals and groups of people with diverse expectations, values, and backgrounds. They must be flexible in their approach—no single best method exists for providing imaging services to a diverse patient population with different ideas about what constitutes "caring." Imaging professionals must be creative and innovative in providing acceptable, high-quality care for diverse patient populations. This chapter is devoted to defining diversity and enhancing understanding of its relationship to ethical and legal problem solving with the ultimate goal of delivering better patient care.

DIVERSITY DEFINED

Within this chapter, **diversity** is not defined merely as a variety of ethnicities. Rather, it includes differences that may be rooted in culture, age, experience, health status, gender, sexual orientation, racial identity, mental abilities, and other aspects of sociocultural organization and socioeconomic position.[4] Issues in diversity may be divided into primary and secondary dimensions.[5] Primary dimensions include physical and mental health, sexual orientation, age, ethnicity, and gender. Secondary dimensions include income, marital status, geographic location, education, and religion.

The encouragement of diversity is an inclusive process of appreciation of the unique contributions different individuals with differing backgrounds bring to an organization.[5] For example, an educational program encouraging diversity values the differences among students and asserts that their uniqueness contributes to the formation of more knowledgeable and experienced professionals who will provide a higher standard of care for imaging patients.

The encouragement of diversity requires individuals to move beyond the Western tradition by broadening their learning and opening their minds to new forms of thought.[6] As teachers mentor students through the educational process, they must also assist the students in moving beyond any self-centered worldviews. Even students from similar geographic locations and of similar races bring unique insights to the class as a result of their differing experiences and backgrounds. As they share these differences, they increase their knowledge base, which provides them with greater empathy for their patients and one another. This intellectual broadening is a crucial component in establishing an appropriate educational and working environment for people of many backgrounds.

Adaptation of resources for people of all backgrounds is termed **multiculturalism**. All the variables identified in issues relating to diversity also must be considered in discussions of multiculturalism.

Interaction Patterns

Imaging professionals should be able to recognize the interaction patterns commonly encountered when issues of diversity are discussed. These interaction patterns are labeled **-isms** because of their common word endings. Each -ism involves a tendency to judge others according to a standard considered ideal or presumed to be "normal." The -isms are grounded in bias, prejudicial in attitude, and discriminatory in their behavioral expression. An -ism is centered on personal judgment, regardless of evidence (Box 9-1).[7]

BOX 9-1 THE -ISMS

ableism The assumption that people who are able bodied and of sound mind are physically or developmentally superior to those who are physically or developmentally disabled or otherwise different. Ableism occurs when medical professionals do not offer choices to patients who are chronically ill because they assume such patients do not want to or cannot make decisions.

adultism The assumption that adults are superior to youths and can or should control, direct, reprimand, and reward them or deprive them of respect. Children in American society are often interrupted or ignored by adults. They may not be given choices that allow them to feel they have some control over a situation.

ageism The assumption that members of one age group are superior to those of others. Young patients and staff members may not be taken as seriously as those who are older; in other circumstances, older persons may be discredited in favor of those who are younger.

classism, or elitism The assumption that certain people are superior because of their social status, economic status, or position in a group or organization. This prejudgment assumes that those with more money or education are superior to people lacking in money or formal schooling. Elitism may occur in medicine if a poorly dressed high school dropout is not given the same treatment options offered to a well-dressed college graduate.

egocentrism The assumption that oneself is superior to others. Egocentrism has occurred if a person (e.g., a staff member) who has never been diagnosed with a mental illness feels superior to a patient with a mental illness.

ethnocentrism The assumption that one's own cultural or ethnic group is superior to that of others. (*Ethnicity* refers to cultural differences other than race.) An organization or country may be ethnocentric if it expects all persons regardless of country of origin to speak a certain language or know a set of implicit rules for conduct that may be peculiar to that organization or country.

heterosexism The assumption that everyone is, or should be, heterosexual and that heterosexuality is superior and expectable. Only recently was homosexuality redefined as a lifestyle rather than a disease.

racism The assumption that members of one race are superior to those of another. (*Race* refers to presumed biologic differences based on skin color.)

sexism The assumption that members of one sex are superior to those of the other. For example, women have historically been viewed as being less rational and more emotional than men.

sizism The assumption that people of one body size are superior to or better than those of other shapes and sizes. Positions involving interaction with the public, for example, may be denied to individuals who are very heavy or otherwise fail to meet arbitrary standards of ideal appearance.

sociocentrism The assumption that one society's intellectual methods or actions are superior to the ways of other societies. For instances, Western medical practitioners may feel that biomedicine is effective and folk medicines are not, even when strong evidence exists that this is not always the case. Many traditional societies have highly effective, community-oriented forms of treatment.

From Creasia J, Parker B: *Conceptual foundations of professional nursing practice*, ed 2, St Louis, 1996, Mosby.

IMAGING SCENARIO

An imaging student from an affluent background is assigned to a clinical rotation providing chest radiographs in an urban medical center. The center provides care to many indigent and homeless people who require imaging services. The student has a great deal of difficulty understanding why these patients are unable to provide homes for themselves and why they are not employed. This lack of understanding affects the student's ability to communicate with patients and project the caring attitude that is essential to high-quality imaging services. After clinical grades have been given for this rotation, the student is dismayed to receive a much lower score than he anticipated. He approaches his instructor and questions the grade.

Discussion questions
- What issues might the instructor discuss with the student?
- In what way do these issues affect ethical problem solving for this student?
- Can the student's attitudes and perceptions be remedied? Should they be?

A Study in Diversity

A study conducted in a midwestern state concerned the incorporation of diversity topics into the imaging sciences curriculum.[8] Researchers gathered information with a survey that asked a variety of questions of the program's directors and students. The majority of respondents answered that topics relating to diversity were important and should be included in the curriculum. A sampling of the comments that were provided in answer to the survey and may be of interest to imaging professionals is included in Boxes 9-2 and 9-3. A small percentage of students enrolled in the programs believed that issues of multiculturalism and diversity are not important to the imaging curriculum. The researcher was concerned about this result. If students do not believe that an understanding of the differences among patients is important, patient care may suffer. Students who do not support multiculturalism may hold that all patients should be treated equally and medicine should be color blind or blind to other differences. This implies that all patients have the same needs. Imaging students would do well to remember that patients are unique and deserve imaging professionals able to recognize individual needs, but they do also all deserve quality imaging services. Program directors need to investigate issues of diversity early in the educational program. Caring requires an identification with and respect for the needs of all patients. When students respect differences, they are better able to care for patients.

Program directors and students should be encouraged to become active in incorporating diversity into the curriculum to enhance patient care and make imaging professionals more sensitive to the needs of others. Sensitivity to the differences among individuals gives imaging professionals a better understanding of patients' differing reactions to the imaging environment, the way patients make choices, and the need to employ ethical decision making. It also allows them to identify a variety of methods to explain imaging procedures to a diverse patient population. These methods may include fluency developed in language courses, visual aids, interpreters, patient advocates, and informational sessions presented as continuing education by a variety of presenters.

| BOX 9-2 | **PROGRAM DIRECTORS' UNEDITED INDIVIDUAL COMMENTS** |

"We are beginning to explore these issues and how to integrate them into the curriculum."

"JCAHO [Joint Commission on Accreditation of Healthcare Organizations] requirements include in-service education involving diversity."

"ASRT [American Society of Radiologic Technologists] educators' group listed diversity issues as important to core curriculum development."

"I believe that if you would add this topic as a part of the curriculum, it would be important to have the class at the start of the first year."

"Multiculturalism and diversity could be interlaced into current patient care classes."

"In patient care there is some discussion about language barriers, age, and ability problems. Also, there are some ethics discussion dealing with sexuality, race, and religion, but no actual unit on cultural differences."

"I agree that multiculturalism and diversity should be included within the program, but may be added to an already existing class."

"We do very little and should do more on this subject. I don't think we have the time to include an entire course but guest lecturers from other cultures would be beneficial. I may incorporate this into our class."

From Towsley D: Assessing the skill requirements for radiographers in the traditional and patient-focused care settings, *Radiol Sci Educ* 2(1), 1995.

Imaging professionals should consider issues of diversity before performing imaging procedures to facilitate a more comfortable environment for communication between them and their patients. They must recognize their responsibility to adapt to the needs of patients from all backgrounds. This adaptation for diversity among patients will increase the reputation of the facility and be an asset for marketing and customer service.

DIVERSITY AND ETHICS

Many ethical issues are involved in dealing with a diverse patient population. By recognizing, accepting, and learning ways to accommodate this diversity, imaging professionals become much more adept at providing care that protects patient autonomy, right to information (informed consent process), and confidentiality.

The ages and mental abilities of patients often have an impact on the ethical challenges faced by imaging professionals. For example, an elderly patient who has Alzheimer's disease and is scheduled to have a barium enema is most likely unable to have a truly informed consent process. Such a patient may require an advocate.

Truthfulness and confidentiality also enter into some diversity challenges. In some cultures the elders of the family make decisions for all family members. This hierarchy may affect the radiologist who is explaining the procedure and discussing alternatives to treatment. Confidentiality may be diminished or lost in situations in which patients are having life decisions made for them by others but need to share information with the radiologist that they do not wish the rest of the family to know.

Many situations require knowledge of the similarities and differences in patients and cultures. The more imaging professionals know about diversity, the more they can ready themselves for these interactions. Certain acceptable approaches are recommended for interactions of imaging professionals with all cultural groups (Box 9-4). In addition,

BOX 9-3 STUDENTS' UNEDITED INDIVIDUAL COMMENTS

"A lot of people don't handle working with diverse people. People have been brought up to stay with their own kind of people, but today people need to learn to interact with different people."

"I think everyone should learn more about how to communicate with different people. I know it would help me."

"Everyone who works in the hospital needs to have a working knowledge of the different cultures. It would be a good idea to teach some beginning Spanish classes as we are in contact with many Hispanics that speak no or little English."

"Since you deal with a variety of people you should be educated about them."

"I believe everyone is different and has different needs. I do the best I can to meet these needs while producing the best possible x-ray."

"I think this is important for people to be multiculturally educated, but it should be in your heart to treat people as if they were all the same."

"I think overall patients have the same basic needs—but learning about specific cultures would be helpful to make the specific patient feel more comfortable."

"Throughout my life I have personally went out to get to know other cultures and I enjoy them so much. But a lot of students maybe have not and I think it would be beneficial to have multicultural education. We need to know some cultural differences to help us communicate with patients better."

"I'm not sure how multiculturalism and diversity relate to radiography except the fact that each radiographer should be able to relate to each patient effectively no matter what the race is. The family style, ability, appearance, etc. really shouldn't matter to the radiographer. Treat each patient equally. We should be informed of the diversity in the radiography field. I agree with that 100 percent."

"Some everyday actions to us can be insulting to people of different cultures. It would be helpful to know these."

"It would probably be beneficial if more staff technologists or students had a basic knowledge of other languages, especially Spanish. This being the more common one that I've run into, there is a definite barrier there if there's no communication—perhaps the hospital needs more interpreters or availability."

"I think multiculturalism issues are important since patients are all unique and as we are placed in other areas of the United States we will be impacted by this. As a student who took classes that dealt with diversity and its issues, I have found much of this knowledge to be more useful than I expected. This is why I think multiculturalism is an important part of all education."

"I think a course dealing with multiculturalism would be very useful in helping both to educate and break down barriers between cultures. Some multicultural education is needed."

IMAGING SCENARIO

> A small child arrives in the radiography department to have an intravenous pyelogram (IVP). The child has been raised in a home in which only German is spoken; he is not of school age and speaks no English. The parent tells the child to behave and leaves the room. Now the radiographer and radiologist, neither of whom speaks German, have to try to help this child understand the procedure and aid him in tolerating it.
>
> **Discussion questions**
> - Why would the parent leave the child?
> - What are the differences in what is expected of children growing up in this culture?
> - In what ways could the imaging professionals have been better prepared to protect the child and make this procedure less traumatic?
> - What are some practical approaches to this situation?

categories for basic cultural assessment enable imaging professionals to provide high-quality imaging services for a variety of patients (Box 9-5).

DIVERSITY AND VALUES

So far this chapter has discussed the importance of respecting the ways in which human beings differ from one another, but imaging professionals also should realize that individuals are more alike than they are different. Every group and individual must manage the same basic requirements of living to survive and thrive; to do so, they choose and follow a set of values. These universal values include orientation toward nature (including the supernatural), time, activity, relationships with other people, and the nature of humankind.[9] Imaging professionals should understand their place and that of the patient in the continua of values. They also should consider the ways in which others' worldviews differ from their own. This consideration enables imaging professionals to understand themselves, their colleagues, and their patients better and in doing so to become more effective in recognizing their own and others' perspectives and the ways in which these perspectives influence relationships.[4]

Imaging professionals must be able to understand their patients' values and worldviews. Ethical decision making requires an acceptance that human beings share values and worldviews, often in spite of other differences. This realization provides a foundation for empathy and truly ethical problem solving.

LEGAL ISSUES

INSTITUTE OF MEDICINE REPORT

According to a report released by the Institute of Medicine (IOM) on Feb. 5, 2004, the United States is rapidly becoming a more diverse nation, as demonstrated by the fact that nonwhite racial and ethnic groups will constitute a majority of the American population later in this century. Statistics show that minority populations are significantly underrepresented in all health professions. Increasing racial and ethnic diversity among health professionals is important because evidence indicates that diversity is associated with improved access to care for racial and ethnic minority patients, greater patient

| BOX 9-4 | **APPROACHES RECOMMENDED FOR ALL CULTURAL GROUPS** |

Provide a feeling of acceptance.

Establish open communication.

Present yourself with confidence. Introduce yourself. Shake hands if appropriate.

Strive to gain your patient's trust, but do not be resentful if you do not receive it.

Understand what "caring" means to members of the cultural or subcultural group, both attitudinally and behaviorally.

Understand the relationship between your patient and authority.

Understand patients' desire to please you and their motivations to comply.

Anticipate diversity. Avoid stereotypes by gender, age, ethnicity, or socioeconomic status.

Do not make assumptions about where people come from. Let them tell you.

Understand the patient's goals and expectations.

Make your own goals realistic.

Emphasize positive points and strengths of minority health beliefs and practices.

Show respect to all family members present, especially to men, even if the patient is a woman or child. Men often are decision makers regarding follow-up care.

Be prepared for the fact that children go everywhere with parents in some cultural groups and in poorer families, who may have few child care options. Include them.

Know the traditional health-related practices common to the group with which you are working. Do not discredit them unless you *know* they are harmful.

Know the folk illnesses and remedies common to the group with which you are working.

Try to make the clinic setting comfortable. Consider colors, music, atmosphere, scheduling expectations, pace, and seating arrangements.

Whenever possible and appropriate, involve the leaders of the local group.

Confidentiality is important, but community leaders know local problems and often can suggest acceptable interventions.

Respect values, beliefs, rights, and practices. Some may come into conflict with your own values or your determination to make changes. Nevertheless, every group and individual deserves to be treated with respect.

Learn to appreciate the richness of diversity as an asset rather than a hindrance in your work.

From Creasia J, Parker B: *Conceptual foundations of professional nursing practice*, ed 2, St Louis, 1996, Mosby.

choice and satisfaction, and better educational experiences for health professions students, among many other benefits.[10]

Many groups have worked to increase the preparation and motivation of students in underrepresented minorities so they can enter the health professions. The IOM report found, however, that less attention has been focused on strategies to reduce institutional- and policy-level barriers to participation by underrepresented minorities in health professions training. Specific policies and programs for increasing diversity in health professions schools, their associations and accreditation bodies, health care systems and organizations, and state and federal governments were examined. The report describes

BOX 9-5   CATEGORIES FOR A BASIC CULTURAL ASSESSMENT

Ethnic origin, identity, affiliation, values (ideas about health and illness, human nature, relationships between humankind and nature, time, activity, and interpersonal relationships), relevant rites of passage, customs, art and symbols, and history

Racial identity (ask, do not assume)

Place of birth; relocation and migration history

Habits, customs, and beliefs associated with health, disease, illness, health maintenance, illness prevention, and health promotion; explanatory models; connections between health and religion

Cultural sanctions and restrictions (behaviors that are encouraged or discouraged)

Language and communication processes (verbal and nonverbal patterns, eye contact, use of and toleration for touching, silence, tempo, styles of questioning and persuasion, styles of decision making)

Gender rules

Healing beliefs and practices (relationships with folk, popular, and professional health systems; symbolism related to health and illness; behaviors that are considered normal or abnormal; care associated with unusual or abnormal behavior; care associated with body fluids, excretions and secretions, and temperature; activities included in tending to one's body; substances and practices used in rituals; myths about health; taboos [substances and events to be avoided]; and ideas and practices related to death, dying, and grief)

Nutritional factors; food preferences, preparation, and consumption patterns (kinds of foods and amounts, schedules and rituals, eating environments, utensils and implements, taboos, changes with illness)

Sleep routines, bedtime rituals, and environment (kinds of covering, sleepwear, comforting materials used, rules for sleeping and awakening)

Environmental resources and strains (the "fit" within the community)

Economic status, resources, and living situation

Educational history and background

Occupational history and background

Social network (types and amount of support available from family, other individuals, and group resources; who and where extended family and significant others are; what is expected and expectable from them; social interaction patterns)

Self-identity or self-concept and sense of well-being

Religious history, background, and beliefs

Other spiritual beliefs and practices

Usual response to stress and discomfort

Meaning of care and caring (expectations, beliefs, and practices related to care; relationships between providers and patients as cultural seekers of health care and between patients and the health care system)

From Creasia J, Parker B: *Conceptual foundations of professional nursing practice,* ed 2, St Louis, 1996, Mosby.

IMAGING SCENARIO

A biker arrives at the emergency room around midnight, severely injured in a collision with a car. He is dressed in leathers, and his arms are covered with tattoos. He is unshaven and badly in need of a bath. He is accompanied by his biker buddies—a scary-looking lot. The computed tomography (CT) imaging specialist is called in to obtain a head CT scan. Not only is she fearful of the bikers, but she is irritated that yet another biker has interrupted her night. She is certain he most likely deserves what he received, and she hopes he had signed a donor card. Her interaction with the biker and his buddies displays her fear and irritation. It is a less than successful patient care situation. She is called into her manager's office after a very negative customer service survey arrives. She is questioned about her feeble attempt to provide a high-quality exam for the biker. At a later date the biker returns to the hospital for a follow-up CT scan. When he introduces himself, the CT technologist is shocked to barely recognize the gentleman in the business suit—who just happens to be one of the hospital's attorneys. He tells her that his passion and diversion from his world of business are to ride his "hog" with his group of weekend biker buddies, who, like him, wear suits during the week and leathers on the weekends. The CT technologist is embarrassed and doesn't know what to say.

Discussion questions
- What should the CT technologist have done differently?
- Why did she act as she did?
- What type of discrimination was this? Was this an "-ism"?
- Should it have made a difference if the CT technologist had known who the "biker" really was?
- How could this have escalated from an ethical dilemma to a legal dilemma?

and assesses the potential benefits of greater diversity among health professionals, as well as strategies that may increase diversity in five areas[10]:
1. Admissions policies and practices of health professions education institutions
2. Public (e.g., state and federal) sources of financial support for health professions training
3. Standards of health professions accreditation organizations pertaining to diversity
4. "Institutional climate" for diversity at health professions education institutions
5. Relationship between community benefit principles and diversity

As mandated by the IOM report, imaging educational programs are now focusing on racially, culturally, and economically diverse populations in efforts to improve the distribution and retention of the health care workforce. In addition, guidelines of the Joint Commission on Accreditation of Healthcare Organizations (JCAHO) are in place to ensure that the recruitment policies are nondiscriminatory with respect to any legally protected status such as race, color, religion, gender, age disability, and national origin.[11] A consideration of discrimination laws is vital in any legal discussion of diversity issues, and such laws are discussed in this chapter. The discussion of diversity also mandates a discussion of linguistic and cultural barriers that may adversely affect quality of health care.

CULTURAL AND LINGUISTIC COMPETENCY

As the U.S. population becomes increasingly diverse, linguistic and cultural competencies take on a more important role in society. Improvement of linguistic and cultural competencies in health care is especially important. Clear and unimpeded communication between patient and health care provider is essential to delivering good health care and achieving positive outcomes.[12]

Cultural competence is defined as a set of congruent, behaviors, attitudes, and policies coming together in a system or agency or among professionals that enables effective interactions in a cross-cultural framework.[13] **Linguistic competence** is defined as providing readily available, culturally appropriate oral and written language services to "limited English proficiency" (LEP) patients through bilingual and bicultural staff, trained medical interpreters, and qualified translators.[13]

Controversy surrounds cultural competency policies and practices. Opponents of these policies say that the United States is an English-speaking country and those who immigrate should learn to adapt. This opinion is based on the "melting pot" view of the United States and the idea that people who immigrated in the past have assimilated into American society.[12] In fact, however, this assimilation did not occur instantly. Furthermore, an assumption that English is the official language of the United States is erroneous. The United States has never adopted an official language at a national level.[12] Regardless of personal feelings on this issue, the truly compassionate position is to aid those who are ailing, regardless of the language they speak.[12]

Language is probably the most significant barrier to cultural competency. The 2000 U.S. census showed significant growth of the LEP population in the United States.[14] According to the 2000 census, approximately 18% of households spoke a language other than English at home, up from 14% in 1990 and 11% in 1980. In the 2000 census 8% of households reported an ability to speak English "less than very well." In California, New Mexico, Texas, Arizona, New York, Hawaii, and New Jersey, more than 25% of households reported that they were LEP households.[12,15]

MANDATES REGARDING DISCRIMINATION AND CULTURAL DIVERSITY

Professional Mandates

The codes of ethics for the imaging professions mandate respectful service to all humankind without discrimination. Communicating and relating to the patient are the most effective means of helping the patient medically and improving outcomes.[12] ASRT has established official positions regarding discrimination and cultural diversity through two position statements. The first, adopted in 1996 and reviewed in 2005, states, "The ASRT supports nondiscrimination in the practice of radiologic sciences in the performance of all procedures and patient care within the scope of practice." The second, adopted in 2005, addresses cultural competency and reads as follows: "The ASRT endorses culturally competent health care education beginning with the entry level curriculum and considers continued cultural-competency education necessary for radiologic technologists."[16]

The ASRT position statements are enforced by the proposed radiography curriculum released in 2006.[17] Specific curriculum goals with regard to diversity and cultural competence include "a focus on providing optimum patient care in a society that is becoming increasingly diverse and experiencing generational, cultural and ethnic

CULTURAL COMPETENCE
Cultural competence is a set of congruent behaviors, attitudes, and policies coming together in a system or agency or among professionals that enables effective interactions in a cross-cultural framework.

LINGUISTIC COMPETENCE
Linguistic competence is providing readily available, culturally appropriate oral and written language services to patients with limited English proficiency through bilingual and bicultural staff, trained medical interpreters, and qualified translators.

shifts."[17] Additionally, under "Radiographic Procedures, General Considerations" is included "Special considerations for: Age; Disability; and Cultural background to include impactors of gender, age, and value systems."[17] Under "Patient Considerations, Establishment of rapport with patient, Patient education," are specifically listed "Communications with regard to type of communication and barriers to communication" and "Cultural awareness."[17]

Health care facilities often rely on bilingual family members or others untrained in the health care field to act as interpreters between the health care provider and the patient. The use of untrained interpreters can result and has resulted in errors in diagnosis and hindered proper care delivery. Examples of erroneous communications include omission of questions about drug allergies, instruction on the dose of medication, frequency and duration of antibiotics, and directions for rehydration fluids. Interpreters have also instructed patients not to answer personal questions asked by the health care provider. It is estimated that two thirds of these mistakes could have serious consequences and that the language barrier may hinder a LEP patient from seeking routine medical care.[12] This can result in less preventive care, more serious illnesses when care is sought, and poorer outcomes.

Federal Mandates

The federal government has taken steps to address linguistic and cultural barriers to health care. By passing Public Law No. 101-527, Congress created the Office of Minority Health (OMH), part of the Department of Health and Human Services, in 1994. This mandate requires OMH to develop the ability of health care professionals to increase access to health care services for LEP individuals. This mandate also directs OMH to support research, demonstrations, and evaluations to test new and innovative models aimed at increasing knowledge and provide a clearer understanding of risk factors and successful prevention strategies for minority populations.[12,18] Congress also encouraged implementation of the Disadvantaged Minority Health Improvement Act of 1990 by encouraging OMH to take steps to improve the ability of health care providers to deliver care in the native languages of LEP populations.[12,18]

Health care language barriers were also addressed in 1990 with the issuance of Executive Order 13166. This order mandated federal agencies to examine the services they provide and develop means for LEP individuals to better access those services. The order also required each federal agency to ensure that any entity receiving federal financial aid (including all federal, state, and local government agencies or any public or private entity) provide meaningful access to LEP applicants and recipients.[12,18,19] Besides English, the most frequently spoken language in the United States is Spanish, followed by a multitude of languages, including Chinese, French, German, Tagalog (official language of the Philippines), Vietnamese, and Italian, and many others not listed here.[14] The executive order requires health care facilities to accommodate LEP individuals when a significant population speaking a particular language resides in the area of service of the facility.[19] Executive Order 13166 brings agencies into compliance with Title VI of the Civil Rights Act of 1964.[12]

State Initiatives

Although English has not been established as the official language nationally, 27 states have adopted some kind of legislation recognizing English as the official language in their state. Interestingly, 3 states have also officially recognized other languages as well, including French in Louisiana, Hawaiian in Hawaii, and Spanish in New Mexico.[20] Some states have taken a leading role in promoting cultural competency training and adopting relevant policies.[12]

An example is the California Department of Health Services (CDHS), which administers Medi-Cal, California's Medicaid program. CDHS is a major health care payer in the state with a budget of over $36 billion per year and 5000 employees in 60 field offices across the state.[12] With these resources, CDHS has the ability to influence and lead public health providers, employees, contractors, and subcontractors concerning health issues.[12] In 1999, CDHS initiated a project to develop a cultural competency curriculum for department training. The components of the program involved a survey to identify steps needed to "achieve a culturally competent department that truly serves all Californians"[12,21] This program resulted in a curriculum for CDHS trainers that focused on skill development to improve staff morale, improved access by diverse populations, and provided a link between the curriculum content and staff responsibilities. This curriculum also draws a distinction between cultural competency training and diversity training.[12] California's effort was a major step in improving cultural competence. Other states are starting to pick up ideas. New Jersey has passed a law requiring that all physicians undergo cultural competency training to obtain a license to practice.[12]

WHAT DOES CULTURAL AND LINGUISTIC COMPETENCY MEAN TO THE RADIOLOGIC TECHNOLOGIST?

Imaging professionals face language challenges every day. An example is an incident that was originally reported in *Medical Economics* in 1984 and is still cited in cultural competency circles today. A patient was brought to an emergency department in Florida, accompanied by his Hispanic mother and girlfriend. The mother and girlfriend told the physicians and staff that he was *intoxicado*, which means nauseated in Spanish. The staff, who spoke no Spanish, assumed he was drunk or on drugs. Two days later, with his condition still undiagnosed, the patient went into respiratory arrest and was found to have multiple hematomas and brainstem compression. Left a quadriplegic, he sued the hospital, paramedics, and physicians involved in his case and was awarded a settlement that could eventually reach more than $70 million.[15]

In addition to linguistic issues, significant cultural issues must be considered. Use of family members to interpret can cause problems not only because of the language issues, but also because of the cultural norms of specific ethnic groups. An example is a female Hispanic patient who needed to sign an informed consent for a hysterectomy. Her son was being used as an interpreter. However, their cultural norms prevented the son from fully explaining what was to be done. Instead he used general terms about a tumor being removed from that area. The women was furious when she later discovered that her uterus had been removed and she could not have more children.

Misconceptions about cultural customs can lead to serious complications. Customs vary tremendously among ethnic groups but also within each ethnicity. In some Asian populations coins are rubbed on the skin for healing. This can leave marks on the skin, which may cause health professionals to suspect abuse. Certain Mexican cultures consider that the health care practitioner who looks at a child without touching the child is putting the "evil eye" on the child. In some Asian cultures, males do not feel they can talk about health issues in front of females from their families. In Saudi Arabian cultures women traditionally care for women and men for men.[22]

The IOM report, JCAHO guidelines, the draft of the new ASRT curriculum, and state and federal mandates require linguistic and cultural competency training for imaging professionals. While this training is important for raising awareness and taking steps toward better understanding, true achievement of cultural competency is a lifelong process. The conscientious imaging professional must make an ongoing effort to learn about the population he or she serves, including their language and culture.[12]

Multilingual technologists will have a competitive edge in the job market. Because translation services can be expensive for a health care facility, hiring multilingual imaging professionals makes good financial sense. Cultural competency training and education will also serve technologists well, since additional standards for these competencies at the federal, state, administrative, and accreditation levels will undoubtedly be adopted. Technologists who understand the cultures and their patients not only will have a professional advantage but also will improve the quality of patient care they deliver.[12]

Discrimination in the Workplace

As discussed earlier, a consideration of discrimination laws is vital in any legal discussion of diversity issues. State and federal laws, JCAHO requirements, the IOM report, the ASRT code of ethics and proposed radiology curriculum, and other sources of standards prohibit discrimination on the basis of race, gender, age, national origin, religion, or disability. The federal statutes most commonly employed in discrimination issues in the workplace are discussed here. State antidiscrimination statutes also often come into play, but because they are diverse and generally similar to federal statutes, they are not discussed. The impact of antidiscrimination laws on the imaging professional is explored with regard to both employment and patient treatment situations.

The federal statutes most commonly invoked in prohibiting discrimination in employment situations are Title VII of the Civil Rights Act of 1964,[23] the Equal Pay Act of 1964,[24] the Age Discrimination in Employment Act (ADEA) of 1967,[25] the Rehabilitation Act of 1973,[26] the Americans with Disabilities Act (ADA) of 1990,[27] and the Family and Medical Leave Act of 1993.[28] The federal statutes most commonly invoked in prohibiting discrimination in patient treatment are the Emergency Medical Treatment and Labor Act,[29] Title VI of the 1964 Civil Rights Act,[30] Section 504 of the Rehabilitation Act of 1974,[31] and the Americans with Disabilities Act.[32]

The Equal Employment Opportunity Commission (EEOC) was established to enforce Title VII of the Civil Rights Act of 1964 (Title VII), the Equal Pay Act (EPA), the Age Discrimination in Employment Act (ADEA), and the Americans with Disabilities Act (ADA).

ANTIDISCRIMINATION STATUTES IN EMPLOYMENT SITUATIONS

Title VII of the Civil Rights Act of 1964[23] prohibits discrimination because of race, color, gender, religion, or national origin. This is the most commonly used statute in employment discrimination cases; it prohibits both discipline and discharge based on any of the reasons previously stated and also prohibits any employer from retaliating against an employee exercising any of these protected rights.

The Equal Pay Act of 1964[24] prohibits discrimination based on gender. It also requires equal compensation for equal work on jobs requiring equal skill, effort, and responsibility when performed under similar working conditions.

The ADEA[25] prohibits discrimination based on age. It protects employees ages 40 and older from discrimination in employment—including discharge based on age—and applies to both private and public employees.

The Rehabilitation Act of 1973[26] and the ADA[27] both protect employees from discrimination based on disability. The Rehabilitation Act applies to federal employers and some private employers performing work for the federal government. The ADA's prohibition of discrimination based on disability is broader than that of the Rehabilitation Act and includes disabled status, perception of disability, or a record of physical or mental impairment. The ADA applies to private employers but specifically excludes the U.S. government. Under the ADA, employers must provide equal employment opportunities for disabled employees by making reasonable accommodations.

The Family and Medical Leave Act of 1993[28] applies to private employers who have 50 or more employees. It also applies to employees who have been employed for 1 year or longer. It allows employees to take as much as 12 weeks of unpaid leave during any 12-month period for several reasons:

- To give birth to a child and provide care for the infant
- To care for a spouse, parent, or child with a serious health condition
- To recover from a serious health condition that prevents the employee from properly performing the job

The act also prohibits employers from discriminating against employees who use such leave and requires that employees returning from such leave be given an equivalent position, pay, and other terms and conditions of employment.

Although each of these laws is complex, some general elements may be extracted to provide a working framework of employment discrimination law. The following section discusses employment discrimination cases in general, sexual harassment cases more specifically, and the legal guidelines that must be followed in the workplace.

Employment Discrimination

Employment discrimination claims are based on statutes. These statutes provide procedures for enforcement of the statutes and time restrictions for filing claims. The procedures must be followed to obtain relief based on these statutes. Many states also allow private lawsuits, but the filing of a complaint with the appropriate agency is generally a prerequisite to a private cause of action, as is filing a timely complaint with the state's enforcement agency (such as the state's civil rights commission).

Many employment discrimination cases involve situations in which employees feel they have been treated differently from other similarly employed individuals. These are called *disparate treatment cases*. Employment discrimination also may be claimed if the policies of an employer have an unfair impact on employees who belong to protected groups (such as women). These are called *disparate impact cases*. Employment discrimination also includes retaliatory actions by employers against employees who exercise their rights under antidiscrimination statutes. Guidance on such cases was established in the landmark 1973 U.S. Supreme Court case of *McDonnell Douglas v Green*[33] and clarified through many other cases.

McDonnell Douglas[33] established that to make a claim of employment discrimination, the employee must first establish a prima facie case. This means that the employee, or complainant, must first show that the following conditions have been met:

- The complainant belongs to a protected class (e.g., woman, ethnic or racial minority, disabled).
- The complainant was qualified for the position.
- Despite the qualifications, the complainant was not hired or was discharged.
- The employer continued to look for an individual with the complainant's qualifications to fill the position or hired an individual less qualified than the complainant who was not a member of that protected class.

The establishment of a **prima facie case** does not prove the complainant was a victim of discrimination. It does, however, establish the proper foundation for the employee to file a claim with the appropriate enforcement agency, such as the Equal Employment Opportunity Commission (EEOC).

Sexual Harassment

Case law has consistently interpreted the prohibition of gender discrimination in Title VII to include the forbidding of **sexual harassment** on the job. Because sexual harassment is the most common employment discrimination claim, imaging professionals will benefit from an understanding of the applicable laws.

The EEOC has established guidelines defining sexual harassment, which the court has recognized[34]:

Harassment on the basis of sex is a violation of Section 703 of Title VII. Unwelcome sexual advances, requests for sexual favors, and other verbal and physical conduct of a sexual nature constitute sexual harassment when (1) submission to such conduct is made either explicitly or implicitly a term or condition of an individual's employment, (2) submission to or rejection of such conduct by an individual is used as the basis for employment decisions affecting such individual, or (3) such conduct has the purpose or effect of unreasonably interfering with an individual's work performance or creating an intimidating, hostile, or offensive working environment.

Two types of sexual harassment claims have been recognized by the courts under these guidelines. They are quid pro quo and hostile work environment claims. In addition, EEOC regulations and numerous federal courts have held that employers can be held liable for sexual harassment perpetrated by persons who are not employees or agents of the employer.[35,36]

Quid pro quo claims assert that initial or continued employment or advancement depends on sexual conduct. A supervisor or manager must necessarily be involved in quid pro quo sexual harassment cases.[37] In **quid pro quo sexual harassment**, the employer is held strictly liable if a supervisor has linked tangible job benefits to the acceptance or rejection of sexual advances. Actual economic loss need not be demonstrated, as it is sufficient to show a threat of economic loss.[38]

Hostile work environment sexual harassment claims argue that the harassment unreasonably interferes with the employee's work performance or creates an intimidating, hostile, or offensive work environment. These cases usually involve conduct such as sexual suggestions, sexually derogatory remarks, and sexually motivated physical contact. Early cases required a finding that the harassment was so severe that it seriously affected

PRIMA FACIE CASE OF EMPLOYMENT DISCRIMINATION
A prima facie case of employment discrimination is what must be proved by a complainant making a claim of employment discrimination. It requires complainants to prove they belong to a protected class, were qualified for the position, were not hired or were discharged, and after their discharge the employer continued to look for an individual with the complainant's qualifications to fill the position or hired an individual less qualified than the complainant who was not a member of that protected class.

SEXUAL HARASSMENT
Sexual harassment includes unwelcome sexual advances, requests for sexual favors, and other verbal and physical conduct of a sexual nature that the employee is required to submit to as a term or condition of employment; that submission to, or rejection of, such conduct is used as the basis for employment decisions; or that such conduct has the purpose or effect of unreasonably interfering with an individual's work performance or creating an intimidating, hostile, or offensive working environment.

the employee's psychological well-being. However, more recent cases have held that if a reasonable person would find the working environment hostile or abusive and the victim perceives the environment to be abusive, a hostile work environment may be found.[39] The loss of tangible job benefits is not a prerequisite to a hostile work environment claim.[40] Actions of supervisors, co-workers, and customers can give rise to hostile work environment claims. Employers are liable if they create or condone a discriminatory work environment.[35,36,41]

Prima Facie Hostile Work Environment

To make a claim for hostile work environment sexual harassment, the complainant must first meet five conditions to establish a prima facie case[39,41]:

1. The employee must be a member of a protected class.
2. The employee must have been subject to unwelcome sexual harassment in the form of sexual advances, requests for sexual favors, or other verbal or physical conduct of a sexual nature, which can include sexually offensive or sexist written material displayed in plain view.[42]

IMAGING SCENARIO

A male technologist is hired to perform computed tomography (CT) by the female director of radiology. The director, as early as the interview, hints to the applicant that she is romantically available and thinks he is attractive. Throughout his first few months of employment, the director pays special attention to him and continues to hint at her availability. The technologist lets the director know that he is currently seeing someone and even introduces his significant other to the director when she comes to meet him for lunch.

Over the next year the director continues to pay special attention to the technologist, makes comments about his attractiveness, and even states that she would like to get together with him. The technologist laughs off these comments as best he can. The position of supervisor of CT opens. The director approaches the male technologist and informs him that the position is his if he will become intimate with her.

Discussion questions
• Is this sexual harassment? If so, what kind of sexual harassment is it?
• Is the hospital liable for the acts of the director?
• What can the technologist do?

Discussion

This is quid pro quo sexual harassment. It is quid pro quo because the advancement of the technologist depends on sexual conduct and the demand is made by his supervisor. Because this is quid pro quo, the employer will be liable for the conduct of its supervisors, whether or not they were aware of the conduct, even if the conduct was not authorized or was forbidden. The facility should have a policy for the technologist to address the harassment internally. The technologist has a right to file a complaint with the Civil Rights Commission and the Equal Opportunity Employment Commission (EEOC). After compliance with the Civil Rights Commission and EEOC procedures, the technologist could file a lawsuit against the director and the facility.

QUID PRO QUO SEXUAL HARASSMENT
Quid pro quo sexual harassment occurs when initial or continued employment or advancement depends on sexual conduct. A supervisor or manager must necessarily be involved in quid pro quo sexual harassment cases.

HOSTILE WORK ENVIRONMENT SEXUAL HARASSMENT
Hostile work environment sexual harassment occurs when sexual behaviors unreasonably interfere with work performance or create an intimidating, hostile, or offensive work environment. Sexual suggestions, sexually derogatory remarks, and sexually motivated physical contact may constitute hostile work environment sexual harassment. Actions of supervisors, co-workers, and customers can give rise to hostile work environment claims. Employers are liable if they create or condone a discriminatory work environment.

3. The complaint of harassment must have been based on gender.
4. The alleged sexual harassment must have had the effect of unreasonably interfering with the employee's work performance and creating a working environment a reasonable person would find intimidating, hostile, abusive, or offensive and the employee perceived as abusive.
5. The employer knew or should have known of the harassment and failed to take appropriate action.

Whether the alleged misconduct is severe enough to be considered hostile or abusive and thus resulting in liability is a question to be determined in light of all the circumstances of the employment relationship.[41] Case law has held that the mere presence of an employee who has engaged in particularly severe or pervasive sexual harassment may create a hostile work environment. EEOC guidelines[43] require investigation of the nature of the sexual advances and the context in which the alleged misconduct occurred; the legality of the actions is determined on a case-by-case basis.[44]

Who Is Protected?

Both men and women are protected by sexual harassment statutes, and harassing conduct toward homosexual and heterosexual individuals is prohibited. However, harassment arising because of a person's sexual preference is not protected under sexual harassment statutes because it is not based on gender.[45] For example, a prima facie case was not established by a male employee who was forced to resign because his co-workers did not approve of his relationship with another man.[45] However, Title VII does protect employees from harassment resulting from terminated consensual relationships.[46]

What Is Unwelcome?

Conduct must be unwanted and offensive to be prohibited under Title VII. As stated previously, the determination of whether conduct is sufficiently hostile or abusive to be actionable must be determined in the light of all the circumstances of the employment relationship.[39,41]

Generally courts must find that the complainant made some effort to indicate that the conduct was unwelcome or offensive. In one case, a court found that because a workplace was one in which sexual horseplay was consensual and the complainant participated in telling sexual jokes, the complainant was not offended to the point of sexual harassment by a sexually explicit cartoon given to her by her supervisor.[47]

Another court found that a personnel director's close attention to a complainant was not unwelcome harassment because the complainant had been giving the personnel director mixed signals by sharing many personal problems with him. In addition, her requests for him to leave her alone were not delivered with any sense of emergency, sincerity, or force.[48] Yet another court found that conduct in a female-run quality-control shop in which sexual innuendo and vulgarity were commonplace and both male and female employees, including the plaintiff, took part in such conduct did not give rise to a Title VII sexual harassment action.[49]

When Are Employers Liable?

Generally, employers are liable for any quid pro quo sexual harassment committed by their supervisory personnel, even if the conduct was not authorized or was even forbidden.[41] This is generally true regardless of whether the employer knew or should have known of the conduct.[50]

In hostile work environment cases, employer liability is not as clear. Most courts have imposed liability if the employer knew or should have known that a supervisor's

IMAGING SCENARIO

A female technologist is hired just after graduation at a hospital across town from where she trained. This hospital does a great deal of orthopedic work, and the majority of her time is to be spent taking radiographs in surgery. The first day she is shocked by the language used in the surgical suite and the subject matter of the discussions. She soon realizes that it is normal procedure for the physicians and surgery staff to tell off-color jokes about sex and even to discuss each other's sexual adventures. She is embarrassed by this behavior but says nothing. Within a few weeks they start teasing her about her sexual behavior and making sexual suggestions to her. She complains to her supervisor. Her supervisor meets with the surgery supervisor, who brushes the behavior off as insignificant. Within a few months the technologist dreads going to work and has even called in sick several times just to avoid the situation.

Discussion questions
- Is this sexual harassment? If so, what kind of sexual harassment is it?
- Is the hospital liable for the acts of the director?
- What can the technologist do?

Discussion

This is hostile work environment sexual harassment. The technologist is a member of a protected class, a woman. Whether the conduct is severe enough to be considered hostile or abusive and thus actionable must be determined in light of all the circumstances of the employment relationship. The technologist made some efforts to communicate that the conduct was offensive and unwelcome by complaining to her supervisor. In addition, the technologist did not participate in the behavior. The fact that the technologist called in sick to avoid the situation also supports her claim that she perceived the environment as abusive or offensive and that it interfered with her work performance. Finally, the employer, through the technologist's supervisor and the surgery supervisor, knew or should have known of the harassment and failed to take appropriate action. The behavior leading to the complaint must be examined to determine whether a reasonable person would find the working environment hostile or abusive and whether the victim perceived it as hostile or abusive. Clearly the EEOC guidelines requiring an investigation into alleged sexual misconduct were not followed here. If the conduct is found to be severe enough to be actionable, the employer would most likely be liable because it knew or should have known of the behavior and did not take prompt remedial action to prevent it.

A policy should be in place within the facility for the technologist to address the harassment internally. The technologist has a right to file a complaint with the Civil Rights Commission and the Equal Opportunity Employment Commission (EEOC). After compliance with the Civil Rights Commission and EEOC procedures, the technologist could file a lawsuit against the facility.

behavior created a hostile work environment and failed to take prompt remedial action.[41]

Harassment in the workplace by co-workers also may create liability for the employer if the employer or supervisory personnel knew or should have known of the harassing behavior and failed to respond promptly and in a manner likely to prevent recurrent behavior.[50] Employers are generally found liable for hostile environment sexual harassment only if the alleged offensive conduct is severe and pervasive and not if the offensive conduct is sporadic or occurs in isolated incidents.[39] Employers may also be found liable for the sexual harassment perpetrated by persons who are not employees or agents of the employer.[35,36] The employer may be found liable for failing to respond reasonably to acts of sexual harassment of which it is aware or reasonably should be aware. The issue here is whether the employer responded reasonably, not whether the efforts were successful in stopping the harassment.[51]

EEOC guidelines[34] provide direction for employers in preventing sexual harassment. After employers become aware of potential sexual harassment, they must take prompt and adequate remedial action. The EEOC encourages prevention of sexual harassment in the workplace[34]:

> An employer should take all steps necessary to prevent sexual harassment from occurring, such as affirmatively raising the subject, expressing strong disapproval, developing appropriate sanctions, informing employees of their right to raise and how to raise the issue of harassment under Title VII, and developing methods to sensitize all concerned.

Health care facilities should have policies to inform employees of conduct constituting sexual harassment, express disapproval of such conduct, facilitate the handling of sexual harassment complaints, clearly identify procedures for dealing with such complaints, describe the manner in which they will be investigated, and list the sanctions to be expected for harassing behavior. Procedures should be fair to both complainant and accused.

The health care facility's policies and procedures should clearly specify to whom reports of sexual harassment should be made and the correct procedure to be followed. A person who feels sexually harassed has a right to file a complaint with the Civil Rights Commission and the EEOC. As discussed earlier, there are time limitations for filing these complaints. After complying with the Civil Rights Commission and the EEOC procedures, the plaintiff may file a lawsuit against the facility.

Most imaging departments necessitate close work with many individuals, including physicians, nurses, other imaging professionals, students, and patients. Imaging professionals must be aware of conduct constituting sexual harassment and their rights and obligations if such behavior occurs, including the duty to state clearly that the conduct is offensive and unwelcome. They should also work to prevent allegations of sexual harassment by avoiding taking part in sexual jokes, teasing, innuendo, and other situations that may be misinterpreted by others.

ANTIDISCRIMINATION STATUTES IN PATIENT TREATMENT SITUATIONS

The Emergency Medical Treatment and Labor Act[29] (also called the Anti-Dumping Act) requires hospitals covered by its provisions to provide emergency medical screening examinations and treatment to stabilize serious medical conditions of all patients who come to the emergency department. Women in labor are to be delivered if inadequate time for transfer exists. The act applies to all hospitals that participate in the federal Medicare program and have emergency departments.

Title VII of the 1964 Civil Rights Act[30] was passed to prevent discrimination against minorities in federally funded programs. The statute provides that "no person in the United States shall on the ground of race, color, or national origin, be excluded from participation in, be denied the benefits of, or be subjected to discrimination under any program or activity receiving Federal financial assistance." Most hospitals, nursing homes, and health care institutions receive federal funds and therefore must comply with the antidiscrimination provisions of Title VII.

Section 504 of the Rehabilitation Act of 1974[31] and the ADA[27] prohibit discrimination against persons who are disabled. The Rehabilitation Act applies only to facilities receiving federal funds. The ADA, however, applies to public accommodations operated by private entities. Both acts provide for private rights of action. The Department of Justice enforces the public accommodation provisions of the ADA.

Although technical differences between the two statutes exist, violations of one or both are generally alleged in claims of denial of treatment. Both include an exception to the duty to provide services if the disabled person presents a "direct threat" to the health and safety of others. *Direct threat* is defined as a significant risk that cannot be eliminated by a modification of policies, practices, or procedures, or by the provision of auxiliary aids or services.

The ADA[32] more explicitly addresses persons with human immunodeficiency virus (HIV) and acquired immunodeficiency syndrome (AIDS) and identifies more specific duties of providers; however, the ADA's suspension of such duties if a threat to others exists may limit its effectiveness. Some state legislatures have specifically made refusal to treat persons with AIDS illegal, and some statutes prohibiting discrimination against disabled persons may create an obligation to treat persons with AIDS and HIV. Physicians and other health care workers also have an ethical obligation to treat patients in need.

Imaging professionals are bound by the laws previously discussed. They are also bound by the ethical duty enumerated in Principle Three of the ASRT code of ethics[52] to "deliver patient care and service unrestricted by the concerns of physical attributes or the nature of the disease or illness, and without discrimination regardless of sex, race, creed, religion, or socioeconomic status."

SUMMARY

- Imaging professionals at all educational levels must accommodate the needs of a diverse patient population.
- The ASRT developed a position statement on cultural competency, articulating the expectations of the radiation imaging and sciences profession.
- Diversity is defined as differences among individuals that are rooted in culture, age, experience, health, gender, sexual orientation, race and ethnic identity, mental abilities, income, marital status, education, religion, and sociocultural status.
- Students must recognize their own uniqueness to appreciate that of others.

- Students should avoid perpetuating "-isms"—interaction patterns that involve a tendency to judge others according to their correlation with a standard considered ideal or "normal."
- Recognition of the positive impact of making diversity a part of the curriculum needs to be encouraged for program directors to enhance patient care and sensitivity to the needs of others.
- Recognizing, accepting, and dealing with issues of diversity will allow students and imaging professionals to become more adept at providing care that protects patient autonomy, right to information, informed consent processes, right to the truth, and confidentiality.
- Imaging professionals should be aware of the similarities among all people. These similarities may be found in patients' value systems and worldviews and provide a foundation for empathy and the realization that the need for ethical problem solving is universal.
- Cultural and linguistic competence has taken on increased importance as the United States has become increasingly diverse.
- Language is probably the most significant barrier to cultural competency.
- The 2000 census shows an increase in the population having limited English proficiency, with 18% of households speaking a language at home other than English, up from 14% in 1990 and 11% in 1980.
- Cultural competence is defined as a set of congruent behaviors, attitudes, and policies that come together in a system or agency or among professionals, enabling effective interactions in a cross-cultural framework.
- Linguistic competence is defined as providing readily available, culturally appropriate oral and written language services to patients with limited English proficiency through bilingual and bicultural staff, trained medical interpreters, and qualified translators.
- While there is no official national language, 27 states have adopted some kind of legislation recognizing English as the official language in their state.
- The IOM report, JCAHO guidelines, ASRT position statements, ASRT draft curriculum, and state and federal mandates now require linguistic and cultural competency training for imaging professionals.
- An understanding of discrimination law is vital in legal discussions of diversity issues.
- State and federal laws, JCAHO requirements, the IOM report, and the ASRT code of ethics and proposed radiography curriculum, among other sources of standards, prohibit discrimination on the basis of race, gender, age, national origin, religion, and disability.
- Discrimination is prohibited both in employment and in patient treatment situations.
- Statutes prohibiting discrimination in employment include Title VII of the Civil Rights Act of 1964,[23] the Equal Pay Act of 1964,[24] the Age Discrimination in Employment Act (ADEA) of 1967,[25] the Rehabilitation Act of 1973,[26] the Americans with Disabilities Act (ADA) of 1990,[27] and the Family and Medical Leave Act of 1993.[28]
- The federal statutes most commonly invoked in prohibiting discrimination in patient treatment include the Emergency Medical Treatment and Labor Act,[29]

Title VI of the 1964 Civil Rights Act,[30] Section 504 of the Rehabilitation Act of 1974,[31] and the Americans with Disabilities Act.[32]

- Employment discrimination may be claimed if an employee is treated differently from a similarly employed individual because of a protected condition (e.g., race, gender, national origin, religion, disability). These are called *disparate treatment cases.*
- Employment discrimination also may be claimed if a policy has an unfair impact on a protected group. These are called *disparate impact cases.*
- Employment discrimination cases are investigated by the EEOC at the federal level and the Civil Rights Commission at the state level. Time limits for filing claims are rigorously enforced.
- To file a discrimination claim, complainants must establish a prima facie case in which they prove membership in a protected group and qualification for the position, argue that despite qualification, they were not hired or were discharged, and note that the employer continued to look for an individual with similar qualifications to fill the position or hired a less qualified individual who was not a member of the protected class.
- Sexual harassment claims under Title VII are the most frequent employment discrimination claims made. The EEOC has established guidelines for behavior in the workplace, and case law has further defined these guidelines.
- Generally, two types of sexual harassment have been recognized—quid pro quo and hostile work environment.
- Quid pro quo harassment occurs if a supervisor requests sexual favors in return for continued employment or employment advancement.
- Hostile work environment harassment occurs if the sexually related conduct unreasonably interferes with the employee's work performance or creates an intimidating, hostile, or offensive work environment.
- The establishment of a prima facie hostile work environment claim requires the complainant to meet five specific conditions, specifically:
  1. The employee is a member of a protected class.
  2. The employee was subject to unwelcome sexual harassment.
  3. The harassment was based on gender.
  4. The harassment had the effect of unreasonably interfering with the employee's work performance and creating a working environment a reasonable person would find intimidating, hostile, abusive, or offensive and the employee perceived as abusive.
  5. The employer knew or should have known of the harassment and failed to take appropriate action.
- Whether the conduct complained about is unwelcome or severe enough to be considered hostile or abusive is determined in light of all the circumstances of the situation, on a case-by-case basis.
- Employers are liable for the actions of their supervisors in quid pro quo harassment cases.
- Employers are generally liable for harassment in the workplace if they or their supervisors knew or should have known of the hostile environment sexual harassment and failed to take immediate and appropriate corrective action.
- A variety of statutes prohibit discrimination in patient care situations. In addition, the Emergency Medical Treatment and Labor Act requires hospitals that

participate in the Medicare program and have emergency rooms to provide medical screening examinations and treatment to stabilize serious conditions to any patients entering the emergency department. Women in labor must be delivered if insufficient time for transfer exists.
- Other statutes prohibit discrimination because of disability, HIV status, or AIDS. Exceptions to this prohibition may be made if the provision of services to the patient presents a direct threat to the health and safety of others.
- Imaging professionals have duties under these statutes and professional ethical guidelines to deliver patient care unrestricted by concerns of physical attributes or nature of illness and without discrimination regarding gender, creed, religion, or socioeconomic status.

REFERENCES

1. Spector RE: *Cultural diversity in health and illness*, ed 3, Norwalk, Conn, 1991, Appleton & Lange.
2. American Society of Radiologic Technologists National Education Consensus: *Radiography: the second century*, Albuquerque, NM, 1995, Author.
3. American Society of Radiologic Technologists: *Professional issues for clinical practice, radiologic science education and public interaction*, Resolution 95-3.12. Adopted by the House of Delegates, 1995. Amended by the House of Delegates, Resolution 96-1.07, 1996.
4. Kavanagh KH, Kennedy PH: *Promoting cultural diversity: strategies for health care professionals*, Newbury Park, Calif, 1992, Sage.
5. Hill-Storks H: *Dimensions of diversity*, American Health Care Radiology Administrators' 22nd Annual Meeting, Sudbury, Mass, 1994, American Health Care Radiology Administrators.
6. Marcus LR: Diversity and its discontents, *Rev Higher Ed* 17:227, 1994.
7. Brislin R: *Understanding culture's influence on behavior*, Fort Worth, Tex, 1993, Harcourt Brace College.
8. Towsley DM: *The need for incorporating course work in cultural diversity in radiologic technology programs*, thesis, Cedar Falls, Ia, 1996, University of Northern Iowa.
9. Kluckhohn FR: Dominant and variant value orientations. In Kluckhohn C, Murray JA (Eds): *Personality in nature, society and culture*, New York, 1971, Knopf.
10. Institute of Medicine: *In the nation's compelling interest: ensuring diversity in the health care workforce*, Washington, DC, 2004, Author.
11. Joint Review Committee on Education in Radiologic Technology: *Standards for an accredited educational program in radiological sciences*, Adopted January 1996, Revised 2001, Chicago, Author.
12. Shams-Avari P: Linguistic and cultural competency, *Radiol Technol* 76(6):437, 2005.
13. US Department of Health and Human Services, Office of Minority Health: National standards on culturally and linguistically appropriate services (CLAS) in health care, *Fed Reg* 65:80865, 2000.
14. Shin H, Bruno R: Language use and English-speaking ability: census 2000 brief, October 2003. Available at: www.census.gov/prod/2003pubs/c2kbr-29.pdf. Accessed 7/10/2006.
15. Weiss B: Cultural competence: caring for Latino patients, *Med Exam* April 23, 2004. Available at: www.memag.com/memag/article/articleDetail.jsp?id=108876. Accessed 7/10/2006.
16. American Society of Radiologic Technologists, House of Delegates: *Position statements*, 2005, Author. Available at http://www.asrt.org/media/pdf/governance/HODPositionStatement2005.pdf. Accessed 7/13/2006.
17. American Society of Radiologic Technologists, Radiography Curriculum Revisions Project Group: *ASRT draft radiography curriculum*. Available at http://www.asrt.org/media/pdf/radiography_curriculum.pdf. Accessed 7/13/2006.
18. U.S. Department of Health and Human Services, Office of Minority Health: *The origins of the Office of Minority Health and the Center for Linguistic and Cultural Competence in Health Care*. Available at: http://www.omhrc.gov/templates/browse.aspx?lvl=1&lvlID=3. Accessed 7/10/2006.
19. President of the United States: Executive Order 13166: Improving access to service for persons with limited English proficiency, *Fed Reg* 65(159), 2000.
20. Wikipedia: *Languages in the United States*. Available at http://en.wiipedia.org/wiki/Languages_in_the_United_States. Accessed 7/13/2006.

21. Allen C, Mutha S: *Cultural competency for California public health staff: train-the-trainer state partnership project; final report,* San Francisco, 2004, University of California, pp 4-9.
22. Transcultural Nursing: *Case studies: the Hispanic American community.* Available at: www.culturediversity. org/hisp.htm. Accessed 7/10/2006.
23. 42 USCA Section 2000e et seq.
24. 29 USCA Sec 225.
25. 29 USCA Section 621 et seq.
26. 29 USCA Section 701 et seq.
27. 42 USCA Section 12-101 et seq.
28. Pub L 103-3.
29. 42 USCA Section 1395 (1994).
30. 42 USCA Section 2000 (1964).
31. 29 USCA Section 794.
32. 42 USCA Sections 12101-12213.
33. *McDonnell Douglas v Green,* 411 U.S. 792 (1973).
34. *Meritor Savings Bank v Vinson,* 106 S.Ct. 2399 (1986), citing other cases.
35. *Watson v Blue Circle, Inc.,* 324 F.3d 358 (9th Cir. 2002).
36. *Little v Windermere Relocation, Inc.,* 301 F.3d 358 (9th Cir. 2002).
37. 29 CFR Section 1604.11 (a).
38. *Karibian v Columbia University,* 14 F.3d 773 (2nd Cir. 1994).
39. *Harris v Forklift Systems, Inc.,* 111 S.Ct. 367 (1993).
40. *Bundy v Jackson,* 641 F.2d 934 (D.C.Cir. 1981).
41. *Henson v City of Dundee,* 682 F.2d.897 (11th Cir. 1982).
42. *Robinson v Jacksonville Shipyards,* 760 F Supp. 1486 (M.D. Fla. 1991).
43. *Cline v General Electric Capital Auto Lease,* 784 F Supp. 650 (N.D. Ill. 1990).
44. 29 CFR Section 1604.11 (b).
45. *Carreno v IBEW Local No. 226,* 54 F.E.P. Cases 81 (D. Ka. 1990).
46. *Williams v Civiletti,* 487 F Supp. 1387 (D.D.C. 1980).
47. *Tindall v Housing Authority,* 762 F Supp. 259 (W.D. Ark. 1991).
48. *Kouri v Liberian Services,* 55 F.E.P. Cases 124, (E.D. Va. 1991).
49. *Weinsheimer v Rockwell International Corp.,* 54 F.E.P. Cases 828 (M.D. Fla. 1990).
50. 29 CFR Section 1604.11 (d).
51. *Modern Continental v Massachusetts Commission Against Discrimination,* 833 N.E. 2d 1130 (S.C. Mass 2005).
52. American Society of Radiologic Technologists and American Registry of Radiologic Technologists: *Code of ethics,* Albuquerque, NM, 2003, Author.

REVIEW QUESTIONS

1 Define diversity.
2 Define multiculturalism.
3 List the primary dimensions of diversity.
4 List the secondary dimensions of diversity.
5 _____ _____ are grounded in bias, prejudicial in attitude, and discriminatory in their behavioral expression.
6 What is the best time to provide educational opportunities in diversity issues for imaging students?
7 What does sensitivity to differences allow the imaging professional?
8 List three methods that might be employed to help patients from different cultures understand information about the examination.
9 **True or False** Imaging practitioners should participate in establishing care standards for patient care services.

10 True or False   All educational and certificate programs for the imaging and radiation sciences should include linguistic and cultural competency.

11 True or False   English is the official language of the United States.

12 Federal and state statutes prohibit discrimination on what basis?

13 Does anything besides the law prohibit discrimination by imaging professionals?

14 Title VII, the Equal Pay Act, the Age Discrimination in Employment Act, the Rehabilitation Act, and the Family and Medical Leave Act all prohibit discrimination in what area?

15 Employment discrimination in which an employee is treated differently from other similarly situated employees because of a protected condition is called _____ _____.

16 Employment discrimination in which a policy has a negative impact on a protected group is called _____ _____.

17 List the four conditions required for a prima facie case of employment discrimination:
   a. _____
   b. _____
   c. _____
   d. _____

18 What is the most frequent kind of employment discrimination claim brought under Title VII?

19 _____ _____ _____ harassment occurs if continued employment or advancement of employment depends on the provision of sexual favors.

20 _____ _____ _____ harassment occurs if the sexually related conduct unreasonably interferes with the employee's work performance or creates an intimidating, hostile, or offensive work environment.

21 List the five conditions required to establish a prima facie case of hostile work environment:
   a. _____
   b. _____
   c. _____
   d. _____
   e. _____

22 Imaging professionals have a legal and ethical duty to provide care to patients who are HIV positive or have AIDS, with one exception. What is it?

23 True or False   People are more alike than they are different.

24 True or False   Diversity is only an issue of culture.

25 True or False   Learning ways to accommodate diversity increases the patient's autonomy and confidentiality.

26 True or False   The best time for the student to learn about diversity is at the end of the program.

27 True or False   If a prima facie case of discrimination is established, the employee wins the case.

28 True or False   Only the specific language or conduct that gave rise to the complaint is considered during the investigation of cases of sexual harassment.

29 True or False   No duty exists for emergency departments to provide emergency treatment to patients without insurance.

1 Discuss ways in which people are more alike than they are different.

2 Why is diversity important in imaging patient care? Justify your answer.

3 Analyze the ways in which uniqueness contributes to a better organization.

4 Select two -isms and explain the impact they have on imaging services.

5 Do you agree with the findings in the diversity study? Why or why not?

6 Describe educational methods to provide understanding of issues of diversity. Which are most likely to succeed?

7 Discuss the kind of conduct that may be interpreted as sexually harassing. Should you tell a sexually explicit (dirty) joke to your classmates? Should you tease fellow students about their sexual conduct? Should you date a fellow student?

8 Discuss the sexual discrimination policy in your facility. Do you know to whom you should report sexual harassment?

9 Discuss the male mammographer situation. Would a questionnaire truly help minimize embarrassment for patients unwilling to have a male mammographer perform their study? Would it help eliminate embarrassment for the male mammographer as well? Discuss the ways in which a male mammographer may help put a patient at ease.

10 Do female imaging professionals face similar situations? Discuss, for instance, female nuclear medicine technologists who must perform testicular scans. What techniques could female technologists use to help put patients at ease?

11 Prepare a scenario illustrating an ethical imaging challenge that diversity issues influence. Discuss the questions raised by the scenario.

10 OVERVIEW OF NEW TECHNOLOGY AND FUTURE CHALLENGES

Far better it is to dare mighty things, to win glorious triumphs, even though checkered by failure, than to take rank with those poor spirits who neither enjoy much nor suffer much, because they live in the gray twilight that know not victory or defeat.

THEODORE ROOSEVELT

Chapter Outline

Ethical Issues
Imaging's Example for Health Care in the 21st Century
New Technologies
Biomedical Research
Imaging Professionals' Obligation to Research
Ethics of Interpretation of Imaging Procedures and Testing
Ethical Dilemmas of Transplants
New Reproductive Methods
Humane Genome Project

Continuous Quality Improvement and Quality Assurance
Advanced Education and Responsibility
Ethics Committees
Preparing for the Future
Legal Issues
Technologic Advances Causing Legal and Ethical Havoc
Law into the Future
Legal Issues with the Human Genome Project
New Technology and the Law for Imaging Professionals

Learning Objectives

After completing this chapter, the reader will be able to perform the following:

- Name a variety of ethical challenges for imaging professionals arising from the following areas:
  - New technology
  - Imaging's example for health care in the 21st century
  - Research methodology
  - Radiographic interpretation and testing
  - Transplant situations
  - New reproductive methods
  - Human Genome Project
  - Quality assurance
  - Newer levels of imaging professional education and responsibility

- Identify complex legal and ethical issues raised by changing technologies.
- State the liability issues associated with the new level of responsibility of the new position of radiologist assistant.
- Identify the inability of law to act proactively in changing technologic fields.
- Name the guidelines provided by professional organizations to aid in ethical decision making in controversial situations.
- State the importance of participation in professional organizations.

Key Terms

continuous quality improvement
ethics committee
Human Genome Project
radiologist assistant
Uniform Parentage Act

Professional Profile

The most exciting advance in medical imaging in the last decade has been the development of fusion imaging. This advanced application, in which information from imaging modalities is merged, has brought about new challenges and opportunities for imaging professionals. This new technology was developed after the use of computer techniques to fuse an image from two separately acquired imaging procedures failed to provide precise alignment of the two studies. Functional imaging using radiotracer imaging of single photon emission computed tomography (SPECT) and positron emission tomography (PET) has been expanding in use in recent years. Both SPECT/CT and PET/CT have provided unparalleled enhancement to give physicians both high-resolution anatomic images and functional information. When hybrid systems are used to combine SPECT/CT or PET/CT in one procedure, the exact alignment may be achieved. We stand on the threshold of Food and Drug Administration (FDA) approval of new radiotracers, which will bring about the availability of radiolabeled biomarkers that will provide more information about the physiologic status of disease.

As the first commercially available PET/CT and SPECT/CT systems were installed, the immediate questions of operator training, licensure, and competency arose. Who was trained, competent, and authorized to handle and administer the radiopharmaceuticals for the physiologic studies (PET and SPECT), and who was trained and certified and had demonstrated appropriate competencies to perform the CT part of the combined procedures?

Federal regulations administered by the Nuclear Regulatory Commission (NRC) authorize the licensed handling of radiopharmaceuticals for human administration. Such licensure is given to facilities, and administration of the radiopharmaceuticals must be under the authority of an appropriately trained physician. Under the direction of the physician, technologists may be authorized to prepare and administer radiopharmaceuticals. This license in some states is granted directly by the NRC. "Agreement states" administer licensing in compliance with NRC regulations. The control of radioactive materials should be safely provided through either mechanism. However, the training and authorization of technologists are not uniform in all states and currently are not required by federal regulations. In some states there are no license, training, or certification requirements for nuclear medicine technologists, other states impose restrictions on handling of radiopharmaceuticals by any radiologic technologist, and still others limit licensing only to nuclear medicine technologists certified either by the Nuclear Medicine Technology Certification Board (NMTCB) or by the American Registry of Radiologic Technologists (ARRT). Both of these certifying bodies also have specialty examinations; the NMTCB in general nuclear medicine or nuclear cardiology (NCT), or positron emission tomography (PET), and the ARRT with radiologic technology (RT), nuclear medicine (NM), computed tomography (CT), and other specialties. At this time no states require specialty certification in CT in order to perform CT studies. All states allow the performance of CT by radiologic technologists, as long as they have appropriately demonstrated competency that has been documented by their institution.

Most states have allowed nuclear medicine technologists to perform PET/CT and SPECT/CT as long as the studies are performed as a combined procedure. This is permitted because the nuclear medicine technologist has appropriate training in radiation safety and minimal training and competency measures are required to appropriately operate the CT portion of the system. Furthermore, the nuclear medicine technologist is not allowed to perform a diagnostic CT procedure by itself. Most nuclear medicine technologists are trained in college-based programs to be only nuclear medicine technologists and are not radiologic technologists before training in nuclear medicine. At this writing there has been a recent trend in a few states to prohibit nuclear medicine technologists from operating the CT, even for combined procedures, thus requiring either two people (a nuclear medicine technologist and a radiologic technologist) or one

Continued

individual with dual credentialing. This limits opportunities for nuclear medicine technologists or may require additional training and certification.

A 2002 Consensus Conference of several professional organizations determined that the number of dual-credentialed technologists was limited. The organizations formed a taskforce that developed a curriculum for core competencies for PET and CT. They also determined that credentialing pathways should be developed to allow nuclear medicine technologists to become eligible for the CT examination administered by the ARRT and for the CT and Radiation Therapy Technologist ARRT(T) to be eligible for the NMTCB(PET) examination. The shortest pathway for technologists to become dual credentialed was for the CNMT technologists to become CT certified. It was also recognized that the CNMT technologists have the most comprehensive scientific training.

Although dual certification pathways have been developed, few technologists have taken advantage of these opportunities to date. The limitation is most likely the time available in busy work schedules to create these opportunities, since few formal programs are available for full-time employees. However, state regulations continue to change rapidly, and practical and cost-effective utilization of appropriately qualified personnel is often not a consideration as rules are implemented.

The impact on patients from these regulatory changes has varied widely. In some states two technologists must be present to perform the procedure, one nuclear medicine/PET technologist and one radiologic technologist. The sole purpose of the radiologic technologist is to set up and start the CT portion of the study. This affects the cost of patient care because of the increased personnel requirement and makes the whole imaging procedure less time efficient, since the radiologic technologist will also have other duties.

The technology of hybrid SPECT/CT and PET/CT is expanding at a rapid rate. There is a continued increase in the number of these imaging devices being installed as institutions want the latest systems and technology. In all of the complex facets that drive hybrid imaging, the bottom line is that appropriately trained, certified, and competent individuals should provide safe and technically accurate imaging procedures.

Note: Current examination criteria are defined on the websites www.arrt.org and www.nmtcb.org.

Paul E. Christian, BS, CNMT, FSNMTS, PET
Director
Cyclotron Radiochemistry Laboratory
and PET/CT Imaging
Huntsman Cancer Institute
University of Utah

ETHICAL ISSUES

The previous chapters of this text have discussed ethical concepts, theories, and common problems faced by imaging and radiation science professionals. However, the problems discussed are not the only ethical dilemmas encountered by these health care professionals. Moreover, as the imaging profession and medical technology evolve, imaging professionals will face intense new ethical problems requiring strong problem-solving skills. Considerations of new technologies, research methodology, new reproductive methods, testing, transplant situations, quality assurance, and advanced levels of education and responsibility require that professionals have ethical awareness of the possible abuses and controversies so they can provide the best possible patient care.

Imaging and radiation science professionals should be prepared to encounter a variety of new difficulties on the path to ethical problem solving. This chapter offers a brief overview of ethical areas in which they may become involved.

IMAGING'S EXAMPLE FOR HEALTH CARE IN THE 21ST CENTURY

Former Speaker of the House Newt Gingrich, founder of the Center for Health Transformation, and Robert Egge, director of the Accelerating Health Innovation Project at the center, recognize the need for transforming the American health system for the 21st century. They explain that Hurricane Katrina is an example of how ineffectively the health care system functioned and that rebuilding a better system is imperative. Gingrich and Egge further explain[1]:

> Radiology is one area where new technologies are rapidly emerging that could dramatically impact the rebuilding effort. Take, for example, the interventional radiology, in which scalpels are replaced by imaging-based procedures. These procedures typically require little or no anesthesia and much less cutting of skin, muscle or other tissues, resulting in less blood loss, shorter hospital stays, shorter recovery time and less expense.

Radiologic imaging is central to another health care trend that should be strongly encouraged: the move toward a greater emphasis on prevention and early detection. Steadily improving imaging technologies will allow health care professionals to identify emerging conditions earlier and with greater accuracy than ever before, enabling intervention when it is least costly and least invasive and has the greatest likelihood of success. These innovations in radiology and imaging are the kinds of development that will transform the health system.

NEW TECHNOLOGIES

Numerous new technologies have been developed and have become valuable tools in diagnosis and treatment. No sooner has a new technique, a new modality, or a new combination of existing modalities hit the headlines than yet another exciting imaging innovation has claimed its place. As a new technology is born, so are the ethical and sometimes legal complications (Table 10-1). These complications or dilemmas will call for critical thinking and problem solving as imaging professionals recognize that new technologies provide new information that requires new and sometimes difficult decisions for the professional and the consumer. Decisions concerning wellness, research, early detection, archiving, monitoring of disease processes, prediction of future health problems, and lulling of consumers into a false sense of security may complicate ethical and legal issues.

BIOMEDICAL RESEARCH

Imaging professionals may be employed by institutions that conduct research on human beings. Certain imaging examinations such as chest radiographs, high-speed radiographs, and nuclear scans may be performed on experimental subjects to ascertain the effect of experimental drugs or treatments. Ethical dilemmas may arise if imaging specialists are concerned about the ways in which subjects are influenced to consent to the research study. Imaging specialists may also wonder whether the risks taken by experimental subjects are justified by the possible benefits to society.

Research can be expensive. To be considered ethical and justified, the expense involved should produce good proportionate to the evils risked.

TABLE 10-1 **NEW TECHNOLOGY OR NEW USES FOR OLDER TECHNOLOGY**

New Technology or New Use	Imaging Ability
Positron emission tomography	Detection of Alzheimer's disease
Magnetic resonance imaging	
Real time	Assessment of beating fetal heart
3D	Detection of pancreatic cancer
Diffusion	Prediction of cancer progress
Contrast enhanced	Detection of breast cancer
Computed tomography	
Full body	Diagnostic overview
Multislice	Complement to coronary angiography
Ultrasound	
Obstetric	Diagnostic and commercial
High intensity focused	Gene therapy and tumor destruction
Multimodality fusion imaging (positron emission tomography and single photon emission computed tomography)	Stem cell tracking and monitoring
Virtual colonoscopy	Diagnostic
Molecular imaging	Monitoring of disease treatments; detection of diseases in early development; tracking of effectiveness of new drugs
Nuclear medicine/cardiovascular	Visualization of heart damage up to 30 hours after brief interruption of blood or oxygen
Fusion picture archiving and communications (PACs)	Archiving of imaging information; multiple media options; more effective information access for health care providers and consumers

IMAGING PROFESSIONALS' OBLIGATION TO RESEARCH

Imaging professionals have an obligation to the profession to maintain current knowledge and be critically aware of future technology and trends. Such maintenance and education require imaging professionals to read scientific journals and practice proper research methods. While reviewing various research materials, imaging professionals must analyze the data and practice critical thinking (see Box 1-2).

Imaging professionals concerned with respect and stature in the health care community should consider the options available to them to encourage others to perceive them more positively. They should educate others about the profession and describe the creative and innovative processes they have undertaken and completed. Moreover, they should expend the extra effort to describe their findings and experiences in established journals. Imaging educators should encourage or even require their students to perform and present research; unfortunately, the imaging sciences lag behind medicine and nursing in research and publishing. Professional journals, periodicals, and organizations are eager for imaging professionals and students to submit work. Given this desire for information and education, imaging professionals must look to the future and promote the recognition of the imaging sciences.[2]

ETHICS OF INTERPRETATION OF IMAGING PROCEDURES AND TESTING

Imaging procedures in all modalities require interpretation. Many imaging professionals have observed differences of opinion between radiologists and physicians concerning the characteristics of a high-quality image. A physician in the urgent care clinic may see a fracture and begin treatment for it. A radiologist may look at the same image and read it as negative. Such fallibility of interpretation may cause technologists to become involved in litigation.

Other imaging professionals may be asked by physicians or emergency personnel to make judgment calls concerning the outcome of tests or imaging procedures. Although the imaging technologist may believe that an image clearly shows a fractured bone, basing treatment for a fracture on the opinion of a professional who is not a radiologist may be unfair to the patient and become the source of litigation.

A less common dilemma encountered by imaging professionals occurs when they know or at least perceive that a test has been misinterpreted. Such a situation raises the question of the responsibilities a technologist has to a patient who has an unrecognized condition, perhaps a fracture, and is being sent home from the emergency

IMAGING SCENARIO

A radiographer who was hired only recently is called to the morgue to take a series of skull radiographs on a body for forensic evaluation. The county medical examiner is present and remarks that no evidence on the films indicates foul play. The radiographer, however, notes an unnatural line on the basal skull projection. The new employee is afraid to say anything to the medical examiner and thus waits until the next day to talk to the radiologist. The radiologist reads the examination as positive for fracture, but he is not inclined to call the medical examiner because they have had a previous confrontation. He does ask why the radiographer did not point out the suspicious line to the examiner. The radiographer explains that he did not believe he was qualified to interpret films. After the medical examiner receives the radiologist's report, he is furious because he has already released the body and it has been cremated. The medical examiner corners the radiographer later that same day and asks him directly if he noticed the fracture line. The radiographer admits with a great deal of hesitation that he saw the fracture. The medical examiner accuses the radiographer of negligence and explains that if the person had been killed, the murderer would go unpunished. The family of the deceased, after being informed by an anonymous source, later sues the medical examiner, radiologist, and radiographer.

Discussion questions
- Who was to blame?
- What alternatives were available to the individuals involved?
- Should all three health care providers have been sued?
- What ethical theory would provide the best tool for answering these ethical questions? Why?
- What would you have done? (Remember, this person was a new employee.)

IMAGING SCENARIO

An imaging professional employed by a major oil company is responsible for producing radiographic images of a newly placed pipeline. As the professional surveys the results of his latest work, he notices a crack in the pipeline along with several other imaging artifacts. He approaches his supervisor with the information. The supervisor, who is being pressured by the company's owners to expedite the process to save time and money, questions the results of the study.

The questionable findings are pigeonholed on the supervisor's desk. The imaging professional decides to go to the company's owners and share his concerns. Before he can keep this appointment, his employment is terminated because of the quality of his work and he is denied references.

Discussion questions
- What would the next step be for the industrial technologist?
- What values are in conflict?
- In what way do ethical and legal issues influence this situation?

room. The risks to the patient outweigh the risks to the imaging professional, indicating that the professional should intervene. This intervention may require little more than questioning a line on the cervical body. Imaging professionals who intervene on behalf of a patient in what they believe is the patient's best interest may put themselves at risk. If the benefits outweigh the risks, however, imaging professionals may choose to intervene.

Imaging has a role in nonmedical testing and industrial testing as well. These noninvasive tests involve evaluating pipelines, casting, and fittings for their strength and structure. Other types of radiographic testing include forensic radiography on human subjects or objects to solve crimes. Archaeological imaging has been used in examining mummified remains and exploring artifacts of previous civilizations. Imaging studies of art objects have proved invaluable in discovering forgeries. Truthfulness and disclosure are as important in these nonmedical imaging areas as they are in medical imaging practice.

ETHICAL DILEMMAS OF TRANSPLANTS

Imaging professionals may find themselves involved with patients and families awaiting organ transplants; they may also have contact with donors and their families. The events surrounding organ transplantation are often emotional and must be handled with empathy and ethical awareness (Box 10-1).

BOX 10-1   **CONSIDERATIONS IN TRANSPLANT ETHICS**

Obtaining of appropriate informed consent
Respectful empathy for the precarious emotional state of patients and families
Provision of high-quality care to donor and recipient

The AMA Council on Ethical and Judicial Affairs has outlined three principal ethical concerns of the physician and health care team—including the radiographer[2]:

1. Full discussion of the proposed procedure with the donor and recipient or responsible relatives or representatives is mandatory. The physician should be objective in discussing the procedure, disclosing known risks and possible hazards, and advising of the alternative procedures available. The physician should not encourage expectations beyond those justified by the circumstances. The physician's interest in advancing scientific knowledge must always be secondary to the primary concern for the patient.
2. The transplantation of body organs should be undertaken only by physicians who possess special medical knowledge and technical competence developed through special training, study, and laboratory experience and practice. Transplants must take place in medical institutions with facilities adequate to protect the health and well-being of the parties to the procedure.
3. Transplantation of body organs should be undertaken only after careful evaluation of the availability and effectiveness of other possible therapy.

Ethical concerns raised by transplant situations involve the obtaining of informed consent, the avoidance of playing on the emotions of the families and patients involved, the proposal of any viable alternatives, the provision of appropriate care to brain-dead

IMAGING SCENARIO

A young man suffering massive head trauma from a motorcycle accident is brought to the emergency room. He is unresponsive and has a flat electroencephalogram. A nuclear study is ordered as a necessary criterion to determine brain death.

In the same hospital a young woman lies in dire need of a liver. She may die within the next few days if she does not receive a transplant. The family of the young man wants to do everything possible to keep him alive, but the nuclear study reveals an absence of brain function. The family is approached by various hospital personnel to consider donating the young man's organs. The family, however, is unwilling to suspend life support and donate the organs. The nuclear technologist feels comfortable enough with the young man's family to discuss organ donation with them. When family members question the technologist, she is tempted to use every method possible to convince them that their son will not recover and they should donate his organs.

Discussion questions
- Whose purpose is the nuclear technologist serving—that of the patient, the woman needing a liver, or her own conscience?
- What are ethical implications of harvesting the organs from a body still functioning on life support?
- When does death occur?
- When has all hope been exhausted?
- Whose hope is more important—that of the family of the potential donor or that of the potential recipient?

donors even if a transplant is anticipated, and above all the maintenance of basic protections for donors and patients[3]:

> In the face of the shortage of organs and the urgency of many situations, there are proposals to increase the supply of organs by improving the recruitment of volunteers and by changing the legal requirements for surrogate consent. The methods proposed pose their own ethical problems.

Nuclear medicine personnel may certainly find themselves involved in transplant situations. Nuclear medicine involves the injection of radioactive materials into the body. Pathologic changes may be discovered through the observation of images of the radioactive material's uptake, use, and excretion by the body. Nuclear medicine technologists are often involved in obtaining images of brain function and may be involved in the determination of brain death.

NEW REPRODUCTIVE METHODS

Ultrasonographers tend to be more involved with the ethical dilemmas presented by new reproductive methods than are other imaging specialists. Infertility treatments have progressed tremendously over the past several years, and ultrasonographers currently play an important role in such procedures. Ultrasonography allows the visualization of the follicles. Doppler studies indicate blood flow to the ovum. Other imaging professionals take part in certain procedures used for diagnosing infertility, such as hysterosalpingography and urethrograms.

A number of ethical dilemmas arise from new reproductive methods (Box 10-2). Each of these dilemmas must be studied in depth and addressed on its own merits; this overview does not undertake this task. Imaging professionals involved in these controversies would benefit from a personal study of reproductive method ethics.

Imaging professionals should participate in medically indicated diagnostic procedures as long as the appropriate informed consent procedures have been employed. However, they should be wary of the possible abuses of new technologies, and they have a right to refuse to take part in frivolous or cavalier procedures.

Imaging professionals also have a right not to participate in procedures they do not condone such as abortions. If imaging professionals are aware that part of their employment practice involves providing this type of care, however, they need to determine whether they should provide this service or seek employment elsewhere. In addition, they should not place themselves in the position of deciding whether a patient should have such a procedure.

BOX 10-2 **ETHICAL DILEMMAS IN ASSISTED REPRODUCTION**

Artificial insemination
Surrogate mothers
Risks to mother and child
Donor concealment and the right to privacy
In vitro fertilization
Embryo transfers
Charges of artificiality
Use of frozen embryos and sperm banks
Reimbursement for surrogacy and donation of eggs and sperm

IMAGING SCENARIO

A sonographer has been working with a couple for the treatment of infertility. In the course of their relationship over the preceding 10 months, the sonographer has become close to the couple. Unfortunately, after 10 months of treatment, the couple's chances of pregnancy appear slim.

In the eleventh month of treatment, fertilization is successful and an embryo is formed. The couple and sonographer are overjoyed. The waiting and hoping are over. The thousands of dollars—almost their entire savings—have paid off. If anyone deserves this miracle, they do. They have had an exceptionally difficult time with the procedures and have been emotionally spent for nearly a year.

Genetic testing of the embryo reveals a problem. A few missing chromosomes have left a pattern that indicates the child may be born with Williams' syndrome. This condition produces mild to severe mental retardation, and genetic testing cannot predict the level of impairment. Williams' syndrome also entails health problems such as heart abnormalities and organ dysfunctions.

The physician discusses the situation with the couple, and they are devastated. He encourages them to abort and try again.

When the couple arrives for a sonographic examination to determine fetal age, they share the unhappy news with the sonographer, who is dismayed by their consideration of abortion. The sonographer has a younger brother with Williams' syndrome and loves him very much. His interactions with his brother have made him aware of both the difficulties and the joys of having a special brother. When the couple asks him for his opinion, he must decide whether to share his personal experiences with them.

Discussion questions
- How much of his personal life should the sonographer share?
- Will the couple's care be compromised if the sonographer's remarks contradict those of the physician?
- Can the couple emotionally and financially afford the abortive procedure and another attempt to produce an embryo?
- Should they take their chances with the fetus they have?
- Should they consider adoption?
- How would you deal with this situation if you were the sonographer?

HUMAN GENOME PROJECT

According to the Human Genome Project Information website, the **Human Genome Project** (HGP), completed in 2003, was a 13-year project coordinated by the U.S. Department of Energy and the National Institutes of Health. The project goals were to identify all the approximately 20,000 to 25,000 genes in human DNA, determine the sequences of the 3 billion chemical base pairs that make up human DNA, store this information in databases, improve tools for data analysis, transfer related technologies to the private sector, and address the ethical, legal, and social issues (ELSI) that could arise from the project. Although the HGP is completed, analyses of the data will continue for many years and possibly affect imaging professionals. This may occur through

HUMAN GENOME PROJECT
The Human Genome Project was undertaken to identify human DNA genes, determine the makeup of human genes, store this information, improve tools for data gathering, transfer the information to the private sector, and address ethical, legal, and social issues that may arise from the project.

interaction with patients involved in genetic testing and research or within the biotechnology industry as new medical applications are developed.[4]

The U.S. Department of Energy (DOE) and the National Institutes of Health (NIH) devoted 3% to 5% of their annual HGP budgets toward studying the ELSI surrounding availability of genetic information. This represents the world's largest bioethics program, which has become a model for ELSI programs around the world. This bioethics program will consider fairness in the use of genetic information, who owns and controls this information, the psychologic impact and stigmatization resulting from an individual's genetic differences, reproductive issues, clinical issues, uncertainty of gene tests, conceptual and philosophical implications, health and environmental issues, and the commercialization of products developed as a result of the HGP.[4]

CONTINUOUS QUALITY IMPROVEMENT AND QUALITY ASSURANCE

Continuous quality improvement and quality assurance are important terms for the imaging professional to remember. The growing emphasis on the maintenance and improvement of quality of care has influenced the ethics of problem solving. The incorporation of problem-solving methods into quality assurance programs has produced the management philosophy of total quality improvement. By gathering data and analyzing trends, **continuous quality improvement** programs seek to anticipate problems and improve the environment before problems arise.

The need for quality improvement programs is clear[5]:

> A test result lost, a specialist who cannot be reached, a missing requisition, a misinterpreted order, duplicate paperwork, a vanished record, a long wait for the CT scan, an unreliable on-call system—these are all-too-familiar examples of waste, rework, complexity, and error in the doctor's daily life. … For the average doctor, quality fails when systems fail.

The same holds true for all health care providers, including imaging professionals. Quality assurance and quality improvement programs focus on the best interests of patients. Imaging professionals can aid in this patient-focused striving for quality care by enhancing their ethical awareness and problem-solving skills. The combination of quality improvement programs with professional ethics allows imaging departments to serve the needs of both patients and organizations. For more information and practical methods, Dr. Jeffrey Papp's *Quality Management in the Imaging Technologies* offers an in-depth examination of continuous quality as it applies to all modalities in the imaging sciences.[6] The Joint Commission on Accreditation of Healthcare Organizations has established quality assurance guidelines that are not only appropriate and useful for the health care organization at the administrative level, but also valuable for the imaging department and the imaging professional. These guidelines serve as a model for critical thinking and problem solving (Box 10-3).

ADVANCED EDUCATION AND RESPONSIBILITY

Not only is the technology of imaging and the radiation sciences growing, changing, and evolving, but imaging and radiation sciences professionals are also experiencing growth, change, and evolution. To meet the demands of such a rapidly changing health care environment, more and more imaging professionals are seeking advanced certifications and advanced degrees. The **radiologist assistant** (RA) position has taken its place

CONTINUOUS QUALITY IMPROVEMENT
The aspect of quality assurance that monitors technical equipment to maintain quality standards.

RADIOLOGIST ASSISTANT
A radiologist assistant is an advanced level radiologic technologist who works under the supervision of a radiologist to enhance patient care by assisting the radiologist in a diagnostic imaging environment.

BOX 10-3	JCAHO QUALITY ASSURANCE GUIDELINES

Assign responsibility
Delineate scope of care and services
Identify important aspects of care and services
Identify indicators of outcome (no less than two; no more than four)
Establish thresholds for evaluation
Collect data
Evaluate data
Take action
Assess action taken
Communicate

From Joint Commission on Accreditation of Healthcare Organizations: *The accreditation manual for hospitals,* Oak Brook, Ill, 1991, Author.

in the imaging environment. The RA will be the physician's assistant in the imaging environment. According to the American Society of Radiologic Technologists (ASRT), the RA has three main areas of responsibility[7]:

First, the RA takes a leading role in patient management and assessment. Duties in this area might include determining whether a patient has been appropriately prepared for a procedure, obtaining patient consent prior to beginning the examination, answering questions from the patient and his or her family, and adapting exam protocols to improve diagnostic quality. The radiologist assistant also is expected to serve as a patient advocate, ensuring that each patient receives quality care while in the radiology department or clinic.

Second. The radiologist assistant performs selected radiology examinations and procedures under the supervision of a radiologist. The level of radiologist supervision varies, depending on the type of exam.

And third, the RA may be responsible for evaluating image quality, making initial image observations and forwarding those observations to the supervising radiologist. The supervising radiologist remains responsible for providing a final written report, an interpretation or a diagnosis.

As imaging professionals assume more responsibility for diagnostic examinations and patient care, it is easy to recognize the many ethical and legal dilemmas in which they may become entangled. The patient may look to these professionals as "the doctor" and have certain expectations. The imaging professional may not ethically or legally be able to meet these expectations. Issues regarding reports, informed consent, diagnosis, and ordering of examinations may be areas of concern.

ETHICS COMMITTEES

Many institutions have an **ethics committee** composed of physicians, chaplains, administrative personnel, and employees from various departments. Legal representatives may also be involved. These committees serve as problem-solving and decision-making bodies. When an ethical dilemma arises that cannot be resolved at a personal or departmental level, the committee chooses a course of action based on its best

ETHICS COMMITTEE
An ethics committee is composed of a variety of institutional personnel who identify values and make the best decision possible for all parties involved.

IMAGING SCENARIO

The year is 2026, and the imaging center is bustling with activity. As the imaging supervisor reviews the day's procedures and determines the units to activate, the patients are aligned for entrance into the imaging dome. The dome was recently leased from the sole provider of imaging equipment. After managed care led to monopolies for technology providers and the federal government intervened to regulate health care costs, equipment purchases became much less time consuming and often less expensive.

Robotic units gently transport the patients as their audio programs explain the procedures, obtain informed consent, and install the patients in the imaging dome, a small room containing all the necessary scanning and recording equipment. As patients enter the room, their vital signs are recorded. Within 60 seconds the machinery performs a total-body scan, including laboratory scanning. The scanned images are relayed to the master reader at the state capital, and the images and reports are sent to the physicians' and patients' personal modems within a few seconds.

All imaging is noninvasive and nonionizing. Thermal, ultrasound, and magnetic imaging are used simultaneously as patients revolve on a platform in the imaging dome, and projections are made at every conceivable angle. All procedures involve total-body imaging so that all patient information is provided and patients do not have the ability to conceal any health information the federal imaging center might find useful to determine the patient's treatment needs.

The first group of patients for the day are cloned specimens to be evaluated for transplant fitness. The second group are geriatric patients. Because the prescribed life expectancy is 120 years, geriatric patients are evaluated for the euthanasia program. The next group of patients are pregnant women whose fetuses are to be studied to determine viability. Fetuses determined to be unfit for mental or physical reasons are aborted and used for organ transplants. Patients with traumatic injuries are evaluated with portable domes and triaged to determine cost benefits.

As the imaging supervisor completes the last of the day's procedures, she remembers that she has a meeting of the ethical and legal issues committee at the capital center.

Discussion questions
- What sort of issues would be discussed at such a meeting?
- In what ways have the ethical and legal issues changed since the 20th century?
- Why have these changes occurred?
- In what ways do ethics and law change with technology?

collaborative judgment of what ought to be done. This decision takes into account institutional values, personal values, and the moral meaning of the situation to all parties involved.

Imaging professionals may become involved in ethics committees, especially when ethical dilemmas present themselves in the imaging environment.

PREPARING FOR THE FUTURE

The future of the imaging and radiation sciences holds immense promise and challenge. The professional must be able to adapt and meet change as an opportunity. Ceela McElveny, ASRT Director of Communication, addresses this issue in a special report in the November/December 2005 issue of *Radiologic Technology*[8]:

> By now, radiologic technologists have become experts at incorporating change into their workplaces. All-digital workflow? Check. Sixty-four slice CT? Check. ACR facility accreditation? Check and double check. But the more rapid the rate of change, the more difficult it becomes to adapt. The introduction of molecular Imaging and fusion technology has accelerated the pace of change in the radiologic sciences and soon could leave technologists racing to keep up.
>
> To succeed in this chaotic environment, the R.T. workforce must be able to foresee change, be willing to make adjustments and be willing to evolve. As Charles Darwin wrote, "It is not the strongest species that survive, nor the most intelligent, but the ones most responsive to change." Substitute the word "professions" for "species," and you have a powerful argument for why the R.T. work force must continuously anticipate and adapt to change. It is a matter of survival.

LEGAL ISSUES

The effect of new technologies on imaging professionals will be varied and currently is largely unknown. Imaging professionals are and will continue to be involved in new developments in technology, although the nature of that involvement is difficult to predict.

Recently developed technologies are increasingly becoming the standard for diagnosis and treatment. These include "virtual" CT colonoscopy,[9] 64-slice CT,[10] coronary CT angiography,[10] hybrid PET/CT angiography,[11] PET brain amyloid imaging for diagnosis of presymptomatic dementia (particularly Alzheimer's disease),[12] prenatal ultrasound for detection of chromosomal abnormalities,[13] imaging used in the assessment of therapeutic drug research,[14] genetic testing and its impact on breast cancer detection by mammography and other imaging procedures,[4] and the use of sonography in the ever-changing arena of assisted reproduction, to name a few. As readers may gather from this list, the possibilities in the imaging field are ever expanding. This section discusses the current state of law surrounding some of these advances, how the courts deal with new and uncharted ground with these new technologies, and how these advances will affect imaging professionals.

TECHNOLOGIC ADVANCES CAUSING LEGAL AND ETHICAL HAVOC

The implications of emerging technologies for humankind could be profound. Examples are cloning, genetic testing that reveals everything about a person's present and future physical condition, the ability to choose whether a child will have green eyes or will be a superior athlete, and solutions for the shortage of transplantable organs.

The legal and ethical issues are astounding. What legal rights would a human clone have? Is he or she able to give informed consent? Should people be cloned to supplement the supply of transplantable organs? Do employers and insurance companies have a right to the results of genetic testing that may show that a person is prone to disease? Do human beings have the right to genetically engineer a child with certain physical attributes or talents? Do they have the right to dispose selectively of preembryos or abort embryos that do not have the desired characteristics?

Should it make a difference to the nuclear medicine technologist that the patient is a clone? Does a clone have a right to informed consent? Does it bother the ultrasonographer that he or she is assisting in the abortion of a fetus because it does not have the genes to excel in sports, be a rocket scientist, or have green eyes?

The future, the unknown world of advancing technology, may be a frightening place. It is a place in which ethics and law need to interact to make some difficult choices. The law cannot be proactive to determine what is right for humankind in this world of advancing technology. Instead, imaging professionals must rely on themselves as members of the scientific community and professional organizations to examine the ethical issues created by each advance and give professional groups input to help make those tough choices.

Future changes in technology will have a great impact on imaging professionals (Figure 10-1). They must look to the scientific community and its professional organizations to help form laws protecting the dignity of human life. The professional organizations that represent the imaging sciences are an important part of this scientific community.

Imaging professionals have the responsibility to remain aware of advances in technology. They must take an active role in the organizations representing the profession to address the legal and ethical implications of new technologies. All the answers for the future are not available. The next section, however, attempts to explain how the law is formed for future technologies and the proactive role the imaging professional should play in this process.

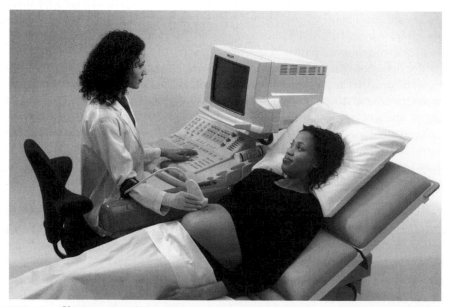

FIGURE 10-1 Keeping up with technologic advances is every imaging professional's responsibility. Courtesy Sound Ergonomics, Kenmore, Wash.

LAW INTO THE FUTURE

Technology is changing at such a rapid rate that the scenario described below may not be all that implausible. With these ever-changing technologies come legal dilemmas that are difficult to deal with on the future level. Where does the law of the future originate? With technology advancing rapidly, legislatures cannot possibly foresee all the consequences of that technology and make appropriate statutory changes to deal with them. Judicial decisions are always based on a set of facts that have *already* occurred and so are of little assistance in evaluating new technologies and the influence they have on human life. Where then, do the courts look for guidance? If clear legal opinions are not available, policies developed by professional medical organizations are often used as guidelines.

Many professional organizations exist within the medical community. These include national, state, and local organizations, made up almost exclusively of volunteers from their profession who dedicate tremendous amounts of their time for the betterment of patients. Members of these organizations spend countless hours grappling with ethical and legal consequences of the technological advances of their particular specialties. Legislatures turn to these organizations for guidance in drafting legislation, and courts often look to them for guidance when attempting to sort out issues that never before existed.

Reproductive Law and the Future

One such example of the guidance available to legislators is the **Uniform Parentage Act**, drafted in 2000 and amended in 2002.[15] This act was a combination of the Uniform Parentage Act of 1973, which was adopted in some form in most states, and the Status of Children of Assisted Conception Act. The new act, although highly controversial, has been adopted in some form in many states. The purpose of this model act was to give guidance for the many legal issues associated with assisted reproduction.

It is now technologically possible to take the sperm from one source and the ovum from another, place the subsequently developed embryo in the uterus of a third person, and have the child brought up by two biologically unrelated persons. This raises the possibility of the child's having five parents.[15] The goal of the act is to provide such a child with certainty as to his or her legal parentage (Box 10-4).

UNIFORM PARENTAGE ACT
The Uniform Parentage Act was drafted in 2000, amended in 2002, and adopted in some form in many states, with the purpose of giving guidance for the many legal issues associated with assisted reproduction.

IMAGING SCENARIO

An ad in a metropolitan paper announces the new body scan available at a local imaging facility. This "total-body scan" would provide a "total picture" of the participant's health status. One of the persons responding to this ad believes he has been given a "clean bill of health." Several months later, this person receives a diagnosis of pancreatic cancer. The consumer files suit against the imaging facility, physicians, and imaging specialists involved.

Discussion questions
- What are the ethical and legal dilemmas involved in this situation?
- Is this total-body scan a step toward wellness imaging, or is it providing a less than sound "clean bill of health"?

BOX 10-4 **REPRODUCTIVE LAW IN THE COURTS**

An example of the guidance used by the courts is the case of *Davis v Davis*.[16] This was the first case involving a preembryo (the product that results when an egg is fertilized by a sperm in a laboratory setting). In this case the preembryos were frozen, the couple subsequently divorced, and a battle ensued over who, if anyone, should have custody of the frozen preembryos. The court sought guidance from the American Fertility Society and adopted their view that because of the potential of a preembryo to become a person, special respect is due.[16] The court thus recognized that the donors of the genetic material have an interest in the preembryos to the extent that they have decision-making authority concerning the disposition of the preembryos.

The guidance of the medical community is invaluable to legislators and courts. In the legal arena of the future, where the usual statutes and precedents have little application, the knowledge and input of the medical community are the best source of information available. Professional organizations, most of which involve physicians and other health care workers who voluntarily give their time to these efforts, have the burden of monitoring technologic advances from an ethical standpoint to ensure that technology is used for good.

LEGAL ISSUES WITH THE HUMAN GENOME PROJECT

As discussed earlier, because of the research of the Human Genome Project, genetic disposition to various diseases and conditions can now be anticipated. While this is a wonderful breakthrough in medicine, it creates enormous ethical and legal issues. A few issues are discussed here, such as whether genetic testing can be required by employers, employment decisions can be based on this information, and insurance companies can require and use this information as a basis for coverage decisions.

In an effort to deal with some of the issues, the National Action Plan on Breast Cancer (NAPBC) and the National Institute of Health (NIH)–Department of Energy (DOE) Working Group on the Ethical, Legal, and Social Implications (ELSI) of human genome research issued a report in 1998. After this report the Clinton administration announced recommendations for future legislation to ensure that discoveries made possible by the Human Genome Project are used to improve health and not to discriminate against workers or their families. These recommendations include the following[4]:

- Employers should not require or request that employees or potential employees take a genetic test or provide genetic information as a condition of employment or benefits.
- Employers should not use genetic information to discriminate against, limit, segregate, or classify employees in a way that would deprive them of employment opportunities.
- Employers should not obtain or disclose genetic information about employees or potential employees under most circumstances.

While these recommendations sound reasonable, legislation at the federal level is necessary to make sure that they are carried out, in particular to ensure that discrimination in the workplace based on genetic information cannot occur. The possibility exists for employers to avoid hiring workers who they believe are likely to take sick leave, resign, or retire early for health reasons. Cost consequences are generally the consideration with

IMAGING SCENARIO

You are a mammographer in a busy metropolitan hospital. Your current patient, a 35-year-old woman, tells you that she is very concerned about breast cancer, enough to refer herself and pay out of pocket for this mammogram even though her doctor said she did not need one yet because of her age, the absence of physical symptoms of a problem, and her having no family history of breast cancer. Her concern is based on the breast cancer that devastated and eventually took the life of her best friend from high school. Her question to you is whether or not she should have genetic testing to determine if she has the gene to predispose her to breast cancer.

Discussion questions
• Do you answer the patient's question? If so, how?
• What are the possible implications if she has this testing?
• Is it your responsibility to share that information with her?

the incentive to discriminate based on genetic information likely to increase with future advances in genetic research.[4]

In addition, although some federal and state legislation applies to employment discrimination based on genetic testing, there are substantial gaps at both levels. Therefore federal legislation is needed to ensure that advances in genetic technology and research are used to address the health needs of the nation—and not to deny individuals employment opportunities and benefits. Federal legislation would establish minimum protections that could be supplemented by state laws.[4]

At this time insurers can use genetic information in the individual market to make decisions about coverage, enrollment, and premiums. Insurers can still require individuals to take genetic tests, and individuals are not protected from the disclosure of genetic information to insurers, plan sponsors (employers), and medical information bureaus, without their consent. While statutes of the Health Insurance and Accountability Act (HIPAA) contain penalties for discrimination and disclosure, they should be strengthened to ensure individuals of the protections intended by the HIPAA legislation.[4]

NEW TECHNOLOGY AND THE LAW FOR IMAGING PROFESSIONALS

Without doubt, technologic advances will affect imaging professionals. Some imaging fields will become obsolete, and some may be absorbed into other imaging fields. Examples include nuclear medicine and the fusion between PET imaging and CT,[10] as well as between coronary angiography and CT.[11] To survive in this constantly changing world of imaging, the imaging professional must be open to change.

Imaging professionals must be cautious about the standards of care of evolving technologies. They must be concerned with whether the new technologies and associated duties expected from imaging professionals fit within their scope of practice. The most reliable source for this information is the professional organization, easily accessible on the Web and providing a wealth of up-to-date information. Imaging professionals have the responsibility to be proactive when new technologies are introduced. They should read about new technologies and equipment, ask questions of vendors and radiologists,

IMAGING SCENARIO

Your busy department was the first in the city to hire a certified radiologist assistant (RA). She has been on the job for almost a year, and although it took some time with some of the radiologists, they now depend on her to help the department operate more efficiently. The RA fields patients' questions, makes sure patients are properly prepped, checks the quality of films before they go to the radiologist for reading, and generally makes things flow more smoothly so the technologists can do their jobs and the radiologists can do theirs. Sometimes the RA performs nasogastric tube placements, does some fluoroscopic examinations for noninvasive procedures, and performs some venous sticks for contrast injection. Her job is particularly important in making the department run smoothly, and she is quite busy when one of the radiologists is on vacation, as one is now.

The RA unfortunately has contracted food poisoning at a local seafood restaurant, causing her and several other patrons to become emergency room patients the previous night. It is obvious that she cannot perform her job, and the department is swamped. You have been a technologist in the department for several years, and the radiologist on duty insists that because you have assisted both him and the RA numerous times, you can place a nasogastric tube under fluoroscopic guidance.

Discussion questions
- What do you do?
- What are the legal implications of your performing this procedure?
- What issues should concern you?

and seek out the information they need to ensure that they know the standards of care and are properly trained. They must also be aware of whether performing a new technology is within their scope of practice.

The new position of radiologist assistant (RA) is an area of concern. As discussed previously, the RA is an advanced-level radiologic technologist who works under the supervision of a radiologist to enhance patient care by assisting the radiologist in a diagnostic imaging environment.[17] The RA must have completed an academic program (bachelor's degree or higher) that teaches an RA curriculum endorsed by the American College of Radiology (ACR) and the ASRT and have passed the certification examination administered by the ASRT. Many states have now recognized the designation of RA and have defined the RA's scope of practice in accordance with the guidelines adopted by the ACR, ASRT, and ARRT. Certified RAs must know their scope of practice and be careful to stay within that scope.

Imaging professionals not certified as RAs may be asked to perform some of the same duties for which a certified RA is qualified. They should remember that when performing any duty with regard to imaging, they will be held to the same standard as a person trained for that specialty.

This is indeed an exciting and changing time for the imaging profession. Imaging professionals should embrace the changes but must be vigilant because imaging as previously known has been and will be forever altered by new technology.

SUMMARY

- Rapid technologic development presents imaging professionals with a variety of ethical dilemmas, such as those arising from research methodology, new reproductive methods, radiographic interpretation and testing, transplant situations, quality assurance, and advanced educational levels.
- New technologies and new uses for already existing technologies and modalities have arisen, and research continues into diagnostic radiography, high-speed radiography, nuclear medicine, and other areas.
- New reproductive methods have created a host of ethical dilemmas. Ultrasonographers are confronted with these situations more often than are other imaging professionals.
- Radiographers performing diagnostic radiography may become involved in situations involving physicians' misinterpretation of radiographic examinations.
- Organ transplant situations produce ethical dilemmas involving death and dying, informed consent, the offering of alternative treatments, the appropriate expression of empathy for families, and protection and adequate treatment for patients and donors.
- The goals of the Human Genome Project were to identify human DNA genes, determine the makeup of human genes, store this information, improve tools for data gathering, transfer the information to the private sector, and address the ethical, legal, and social issues that may arise from the project.
- Quality control and continuous quality improvement focus on the ethics of problem solving.
- Quality improvement involves anticipation of the future needs of patients and consumers, the proper performance of procedures, and the correction of problems before they become serious.
- The JCAHO quality assurance guidelines provide a critical thinking and problem-solving model for imaging professionals and departments.
- Radiologist assistant is a new medical imaging job that includes taking a leading role in patient management, performing selected radiologic examinations under the supervision of a radiologist, and evaluating and observing images.
- Ethics committees may become involved in ethical problem solving. These committees are composed of a variety of institutional personnel who identify values and make the best decision possible for all parties involved.
- Imaging professionals must take an active role in the organizations representing the profession so that they can remain aware of technologic advances and help their organizations examine those that will affect the profession.
- The law cannot be proactive to determine what is right for humankind in this world of advancing technology. Legislatures cannot possibly foresee all the consequences of future technology and make appropriate statutory changes to deal with them. Judicial decisions are always based on a set of facts that have *already* occurred and so are of little assistance in evaluating new technologies and the influence they have on human life.
- When clear legal opinions are not available, policies developed by professional medical organizations are often used by legislatures for guidance in drafting legislation and by courts when attempting to sort out issues that never before existed.

- Research by the Human Genome Project has allowed the discovery of genetic disposition to various diseases and conditions but creates enormous ethical and legal issues, including employment discrimination and refusal of coverage by insurance companies.
- Imaging professionals must take an active role in their professional organizations to have input into the ethical and legal implications of future technologies.
- Imaging professionals must be open to change but cautious about the standards of care of evolving technologies and whether a new technology is within their scope of practice.
- Radiologist assistants (RAs) must know their scope of practice and stay within that scope.
- Imaging professionals not certified as RAs must also be cautious if asked to perform some of the duties for which a certified RA is qualified, since they will be held to the same standard as a person trained for that specialty.

REFERENCES

1. Gingrich N, Egge R: From disaster to opportunity—transforming the American health system for the 21st century, *RT Image* 18(46): 2005.
2. Towsley-Cook D: An educator's voice—pride in the profession, *RT Image* 10(10):20, 1997.
3. American Medical Association, Council on Ethical and Judicial Affairs: Current opinions of the Council on Ethical and Judicial Affairs of the American Medical Association, Chicago, 1986, American Medical Association.
4. U.S. Department of Energy Office of Science, Office of Biological and Environmental Research, Human Genome Program website. Available at www.doegenomes.org. Accessed July 31, 2006.
5. Joint Commission on Accreditation of Healthcare Organizations: *Transitions: from QA to CQI,* Oakbrook Terrace, Ill, 1991, Author.
6. Papp J: Quality management in the imaging sciences, St Louis, 1998, Mosby.
7. American Society of Radiologic Technologists: *The radiologist assistant—the new member of the health care team.*
8. McElveny C: Scanning the future—special report, *Radiol Technol* 77(2):91, 2005.
9. Trevino M: CT colonography gets ready for its close-up, *Diagn Imag,* February 2006.
10. Silver M, Farr C, Sharma A: Coronary CTA establishes new markets, standards, *Diagn Imag,* March 2006.
11. Kaiser C: Hybrid PET/CT angiography strikes at clinical mainstream, *Diagn Imag,* March 2006.
12. Kaiser C: Study taps cerebrospinal fluid to identify dementia, *Diagn Imag,* March 2006.
13. Oyler M, Long BW, Cox LA: Sonographic markers used to detect frequent trisomies, *Radiol Technol* 76(1):13, 2004.
14. Brice J: Imaging assumes broader role in assessing therapy, *Diagn Imag,* February 2006.
15. Furrow B, Creasey TL, Johnson SH, et al: *Health law: cases, materials and problems,* ed 5, St Paul, Minn, 2004, West.
16. *Davis v Davis,* 842 S.W.2d 588 (Tenn. 1992).
17. Patti J: Hot issue: radiologic assistant, *ACR Advocate, ACR Bulletin* 61(6): 2006.

REVIEW QUESTIONS

1 The radiographer may become involved in ethical dilemmas concerned with which of the following?
a. Biomedical research
b. Reproduction methods
c. Quality improvement
d. All the above

2 Transplant situations require appropriate care for both the _____ _____ and the _____.

3 Why should imaging professionals be personally responsible for certain types of research? How does this display professionalism?

4 What are the attributes of a critical thinker? What skills do you need to develop to become a higher level thinker?

5 Quality improvement addresses issues of ethics and patient care. Explain the ways in which the establishment of health care trends may improve patient care.

6 Why do imaging professionals need to anticipate and prepare for the ethical dilemmas of transplant procedures?

7 **True or False**   Research methods involve critical thinking.

8 **True or False**   Reading scientific journals is not a research method.

9 **True or False**   The law is very clear on all reproductive issues.

10 **True or False**   Laws are generally written for new technologies when those technologies are being developed.

11 **True or False**   A good source of guidance in evolving technologic areas is the professional medical organization associated with that technology.

12 **True or False**   The imaging professional has an obligation to stay abreast of technologic advances.

13 List three newer technologies and identify their use:

　　a. _____

　　b. _____

　　c. _____

14 The _____ is an accrediting commission for health care organizations.

15 **True or False**   Radiology/imaging is not a good example of how health care in the United States should progress in the future.

16 _____ _____ may be used to track stem cells.

17 _____ _____ _____ _____ may be used to monitor the fetal heart.

18 Pancreatic cancer diagnosis may be aided by _____ _____ _____ _____.

19 The _____ _____, an advanced level to which the imaging professional may aspire, includes certain duties once performed only by imaging physicians.

20 **True or False**   The imaging professional who survives in the profession is able to deal with change.

21 **True or False**   The introduction of molecular imaging and fusion technology has accelerated the pace of change in the radiologic sciences.

22 List three duties of the radiologist assistant:

　　a. _____

　　b. _____

　　c. _____

23 The Joint Commission on Accreditation of Healthcare Organizations _____ _____ _____ provides a critical thinking and problem-solving model.

24 **True or False**   The American Society of Radiologic Technologists encourages the imaging professional to foresee change and be willing to adapt.

25 **True or False** The Human Genome Project includes the goal of transferring related genetic technologies to the private sector.
26 **True or False** Judicial decisions can be made based on future facts.
27 Imaging professionals faced with changes associated with new technologies should:
   a. Read about the new technology
   b. Ask questions of the radiologist involved
   c. Ask questions of the vendor of the technology
   d. All of the above
28 **True or False** The imaging professional has no responsibility for researching the standards of care or scope of practice issues for new technologies.
29 **True or False** Radiologist assistants can do anything the radiologist asks them to as long as they are under the radiologist's supervision.
30 **True or False** An imaging professional can perform the duties of a radiologist assistant when the radiologist assistant calls in sick.
31 **True or False** Professional organizations are the best source of information for imaging professionals faced with new technologies.

CRITICAL THINKING *Questions & Activities*

1 Who should pay for the new methods of reproduction? Defend your answer.
2 How is the "good" of society helped or hindered by new methods of reproduction and imaging procedures and testing?
3 Analyze your own education and experience and the ways in which they prepared you for ethical awareness and decision making.
4 Examine your ethical strengths and weaknesses and the ways in which they aid and interfere with your ethical problem solving.
5 Interview an ethics committee member.
6 Establish an ethical awareness committee in your imaging area.
7 Describe imaging areas that are evolving and may lead to controversial ethical situations. Explain the situations.
8 Discuss a futuristic scenario in which you must perform an imaging procedure on a human clone to evaluate the donor liver before a liver transplant. Do you need to obtain informed consent? Is a clone a person?
9 Discuss a surrogacy situation in which the intended mother and father (whose ovum and sperm were used), the patient (the surrogate), and her husband all want to come in and view a sonographic examination of the surrogate. What should the sonographer do?
10 Discuss a scenario in which an ultrasonographer provides imaging services for a selective abortion because the parents want a child with the ability to become a concert pianist. Genetic testing has indicated that only the female of the three embryos has the concert pianist gene. Describe the ethical and legal problems with performing this procedure.

GLOSSARY

abortion Expulsion or removal of a usually nonviable fetus (a fetus that cannot live outside the uterus at that time).

active euthanasia The ending of another person's life by an aggressive method to end suffering.

active suicide The taking of one's own life through a conscious act.

administrative law Law determining the licensing and regulation of the practice of imaging professionals and regulating some employer-employee relations.

advance directive A predetermined (usually written) choice made to inform others of the ways in which the patient wishes to be treated while incompetent. Also, a living will that contains written instructions for future health care.

ALARA The approach to radiation protection with the goal to keep radiation exposure as low as reasonably achievable.

apology statutes Statutes in many states that allow a physician or other health care provider to have an honest and open dialog when a medical error, accident, or unanticipated outcome occurs without that apology's being taken as an admission of guilt.

artificial insemination The depositing of seminal fluid within the vagina or cervix by means other than a penis.

assault A deliberate act wherein one person threatens to harm another without consent and the victim believes the attacker has the ability to carry out the threat.

autonomy The concept that patients are to be treated as individuals and informed about procedures to facilitate appropriate decisions.

battery Touching to which the victim has not consented.

beneficence Performance of good acts.

caring A function of the whole person in which concern for the growth and well-being of another is expressed in an integrated application of the mind, body, and spirit that seeks to maximize positive outcomes.

case law Law developed from precedents set during civil and criminal trials.

civil law Law that addresses wrongs committed by one party harming another. Penalties for violation can include monetary damages to compensate for loss and to punish.

collegial model A cooperative method of providing health care for the patient involving sharing, trust, and the pursuit of common goals. This model may be helpful in addressing patients' emotional needs and engaging their cooperation.

common law Law encompassing principles and rules based on ancient usages and customs.

communication A symbolic interaction in which a message is sent and responded to.

competence The ability to make choices.

complaint The written allegation of wrongdoing filed to initiate a lawsuit. It also may be called a claim or petition, depending on the court in which it is brought.

confidentiality The duty owed by health care providers to protect the privacy of patient information.

consequentialism An ethical school of thought in which decisions are based on the consequences or outcomes of a given act; the good of an activity is evaluated based on whether immediate harm is balanced with future benefits.

consent forms Useful tools to help inform patients about procedures and document consent.

continuous quality control The aspect of quality assurance that monitors technical equipment to maintain quality standards.

continuous quality improvement Programs that seek to anticipate problems by data gathering and trend analysis and to improve the environment before problems arise.

contractual model A health care model that defines health care as a business relationship between the provider and patient. A contractual arrangement serves as the guideline for decision making and provision of services.

criminal law Law that seeks to redress wrongs against the state.

critical thinking Purposeful, self-regulatory judgment resulting in interpretation, analysis, evaluation, and inference.

cultural values Values specific to a people or culture.

cultural competence A set of congruent behaviors, attitudes, and policies coming together in a system or agency or among professionals that enables effective interactions in a cross-cultural framework.

death Cessation of life; lack of biologic function.

defamation The making of a false statement to a third party that is harmful to another's reputation. Defamatory statements may concern patients, family members, visitors, other employees, or physicians.

defendant The party called to answer the allegations made in a lawsuit or criminal case.

deontology An ethical school of thought that bases decision making on individual motives and morals rather than consequences and examines the significance of actions themselves. Deontologic problem solving uses personal rules of right and wrong derived from individual actions, relationships of all kinds, and society.

deposition Oral testimony given under oath during the discovery phase of a trial.

development Ability to grow and continue the life process.

digital imaging Electronic image detection, storage, and display.

discovery phase The phase of a trial in which attorneys seek to ascertain the truth concerning an incident. During the discovery phase, questions may be asked of any of the parties (including employees and students of a party) either in writing (interrogatories) or orally (depositions). Parties are under oath regardless of whether questions are oral or written. Their statements may be used at trial if testimony contradicts or does not agree with earlier statements.

dismissal The ending of a trial before it goes to the jury or the judge; this may occur because of lack of evidence or lack of legal grounds to pursue a lawsuit.

distribution allocation groups Health care allocation questions are divided into three groups: macro-allocation questions ask how big the health care budget will be, meso-allocation questions ask how it will be divided, and micro-allocation questions ask who should get what share of the budget.

distribution-making criteria Criteria that will aid the health care professional in ethical problem solving when the dilemma calls for fairness in the distribution of scarce resources.

diversity Differences rooted in culture, age, experience, health status, gender, sexual orientation, racial or ethnic identity, mental abilities, and other aspects of sociocultural description and socioeconomic status.

documentation Standardized recording of information necessary for continuity of patient care and protection from medical negligence litigation.

Dowd Problem-Solving Model An ethical problem-solving model, developed by S. Dowd, that consists of six steps: assessment of the problem, evaluation of the issues, analysis of the data, development of the plan of action, institution of the plan, and analysis of the outcome.

due process The constitutional right that protects individuals from arbitrary decisions by government, including those regarding education, and provides a path of recourse. It requires that specific procedures be followed in bringing charges against a person to ensure fairness.

duty to warn third parties The obligation to disclose information to third parties to warn them of a risk such as violence or contagious disease.

egalitarian theory Health care distribution theory that demands equal distribution of equal opportunities and resources.

employment at will A policy that allows employers and employees to terminate their relationship for no cause, subject to the restrictions of antidiscrimination and other statutes. The concept of an implied contract provides an exception to the policy, as does the public policy exception.

engineering model A health care model that identifies the health care provider as a scientist concerned with facts and defines the patient as a condition or procedure, not a person. A health care professional using the engineering model tends to view a patient as a collection of body systems rather than as a whole.

entitlement theory A system of contracts in which a patient has to pay for the contract.

ERISA Employee Retirement and Security Act, enacted to deal with pension scams, also covers health plans and preempts or sometimes prevents state tort lawsuits and state regulation of managed care organizations.

ethics The system or code of conduct and morals advocated by a particular individual or group.

ethics committee A committee that is composed of a variety of health care professionals and has the mission of helping to address ethical dilemmas in the health care setting.

euthanasia Deliberately ending the life of another to end that person's suffering.

existential care Compassion arising from an awareness of common bonds of humanity and common expressions, fates, and feelings.

fairness theory Health care distribution theory that adjusts the equality of individuals with the inequality of their needs and resources.

false imprisonment The unlawful confinement of a person within a fixed area.

fusion imaging The combining of two modalities to obtain imaging information; for example, PET and SPECT can be combined to track and monitor stem cells.

health care A practice, a commodity, an approach, or a collective responsibility to ensure the wellness of a population.

health communication A subset of human communication that is concerned with how individuals in a society seek to maintain health and resolve health-related issues.

health literacy The ability to read, understand, and act on health care information to make effective health care decisions and follow instructions for treatment.

health management organization Also known as an HMO; a form of organized health care management.

HIPAA Health Insurance Portability and Accountability Act, enacted by the federal government to enhance the rights of consumers regarding access to their records, limit access of others to those records, and improve quality, efficiency, and effectiveness of health care delivery through a national framework.

hostile work environment sexual harassment Harassment that occurs when sexual behaviors unreasonably interfere with work performance or create an intimidating, hostile, or offensive work environment. Sexual suggestions, sexually derogatory remarks, and sexually motivated physical contact may constitute hostile work environment sexual harassment. Actions of supervisors, co-workers, and customers can give rise to hostile work environment claims. Employers are liable if they create or condone a discriminatory work environment.

Human Genome Project A project coordinated by the U.S. Department of Energy and the National Institutes of Health and designed to identify all the genes in human DNA, determine the sequences of the 3 billion chemical base pairs that make up human DNA, store this information in databases, improve tools for data analysis, transfer related technologies to the private sector, and address the ethical, legal, and social issues that may arise from the project.

inappropriate documentation Recording of opinions or derogatory comments that may result in liability.

informed consent The written assent of a patient to receive a proposed treatment; adequate information is essential for the patient to give truly informed consent.

intentional torts Wrongs resulting from acts done with the intention of causing harm to another.

interrogatory Written testimony given under oath during the discovery phase of a trial.

in vitro fertilization The process by which conception takes place in a laboratory medium.

-isms Prejudgments entailing a tendency to judge others according to a standard considered ideal or presumed to be "normal."

judicial decisions Previous cases that either interpret statutes or adopt and adapt common law principles.

law A body of rules of action or conduct prescribed by controlling authority and having binding legal force. Its basis is in common law from England, but it has been molded by statutes and judicial decisions since the founding of the United States.

lawsuit A legal action taken in a court for redress of wrongs; it is generally composed of a pleading phase, discovery phase, and trial.

legislation All the laws and statutes put in place by elected officials in federal, state, county, and city governments.

lie A falsehood told to another who has a reasonable expectation of the truth.

life The entire state of the living thing.

linguistic competence Readily available, culturally appropriate, oral and written language services for patients with limited English proficiency; includes bilingual and bicultural staff, trained medical interpreters, and qualified translators.

managed care Any type of delivery and reimbursement system that monitors or controls types, quality, use, and costs of health care.

medical immobilization Immobilization used to perform effective treatment; not considered restraint; includes mechanisms usually and customarily applied during diagnostic and therapeutic procedures and based on standard practice.

medical indication principle Medically appropriate procedures a physician should follow after the patient grants informed consent; will produce more medical good than evil.

medical negligence A breach of the health care provider's obligation to follow the appropriate standard of care, which results in harm to the patient.

Medicaid A joint and voluntary program between the federal government and the states, with the mission to provide health insurance coverage to the nation's poor, disabled, and impoverished elderly.

Medicare A health insurance program for people 65 years of age and older, some disabled people under 65 years of age, and people with certain other disease processes.

multiculturalism Respect for the diversity of the many ways of knowing beyond the Western model, brought about by a broadening of learning and an opening of the mind to new ways of thought.

National Patient Safety Goals Set of goals to increase patient safety and quality; approved by the Joint Commission on the Accreditation of Healthcare Organizations.

nature of the truth The kind of information expected by the person seeking information.

negligence An unintentional tort involving duty, breach of duty, injury, and causation.

no-code order Order not to resuscitate if the patient's heart stops.

nonmaleficence The avoidance of evil.

passive euthanasia The ending of another person's life by withdrawal of treatment.

passive suicide A person's refusal to be treated when the person knows the refusal will lead to death.

paternalistic (priestly) model A health care model that casts the caregiver in the omniscient, paternalistic role of making decisions *for* patients rather than *with* patients. Those who subscribe to this model generally believe they know best and tend to discount the patient's feelings.

patient care partnership Statement by the American Hospital Association recognizing the importance of patient rights and published materials to help patients understand what they can expect, their rights, and their responsibilities.

patient data sheet A uniform document for the recording of pertinent medical information; crucial for adequate risk management.

patient focused care A health care distribution model that calls for decentralization of patient care services and cross-training of health care professionals.

personal liability insurance Liability insurance that the imaging professional may decide to carry independent of the employer's policy and that may cover things not covered by the employer's policy. In certain circumstances this is a reasonable and even necessary purchase.

personal values Beliefs and attitudes held by an individual that provide a foundation for behavior and the way the individual experiences life. Religious convictions, family, political beliefs, education, life experiences, and culture influence personal values.

place of communication The environment of the expectation of truth.

plaintiff The party making the allegations in a lawsuit or criminal case.

pleading phase The phase of a lawsuit in which the plaintiff files a complaint (also called a claim or a petition, depending on the court in which it is brought) against a defendant with the court. The complaint alleges that the plaintiff has been injured as a result of the action or inaction of the defendant. The defendant must file a written answer to the allegations in the complaint.

point of service plan Also called POS plan; a form of managed care in which patients can get care outside the network for additional cost.

practical wisdom Right reason or virtue ethics that includes a consideration of emotional factors and development of the reason balanced by consideration of the consequences for the individual in society.

prima facie case of employment discrimination What must be proved by a complainant making a claim of employment discrimination. It requires complainants to prove that they belong to a protected class, were qualified for the position, and were not hired or were discharged and that afterward the employer continued to look for an individual with the complainant's qualifications to fill the position or hired an individual less qualified than the complainant who was not a member of that protected class.

principle of double effect A person may perform an act that has or risks evil effects as long as four certain conditions are met.

procedural due process The mechanism by which individuals can refute attempts by government or other bodies to deprive them of their substantive rights.

professional care The application of the knowledge of a discipline, including its science, theory, practice, and art.

professional values The general attributes prized by a professional group.

professionalism An awareness of the conduct, aims, and qualities defining a given profession, familiarity with professional codes of ethics, and understanding of ethical schools of thought, patient-professional interaction models, and patient rights.

provider sponsored organization Also called PSO; includes numerous networks that contract directly with employers for services on a capitated basis, such as IDAs (integrated delivery systems), PHOs (physician hospital organizations), and PSNs (provider sponsored networks).

quality assurance A process to assess quality of patient care that uses hospital committees to oversee the quality of various hospital functions.

quality improvement Performing procedures correctly and anticipating, meeting, or exceeding the needs of customers.

quality of life Essential traits that make life worth living.

quid pro quo sexual harassment Harassment that occurs when initial or continued employment or advancement depends on sexual conduct. A supervisor or manager must necessarily be involved in quid pro quo sexual harassment cases.

radiation protection A set of safety procedures involving appropriate radiation protection education, proper equipment maintenance and calibration, quality control and assurance procedures, consistent shielding and collimation, clear policies concerning pregnant patients, and adequate documentation.

radiologist assistant Physicians' assistant in the imaging environment who will aid the radiologist in patient management and assessment, will perform selected procedures under the supervision of the radiologist, and may evaluate image quality, make initial observations, and forward observations to the supervising radiologist.

rational choice principle A choice made in keeping with the choice the patient would most likely have made had he or she been competent.

reasonable care The degree of care a reasonable person, similarly situated, would use.

res ipsa loquitur Latin term meaning "the thing speaks for itself." It is a legal concept invoked in situations in which a particular injury could not have occurred in the absence of negligence.

right A claim or an entitlement.

rights theory Health care distribution theory that claims individuals have a right to health care because of their human dignity and because society has an obligation to serve those needs.

risk management The system for identifying, analyzing, and evaluating risks and selecting the most advantageous method for treating them. Its goal is to maintain high-quality patient care and conserve the facility's financial resources.

role of communication The relationship between the communicators, which may have an impact on the expectation of truth.

sanctity of human life The ideal underpinning the obligation not to take human life.

secret Knowledge a person has a right or obligation to conceal.

sexual harassment Unwelcome sexual advances, requests for sexual favors, and other verbal and physical conduct of a sexual nature to which the employee is required to submit as a term or condition of employment; submission to or rejection of such conduct as the basis for employment decisions also constitutes sexual harassment, as does behavior having the purpose or effect of unreasonably interfering with work performance or creating an intimidating, hostile, or offensive working environment.

simple consent The assent required of a patient for any procedure.

slippery slope When one act leads to another and then to another at an accelerating rate.

standard of care The degree of skill or care practiced by a reasonable professional practicing in the same field.

statutory duty to report Legal obligation to report a variety of medical conditions and incidents, including venereal disease, contagious diseases such as tuberculosis, wounds inflicted by violence, poisonings, industrial accidents, abortions, drug abuse, and abuse of children, elderly people, and people with disabilities.

statutory law Any law enacted by federal, state, county, or city government.

substantive due process The notion that the rights of individuals and the circumstances under which those rights may be restricted must be clearly defined and regulated.

suicide The act of knowingly ending one's life.

surrogate A person who substitutes for another, often in decision-making processes.

terminal illness A condition that leaves the patient irreversibly comatose or will lead to death within a year.

tort A subdivision of civil law under which actions are filed to recover damages for personal injury or property damage occurring from negligent conduct or intentional misconduct. The types of torts most likely to be encountered by imaging professionals include assault, battery, false imprisonment, defamation, negligence, lack of informed consent, and breach of patient confidentiality.

triage A system of prioritizing that encourages the delivery of treatment to those with the greatest opportunity for a positive outcome.

trial The part of a lawsuit in which the facts of a case are presented to a judge or jury for a decision.

truthfulness Conformity with fact or reality.

Uniform Determination of Death Act Enacted in 1980 and established two tests to determine death: (1) the irreversible cessation of circulatory and respiratory function and (2) the irreversible cessation of all functions of the entire brain, including the brainstem.

unintentional torts Wrongs resulting from actions that were not intended to do harm.

utilitarian theory Health care distribution theory that calls for realizing the greatest good for the greatest number.

values Qualities or standards desirable or worthy of esteem in themselves; they are expressed in behaviors, language, and standards of conduct.

values clarification Developed by Louis Rath; enables the individual to discover, analyze, prioritize, and organize values into a personally meaningful system.

veracity The obligation to tell the truth and not to lie or deceive others.

virtue ethics A new school of ethics that focuses on the use of practical wisdom for emotional and intellectual problem solving. It incorporates elements of teleology and deontology to provide a more holistic approach to solving ethical dilemmas.

whistleblowing Reporting concerns about unsafe conditions or poor-quality care to one's employer, to a national or state agency responsible for regulation of the institution, or in the case of criminal activity, to law enforcement agencies.

APPENDIX A CODES OF ETHICS

Appendix Outline

THE PATIENT CARE PARTNERSHIP

UNDERSTANDING EXPECTATIONS, RIGHTS AND RESPONSIBILITIES

When you need hospital care, your doctor and the nurses and other professionals at our hospital are committed to working with you and your family to meet your health care needs. Our dedicated doctors and staff serve the community in all its ethnic, religious and economic diversity. Our goal is for you and your family to have the same care and attention we would want for our families and ourselves.

The sections explain some of the basics about how you can expect to be treated during your hospital stay. They also cover what we will need from you to care for you better. If you have questions at any time, please ask them. Unasked or unanswered questions can add to the stress of being in the hospital. Your comfort and confidence in your care are very important to us.

WHAT TO EXPECT DURING YOUR HOSPITAL STAY

High Quality Hospital Care

Our first priority is to provide you the care you need, when you need it, with skill, compassion and respect. Tell your caregivers if you have concerns about your care or if you have pain. You have the right to know the identity of doctors, nurses and others involved in your care, and you have the right to know when they are students, residents or other trainees.

A Clean and Safe Environment

Our hospital works hard to keep you safe. We use special policies and procedures to avoid mistakes in your care and keep you free from abuse or neglect. If anything unexpected and significant happens during your hospital stay, you will be told what happened, and any resulting changes in your care will be discussed with you.

Involvement in Your Care

You and your doctor often make decisions about your care before you go to the hospital. Other times, especially in emergencies, those decisions are made during your hospital stay. When decision-making takes place, it should include:

Discussing Your Medical Condition and Information About Medically Appropriate Treatment Choices

To make informed decisions with your doctor, you need to understand:

- The benefits and risks of each treatment.
- Whether your treatment is experimental or part of a research study.
- What you can reasonably expect from your treatment and any long-term effects it might have on your quality of life.
- What you and your family will need to do after you leave the hospital.
- The financial consequences of using uncovered services or out-of-network providers.

Please tell your caregivers if you need more information about treatment choices.

Discussing Your Treatment Plan

When you enter the hospital, you sign a general consent to treatment. In some cases, such as surgery or experimental treatment, you may be asked to confirm in writing that you understand what is planned and agree to it. This process protects your right to consent to or refuse a treatment. Your doctor will explain the medical consequences of refusing recommended treatment. It also protects your right to decide if you want to participate in a research study.

Getting Information from You

Your caregivers need complete and correct information about your health and coverage so that they can make good decisions about your care. That includes:

- Past illnesses, surgeries or hospital stays.
- Past allergic reactions.
- Any medicines or dietary supplements (such as vitamins and herbs) that you are taking.
- Any network or admission requirements under your health plan.

Understanding Your Health Care Goals and Values

You may have health care goals and values or spiritual beliefs that are important to your well-being. They will be taken into account as much as possible throughout your hospital stay. Make sure your doctor, your family and your care team know your wishes.

Understanding Who Should Make Decisions When You Cannot

If you have signed a health care power of attorney stating who should speak for you if you become unable to make health care decisions for yourself, or a "living will" or "advance directive" that states your wishes about end-of-life care; give copies to your doctor, your family and your care team. If you or your family need help making difficult decisions, counselors, chaplains and others are available to help.

Protection of Your Privacy

We respect the confidentiality of your relationship with your doctor and other caregivers, and the sensitive information about your health and health care that are part of that relationship. State and federal laws and hospital operating policies protect the privacy of your medical information. You will receive a Notice of Privacy Practices that describes the ways that we use, disclose and safeguard patient information and that explains how you can obtain a copy of information from our records about your care.

Preparing You and Your Family for When You Leave the Hospital

Your doctor works with hospital staff and professionals in your community. You and your family also play an important role in your care. The success of your treatment often depends on your efforts to follow medication, diet and therapy plans. Your family may need to help care for you at home.

You can expect us to help you identify sources of follow-up care and to let you know if our hospital has a financial interest in any referrals. As long as you agree that we can share information about your care with them, we will coordinate our activities with your caregivers outside the hospital. You can also expect to receive information and, where possible, training about the self-care you will need when you go home.

Help with Your Bill and Filing Insurance Claims

Our staff will file claims for you with health care insurers or other programs such as Medicare and Medicaid. They also will help your doctor with needed documentation. Hospital bills and insurance coverage are often confusing. If you have questions about your bill, contact our business office. If you need help understanding your insurance coverage or health plan, start with your insurance company or health benefits manager.

If you do not have health coverage, we will try to help you and your family find financial help or make other arrangements. We need your help with collecting needed information and other requirements to obtain coverage or assistance.

While you are here, you will receive more detailed notices about some of the rights you have as a hospital patient and how to exercise them. We are always interested in improving. If you have questions, comments or concerns, please contact:

AMERICAN SOCIETY OF RADIOLOGIC TECHNOLOGISTS AND THE AMERICAN REGISTRY OF RADIOLOGIC TECHNOLOGISTS CODE OF ETHICS

The radiologic technologist conducts herself or himself in a professional manner, responds to patient needs and supports colleagues and associates in providing quality patient care.

The radiologic technologist acts to advance the principal objective of the profession to provide services to humanity with full respect for the dignity of mankind.

The radiologic technologist delivers patient care and service unrestricted by concerns of personal attributes or the nature of the disease or illness, and without discrimination on the basis of sex, race, creed, religion or socioeconomic status.

The radiologic technologist practices technology founded upon theoretical knowledge and concepts, uses equipment and accessories consistent with the purpose for which they were designed and employs procedures and techniques appropriately.

The radiologic technologist assesses situations; exercises care, discretion and judgment; assumes responsibility for professional decisions; and acts in the best interest of the patient.

The radiologic technologist acts as an agent through observation and communication to obtain pertinent information for the physician to aid in the diagnosis and treatment of the patient and recognizes that interpretation and diagnosis are outside the scope of practice for the profession.

The radiologic technologist uses equipment and accessories, employs techniques and procedures, performs services in accordance with an accepted standard of practice and demonstrates expertise in minimizing radiation exposure to the patient, self and other members of the health care team.

The radiologic technologist practices ethical conduct appropriate to the profession and protects the patient's right to quality radiologic technology care.

The radiologic technologist respects confidences entrusted in the course of professional practice, respects the patient's right to privacy and reveals confidential information only as required by law or to protect the welfare of the individual or the community.

The radiologic technologist continually strives to improve knowledge and skills by participating in continuing education and professional activities, sharing knowledge with colleagues and investigating new aspects of professional practice.

Revised and adopted by the American Society of Radiologic Technologists and the American Registry or Radiologic Technologists, February 2003.

CODE OF ETHICS FOR THE PROFESSION OF DIAGNOSTIC MEDICAL SONOGRAPHY

PREAMBLE

The goal of this code of ethics is to promote excellence in patient care by fostering responsibility and accountability among diagnostic medical sonographers. In so doing, the integrity of the profession of diagnostic medical sonography will be maintained.

OBJECTIVES

To create and encourage an environment where professional and ethical issues are discussed and addressed.

To help the individual diagnostic medical sonographer identify ethical issues.

To provide guidelines for individual diagnostic medical sonographers regarding ethical behavior.

PRINCIPLES

Principle I: In order to promote patient well-being, the diagnostic medical sonographer shall:

A. Provide information to the patient about the purpose of the sonography procedure and respond to the patient's questions and concerns.

B. Respect the patient's autonomy and the right to refuse the procedure.

C. Recognize the patient's individuality and provide care in a non-judgmental and non-discriminatory manner.

D. Promote the privacy, dignity and comfort of the patient by thoroughly explaining the examination, patient positioning and implementing proper draping techniques.

E. Maintain confidentiality of acquired patient information, and follow national patient privacy regulations as required by the "Health Insurance Portability and Accountability Act of 1996 (HIPAA)."

F. Promote patient safety during the provision of sonography procedures and while the patient is in the care of the diagnostic medical sonographer.

Principle II: To promote the highest level of competent practice, diagnostic medical sonographers shall:

A. Obtain appropriate diagnostic medical sonography education and clinical skills to ensure competence.

B. Achieve and maintain specialty specific sonography credentials. Sonography credentials must be awarded by a national sonography credentialing body that is accredited by a national organization which accredits credentialing bodies, i.e., the National Commission for Certifying Agencies (NCCA); http://www.noca.org/ncca/ncca.htm or the International Organization for Standardization (ISO); http://www.iso.org/iso/en/ISOOnline.frontpage.

C. Uphold professional standards by adhering to defined technical protocols and diagnostic criteria established by peer review.

D. Acknowledge personal and legal limits, practice within the defined scope of practice, and assume responsibility for his/her actions.

E. Maintain continued competence through lifelong learning, which includes continuing education, acquisition of specialty specific credentials and recredentialing.

F. Perform medically indicated ultrasound studies, ordered by a licensed physician or their designated health care provider.

G. Protect patients and/or study subjects by adhering to oversight and approval of investigational procedures, including documented informed consent.

H. Refrain from the use of any substances that may alter judgment or skill and thereby compromise patient care.

I. Be accountable and participate in regular assessment and review of equipment, procedures, protocols, and results. This can be accomplished through facility accreditation.

Principle III: To promote professional integrity and public trust, the diagnostic medical sonographer shall:

A. Be truthful and promote appropriate communications with patients and colleagues.

B. Respect the rights of patients, colleagues and yourself.

C. Avoid conflicts of interest and situations that exploit others or misrepresent information.

D. Accurately represent his/her experience, education and credentialing.

E. Promote equitable access to care.

F. Collaborate with professional colleagues to create an environment that promotes communication and respect.

G. Communicate and collaborate with others to promote ethical practice.

H. Engage in ethical billing practices.

I. Engage only in legal arrangements in the medical industry.

J. Report deviations from the Code of Ethics to institutional leadership for internal sanctions, local intervention and/or criminal prosecution. The Code of Ethics can serve as a valuable tool to develop local policies and procedures.

Approved by SDMS Board of Directors, December 6, 2006. © Copyright 1999-2007, Society of Diagnostic Medical Sonography, Plano, Texas.

AMERICAN SOCIETY OF RADIOLOGIC TECHNOLOGISTS RADIATION THERAPIST CODE OF ETHICS

The radiation therapist advances the principal objectives of the profession to provide services to humanity with full respect for the dignity of mankind.

The radiation therapist delivers patient care and service unrestricted by concerns of personal attributes of the nature of the disease or illness, and without discrimination on the basis of sex, race, creed, religion or socioeconomic status.

The radiation therapist assesses situations; exercises care, discretion and judgment; assumes responsibility for professional decisions and acts in the best interest of the patient.

The radiation therapist adheres to the tenets and domains of the scope of practice for radiation therapists.

The radiation therapist actively engages in lifelong learning to maintain, improve and enhance professional competence and knowledge.

Revised and adopted by the American Society of Radiologic Technologists, July 1998.

CODE OF ETHICS FOR THE NUCLEAR MEDICINE TECHNOLOGIST

Nuclear Medicine Technologists, as Certificants of the health care profession, must strive as individuals and as a group to maintain the highest of ethical standards.

The Principles (SNMTS Code of Ethics) listed below are not laws, but standards of conduct to be used as ethical guidelines by nuclear medical technologists. These Principles were adopted by the Technologist Section and the Society of Nuclear Medicine at the 2004 Annual Meeting. They are standards of conduct to be used as a quick guide by nuclear medicine technologists.

Principle 1: The Nuclear Medicine Technologist will provide services with compassion and respect for the dignity of the individual and with the intent to provide the highest quality of patient care.

Principle 2: The Nuclear Medicine Technologist will provide care without discrimination regarding the nature of the illness or disease, gender, race, religion, sexual preference or socioeconomic status of the patient.

Principle 3: The Nuclear Medicine Technologist will maintain strict patient confidentiality in accordance with state and federal regulations.

Principle 4: The Nuclear Medicine Technologist will comply with the laws, regulations, and policies governing the practice of nuclear medicine.

Principle 5: The Nuclear Medicine Technologist will continually strive to improve their knowledge and technical skills.

Principle 6: The Nuclear Medicine Technologist will not engage in fraud, deception, or criminal activities.

Principle 7: The Nuclear Medicine Technologist will be an advocate for their profession.

Reprinted by permission of the Society of Nuclear Medicine from: Kai-Yuan Tzen, Chin-Song Lu, Tzu-Chen Yen, Shiaw-Pyng Wey, and Gann Ting. Differential Diagnosis of Parkinson's Disease and Vascular Parkinsonism by 99mTc-TRODAT-1. J Nucl Med. 2001; 42:408-413. Figure 1.

AMERICAN REGISTRY OF RADIOLOGIC TECHNOLOGISTS STANDARDS OF ETHICS

Last Revised: August 1, 2006
Published: August 1, 2006

PREAMBLE

The *Standards of Ethics* of the American Registry of Radiologic Technologists shall apply solely to persons holding certificates from ARRT who either hold current registrations by ARRT or formerly held registrations by ARRT (collectively, "Registered Technologists" or "Registered Radiologist Assistants"), and to persons applying for examination and certification by ARRT in order to become Registered Technologists ("Candidates"). Radiologic Technology is an umbrella term that is inclusive of the disciplines of radiography, nuclear medicine technology, radiation therapy, cardiovascular-interventional radiography, mammography, computed tomography, magnetic resonance imaging, quality management, sonography, bone densitometry, vascular sonography, cardiac-interventional radiography, vascular-interventional radiography, breast sonography, and radiologist assistant. The *Standards of Ethics* are intended to be consistent with the Mission Statement of ARRT, and to promote the goals set forth in the Mission Statement.

A. CODE OF ETHICS

The Code of Ethics forms the first part of the *Standards of Ethics.* The Code of Ethics shall serve as a guide by which Registered Technologists and Candidates may evaluate their professional conduct as it relates to patients, healthcare consumers, employers, colleagues, and other members of the healthcare team. The Code of Ethics is intended to assist Registered Technologists and Candidates in maintaining a high level of ethical conduct and in providing for the protection, safety, and comfort of patients. The Code of Ethics is aspirational.

1. The radiologic technologist conducts herself or himself is a professional manner, responds to patient needs, and supports colleagues and associates in providing quality patient care.
2. The radiologic technologist acts to advance the principal objective of the profession to provide services to humanity with full respect for the dignity of mankind.
3. The radiologic technologist delivers patient care and service unrestricted by the concerns of personal attributes or the nature of the disease or illness, and without discrimination on the basis of sex, race, creed, religion, or socioeconomic status.
4. The radiologic technologist practices technology founded upon theoretical knowledge and concepts, uses equipment and accessories consistent with the purposes for which they were designed, and employs procedures and techniques appropriately.
5. The radiologic technologist assesses situations; exercises care, discretion, and judgment; assumes responsibility for professional decisions; and acts in the best interest of the patient.
6. The radiologic technologist acts as an agent through observation and communication to obtain pertinent information for the physician to aid in the diagnosis and treatment of the patient and recognizes that interpretation and diagnosis are outside the scope of practice for the profession.

7. The radiologic technologist uses equipment and accessories, employs techniques and procedures, performs services in accordance with an accepted standard of practice, and demonstrates expertise in minimizing radiation exposure to the patient, self, and other members of the healthcare team.

8. The radiologic technologist practices ethical conduct appropriate to the profession and protects the patient's right to quality radiologic technology care.

9. The radiologic technologist respects confidences entrusted in the course of professional practice, respects the patient's right to privacy, and reveals confidential information only as required by law or to protect the welfare of the individual or the community.

10. The radiologic technologist continually strives to improve knowledge and skills by participating in continuing education and professional activities, sharing knowledge with colleagues, and investigating new aspects of professional practice.

B. RULES OF ETHICS

The Rules of Ethics form the second part of the *Standards of Ethics*. They are mandatory standards of minimally acceptable professional conduct for all present Registered Technologists, Registered Technologist Assistants, and Candidates. Certification is a method of assuring the medical community and the public that an individual is qualified to practice within the profession. Because the public relies on certificates and registrations issued by ARRT, it is essential that Registered Technologists and Candidates act consistently with these Rules or Ethics. These Rules of Ethics are intended to promote the protection, safety, and comfort of patients. The Rules of Ethics are enforceable. Registered Technologists, Registered Technologist Assistants, and Candidates engaging in any of the following conduct or activities, or who permit the occurrence of the following conduct or activities with respect to them, have violated the Rules of Ethics and are subject to sanctions as described hereunder:

1. Employing fraud or deceit in procuring or attempting to procure, maintain, renew, or obtain reinstatement of certification or registration as issued by ARRT; employment in radiologic technology; or a state permit, license, or registration certificate to practice radiologic technology. This includes altering in any respect any document issued by the ARRT or any state or federal agency, or by indicating in writing certification or registration with the ARRT when that is not the case.

2. Subverting or attempting to subvert ARRT's examination process. Conduct that subverts or attempts to subvert ARRT's examination process includes, but is not limited to:

   (i) conduct that violates the security of ARRT examination materials, such as removing or attempting to remove examination materials from an examination room, or having unauthorized possession of any portion of or information concerning a future, current, or previously administered examination of ARRT; or disclosing information concerning any portion of a future, current, or previously administered examination of ARRT; or disclosing what purports to be, or under all circumstances is likely to be understood by the recipient as, any portion of or "inside" information concerning any portion of a future, current, or previously administered examination of ARRT;

   (ii) conduct that in any way compromises ordinary standards of test administration, such as communicating with another Candidate during administration of the examination, copying another Candidate's answers, permitting another Candidate to copy one's answers, or possessing unauthorized materials; or

(iii) impersonating a Candidate or permitting an impersonator to take the examination on one's own behalf.

3. Convictions, criminal proceedings, or military court-martials as described below:

(i) Conviction of a crime, including a felony, a gross misdemeanor, or a misdemeanor, with the sole exception of speeding and parking violations. All alcohol and/or drug related violations must be reported. Offenses that occurred while a juvenile and that are processed through the juvenile court system are not required to be reported to ARRT.

(ii) Criminal proceedings where a finding or verdict of guilt is made or returned but the adjudication of guilt is either withheld, deferred, or not entered or the sentence is suspended or stayed; or a criminal proceeding where the individual enters a plea of guilty or nolo contendere (no contest).

(iii) Military court-martials that involve substance abuse, any sex-related infractions, or patient-related infractions.

4. Failure to report to the ARRT that:

(i) charges regarding the person's permit, license, or registration certificate to practice radiologic technology or any other medical or allied health profession are pending or have been resolved adversely to the individual in any state, territory, or country (including, but not limited to, imposed conditions, probation, suspension, or revocation); or

(ii) that the individual has been refused a permit, license, or registration certificate to practice radiologic technology or any other medical or allied health profession by another state, territory, or country.

5. Failure or inability to perform radiologic technology with reasonable skill and safety.

6. Engaging in unprofessional conduct, including, but not limited to:

(i) a departure from or failure to conform to applicable federal, state, or local governmental rules regarding radiologic technology practice; or, if no such rule exists, to the minimal standards of acceptable or prevailing radiologic technology practice;

(ii) any radiologic technology practice that may create unnecessary danger to a patient's life, health, or safety; or

(iii) any practice that is contrary to the ethical conduct appropriate to the profession that results in the termination from employment.

Actual injury to a patient or the public need not to be established under this clause.

7. Delegating or accepting the delegation of a radiologic technology function or any other prescribed health care function when the delegation or acceptance could reasonably be expected to create an unnecessary danger to a patient's life, health, or safety. Actual injury to a patient need not be established under this clause.

8. Actual or potential inability to practice radiologic technology with reasonable skill and safety to patients by reason of illness; use of alcohol, drugs, chemicals, or any other materials; or as a result of any mental or physical condition.

9. Adjudication as mentally incompetent, mentally ill, a chemically dependent person, or a person dangerous to the public, by a court of competent jurisdiction.

10. Engaging in any unethical conduct, including, but not limited to, conduct likely to deceive, defraud, or harm the public; or demonstrating a willful or careless disregard for the health, welfare, or safety of a patient. Actual injury need not be established under this clause.

11. Engaging in conduct with a patient that is sexual or may reasonably be interpreted by the patient as sexual, or in any verbal behavior that is seductive or sexually demeaning to a patient; or engaging in sexual exploitation of a patient or former patient. This also applies to any unwanted sexual behavior, verbal or otherwise, that results in the termination of employment. This rule does not apply to pre-existing consensual relationships.

12. Revealing a privileged communication from or relating to a former or current patient, except when otherwise required or permitted by law.

13. Knowingly engaging or assisting any person to engage in, or otherwise participating in, abusive or fraudulent billing practices, including violations of federal Medicare and Medicaid laws or state medical assistance laws.

14. Improper management of patient records, including failure to maintain adequate patient records or to furnish a patient record or report required by law; or making, causing, or permitting anyone to make false, deceptive, or misleading entry in any patient record.

15. Knowingly aiding, assisting, advising, or allowing a person without current and appropriate state permit, license, or registration certificate or a current certificate of registration with ARRT to engage in the practice of radiologic technology, in a jurisdiction which requires a person to have such a permit, license, or registration certificate or a current and appropriate certification of registration with ARRT in order to practice radiologic technology in such jurisdiction.

16. Violating a rule adopted by any state board with competent jurisdiction, an order of such board, or state or federal law relating to the practice of radiologic technology, or any other medical or allied health professions, or a state or federal narcotics or controlled-substance law.

17. Knowingly providing false or misleading information that is directly related to the care of a former or current patient.

18. Practicing outside the scope of practice authorized by the individual's current state permit, license, or registration certificate, or the individual's current certificate of registration with ARRT.

19. Making a false statement or knowingly providing false information to ARRT or failing to cooperate with any investigation by ARRT or the Ethics Committee.

20. Engaging in false, fraudulent, deceptive, or misleading communications to any person regarding the individual's education, training, credentials, experience, or qualifications, or the status of the individual's state permit, license, or registration certificate in radiologic technology or certificate of registration with ARRT.

21. Knowing of a violation or a probable violation of any Rule of Ethics by any Registered Technologist, Registered Radiologist Assistant, or Candidate and failing to promptly report in writing the same to the ARRT.

22. Failing to immediately report to his or her supervisor information concerning an error made in connection with imaging, treating, or caring for a patient. For purposes of this rule, errors include any departure from the standard of care that reasonably may be considered to be potentially harmful, unethical, or improper

(commission). Errors also include behavior that is negligent or should have occurred in connection with a patient's care, but did not (omission). The duty to report under this rule exists whether or not the patient suffered any injury.

C. ADMINISTRATIVE PROCEDURES

These Administrative Procedures provide for the structure and operation of the Ethics Committee; they detail procedures followed by the Ethics Committee and by the Board of Trustees of ARRT in handling challenges raised under the Rules of Ethics, and in handling matters relating to the denial of an application for certification (for reasons other than failure to meet the criteria as stated in Article II, Sections 2.03 and 2.04 of the *Rules and Regulations* of ARRT, in which case, there is no right to a hearing) or the denial of renewal or reinstatement of a registration. All Registered Technologists, Registered Radiologist Assistants, and Candidates are required to comply with these Administrative Procedures; the failure to cooperate with the Ethics Committee or the Board of Trustees in a proceeding on a challenge may be considered by the Ethics Committee and by the Board of Trustees according to the same procedures and with the same sanctions as failure to observe the Rules of Ethics.

1. Ethics Committee

(a) Membership and Responsibilities of the Ethics Committee

The President, with the approval of the Board of Trustees, appoints at least three Trustees to serve as members of the Ethics Committee, each such person to serve on the Committee until removed and replaced by the President, with the approval of the Board of Trustees, at any time, with or without cause. The President, with the approval of the Board of Trustees, will also appoint a fourth, alternate member to the Committee. The alternate member will participate on the Committee in the event that one of the members of the Ethics Committee is unable to participate. The Ethics Committee is responsible for (1) investigating each alleged breach of the Rules of Ethics and determining whether a Registered Technologist, Registered Radiologist Assistant, or Candidate has failed to observe the Rules of Ethics in the Standards, and determining an appropriate sanction; and (2) periodically assessing the Code of Ethics, Rules of Ethics, and Administrative Procedures in the Standards and recommending any amendments to the Board of Trustees.

(b) The Chair of the Ethics Committee

The President, with the approval of the Board of Trustees, appoints one member of the Ethics Committee as the Committee's Chair to serve for a term of two years as the principal administrative officer responsible for management of the promulgation, interpretation, and enforcement of the *Standards of Ethics.* The President may remove and replace the Chair of the Committee, with the approval of the Board of Trustees, at any time, with or without cause. The Chair presides at and participates in meetings of the Ethics Committee and is responsible directly and exclusively to the Board of Trustees, using staff, legal counsel, and other resources necessary to fulfill the responsibilities of administering the *Standards of Ethics.*

(c) Preliminary Screening of Potential Violation of the Rules of Ethics

The Chair of the Ethics Committee shall review each alleged violation of the Rules of Ethics that is brought to the attention of the Ethics Committee. If in the sole discretion of the Chair (1) there is insufficient information upon which to base a charge of a violation of the Rules of Ethics, or (2) the allegations against the Registered Technologist or Candidate are patently frivolous or inconsequential, or (3) the allegations if true would not constitute a violation of the Rules of Ethics, the Chair may summarily dismiss the matter. The Chair may be assisted by staff and/or legal counsel of ARRT. The Chair shall report each such summary dismissal to the Ethics Committee.

(d) Alternative Dispositions

At the Chair's direction and upon request, the Executive Director of ARRT shall have the power to investigate allegations and to enter into negotiations with Registered Technologist, Registered Radiologist Assistant, or Candidate regarding the possible settlement of an alleged violation of the Rules of Ethics. The Executive Director may be assisted by staff members and/or legal counsel of ARRT. The Executive Director is not empowered to enter into a binding settlement, but rather may recommend a proposed settlement to the Ethics Committee. The Ethics Committee may accept the proposed settlement, make a counterproposal to the Registered Technologist, Registered Radiologist Assistant, or Candidate, or reject the proposed settlement and proceed under these Administrative Procedures.

(e) Summary Suspensions

If an alleged violation of the Rules of Ethics involves the occurrence, with respect to a Registered Technologist, of an event described in paragraph 3 of the Rules of Ethics, or any other event that the Ethics Committee determines would, if true, potentially pose harm to the health, safety, or well being of any patient or the public, then, notwithstanding anything apparently or expressly to the contrary contained in these Administrative Procedures, the Ethics Committee may, without prior notice to the Registered Technologist or Registered Radiologist Assistant and without prior hearing, summarily suspend the registration of the Registered Technologist or Registered Radiologist Assistant pending a final determination under these Administrative Procedures with respect to whether the alleged violation of the Rules of Ethics in fact occurred. Within five working days after the Ethics Committee summarily suspends the registration of the Registered Technologist or Registered Radiologist Assistant in accordance with this provision, the Ethics Committee shall, by certified mail, return receipt requested, give to the Registered Technologist or Registered Radiologist Assistant written notice that describes (1) the summary suspension, (2) the reason or reasons for it, and (3) the right of the Registered Technologist or Registered Radiologist Assistant to request a hearing with respect to the summary suspension by written notice to the Ethics Committee, which written notice must be received by the Ethics Committee not later than 15 days after the date of the written notice of summary suspension by the Ethics Committee to the Registered Technologist or Registered Radiologist Assistant. If the Registered Technologist or Registered Radiologist Assistant requests a hearing in a timely manner with respect to the summary suspension, the hearing shall be held before the Ethics Committee or panel comprised of no fewer than three members of the Ethics Committee as promptly as practicable, but in any event within 30 days after the Ethics Committee's receipt of the Registered Technologist's or Registered Radiologist Assistant's request for the hearing. The applicable provisions of paragraph 2 of these Administrative Procedures shall govern all hearings with respect to summary suspensions, except that neither a determination of the Ethics Committee, in the absence of a timely request for a hearing by the affected Registered Technologist or Registered Radiologist Assistant, nor a determination by the Ethics Committee or a panel following a timely requested hearing is appealable to the Board of Trustees.

2. Hearings

Whenever the ARRT proposes to take action in respect to the denial of an application for certification (for reasons other than failure to meet the criteria as states in Article II, Sections 2.03 and 2.04 of the *Rules and Regulations* of ARRT, in which case there is no right to a hearing) or of an application for renewal or reinstatement of a registration, or in connection with the revocation or suspension of a certificate or registration, or the censure of a Registered Technologist or Registered Radiologist Assistant for an alleged violation of the Rules of Ethics, it shall give written notice thereof to such person, specifying the reasons for such proposed action. A Registered Technologist, Registered Radiologist Assistant, or Candidate to whom such notice is given shall have 30 days from the date the notice of such proposed action is mailed to make a written request for a hearing. The written request for a hearing must be accompanied by a nonrefundable hearing fee in the amount of $100. In rare cases, the hearing fee may be waived, in whole or in part, at the sole discretion of the Ethics Committee.

Failure to make a written request for a hearing and to remit the hearing fee (unless the hearing fee is waived in writing by the ARRT) within such period shall constitute consent to the action taken by the Ethics Committee or the Board of Trustees pursuant to such notice. A Registered Technologist, Registered Radiologist Assistant, or Candidate who requests a hearing in the manner prescribed above shall advise the Ethics Committee of his or her intention to appear at the hearing. A Registered Technologist, Registered Radiologist Assistant, or Candidate who requests a hearing may elect to appear by a written submission which shall be verified or acknowledged under oath.

Failure to appear at the hearing or to supply a written submission in response to the charges shall be deemed a default on the merits and shall be deemed consent to whatever action or disciplinary measures which the Ethics Committee determines to take. Hearings shall be held at such date, time, and place as shall be designated by the Ethics Committee or the Executive Director. The Registered Technologist or the Candidate shall be given at least 30 days' notice of the date, time, and place of the hearing.

The hearing is conducted by the Ethics Committee with any three or more of its members participating, other than any member of the Ethics Committee whose professional activities are conducted at a location in the approximate area of the Registered Technologist, Registered Radiologist Assistant, or Candidate in question. In the event of such disqualification, the President may appoint a Trustee to serve on the Ethics Committee for the sole purpose of participating in the hearing and rendering a decision. At the hearing, ARRT shall present the charges against the Registered Technologist, Registered Radiologist Assistant, or Candidate in question, and the facts and evidence of ARRT in respect to the basis or bases for the proposed action or disciplinary measure. The Ethics Committee may be assisted by legal counsel. The Registered Technologist, Registered Radiologist Assistant, or Candidate in question, by legal counsel or other representative if he or she desires (at the sole expense of the Registered Technologist, Registered Radiologist Assistant, or Candidate in question), shall have the right to call witnesses, present testimony, and be heard in his or her own defense; to hear the testimony of and cross-examine any witnesses appearing at such hearing; and to present such other evidence or testimony as the Ethics Committee shall deem appropriate to do substantial justice. Any information may be considered which is relevant or potentially relevant. The Ethics Committee shall not be bound by any state or federal rules of evidence. A transcript or an audio recording of the hearing is made. The Registered Technologist, Registered Radiologist Assistant, or Candidate in question shall have the right to submit a written statement at the close of the hearing.

In a case where ARRT proposes to take action in respect to the denial of an application for certification (for reasons other than failure to meet the criteria as stated in Article II, Sections 2.03 and 2.04 of the *Rules and Regulations* of the ARRT) or the denial of renewal or reinstatement of a registration, the Ethics Committee shall assess the evidence presented at the hearing and make its decision accordingly, and shall prepare written findings of fact and its determination as to whether grounds exist for the denial of an application for certification or renewal or reinstatement of a registration, and shall promptly transmit the same to the Board of Trustees and to the Registered Technologist, Registered Radiologist Assistant, or Candidate in question.

In the case of alleged violations of the Rules of Ethics by a Registered Technologist or Registered Radiologist Assistant, the Ethics Committee shall assess the evidence presented at the hearing and make its decision accordingly, and shall prepare written findings of fact and its determination as to whether there has been a violation of the Rules of Ethics and, if so, the appropriate sanction, and shall promptly transmit the same to the Board of Trustees and to the Registered Technologist or Registered Radiologist Assistant in question. Potential sanctions include denial of renewal or reinstatement of a registration with ARRT, revocation or suspension of a certification or registration or both with ARRT, or the public or private reprimand of a Registered Technologist or Registered Radiologist Assistant.

Unless a timely appeal from any findings of fact and determination by the Ethics Committee is taken to the Board of Trustees in accordance with paragraph 3 below, the Ethics Committee's findings of fact and determination in any matter (including the specified sanction) shall be final and binding upon the Registered Technologist, Registered Radiologist Assistant, or Candidate in question.

3. Appeals

Except as otherwise noted in these Administrative Procedures, the Registered Technologist, Registered Radiologist Assistant, or Candidate may appeal any decision of the Ethics Committee to the Board of Trustees by submitting a written request for an appeal within 30 days after the decision of the Ethics Committee is mailed. The written request for an appeal must be accompanied by a nonrefundable appeal fee in the amount of $250. In rare cases, the appeal fee may be waived, in whole or in part, at the sole discretion of the Ethics Committee.

In the event of an appeal, those Trustees who participated in the hearing at the Ethics Committee shall not participate in the appeal. The remaining members of the Board of Trustees shall consider the decision of the Ethics Committee, the files and records of ARRT applicable to the case at issue, and any written appellate submission of the Registered Technologist, Registered Radiologist Assistant, or Candidate in question, and shall determine whether to affirm or to overrule the decision of the Ethics Committee or to remand the matter to the Ethics Committee for further consideration. In making such determination to affirm or to overrule, findings of fact made by the Ethics Committee shall be conclusive if supported by any evidence. The Board of Trustees may grant re-hearings, hear additional evidence, or request that ARRT or the Registered Technologist, Registered Radiologist Assistant, or Candidate in question provide additional information in such manner, on such issues, and within such time as it may prescribe.

All hearings and appeals provided for herein shall be private at all stages. It shall be considered an act of professional misconduct for any Registered Technologist, Registered Radiologist Assistant, or Candidate to make an unauthorized publication or revelation of the same, except to his or her attorney or other representative, immediate superior, or employer.

4. Publication of Adverse Decisions

Final decisions that are adverse to the Registered Technologist, Registered Radiologist Assistant, or Candidate will be communicated to the appropriate authorities of all states and provided in response to inquiries into a person's registration status. ARRT shall also have the right to publish any adverse decisions and the reasons therefore. For purposes of this paragraph, a "final decision" means and includes: a determination of the Ethics Committee relating to a summary suspension, if the affected Registered Technologist does not request a hearing in a timely manner; a non-appealable decision of the Ethics Committee or a panel relating to a summary suspension that is issued after a hearing on the matter; an appealable decision of the Ethics Committee from which no timely appeal is taken; and, in a case involving an appeal of an appealable decision of the Ethics Committee in a matter, the decision of the Board of Trustees in the matter.

5. Procedure to Request Removal of a Sanction

Unless a sanction imposed by ARRT specifically provides for a shorter or longer term, it shall be presumed that a sanction may only be reconsidered after at least three years have elapsed since the sanction first became effective. At any point after a sanction first becomes eligible for reconsideration, the individual may submit a written request ("Request") to ARRT asking the Ethics Committee to remove the sanction. The Request much be accompanied by a nonrefundable fee in the amount of $250. A Request that is not accompanied by the fee or which is submitted before the matter is eligible for reconsideration will be returned to the individual and will not be considered. In rare cases, the fee may be waived, in whole or in part, at the sole discretion of the Ethics Committee.

The Request, the fee, and all documentation in support of the Request must be received by ARRT at least 45 days prior to a meeting of the Ethics Committee in order to be included on the agenda of that meeting. If the Request is received less than 45 days before the meeting, the Request will be held until the following meeting. The Ethics Committee typically meets three times a year. The individual is not entitled to make a personal appearance before the Ethics Committee in connection with a request to remove a sanction.

Although there is no required format, the Request must include compelling reasons justifying the removal of the sanction. It is recommended that the individual demonstrate at least the following: (1) an understanding of the reasons for the sanction, (2) an understanding of why the action leading to the sanction was felt to warrant the sanction imposed, and (3) detailed information demonstrating that his or her behavior has improved and similar activities will not be repeated. Letters of recommendation from individuals who are knowledgeable about the person's current character and behavior, including efforts at rehabilitation, are advised. If a letter of recommendation is not on original letterhead or is not duly notarized, the Ethics Committee shall have the discretion to ignore that letter of recommendation.

Removal of the sanction is a prerequisite to applying for reinstatement of certification and registration. If the Ethics Committee, in the exercise of its sole discretion, removes the sanction, the individual will be allowed to pursue reinstatement via the policies and procedures in place at that time, which may require the individual to take and pass the current certification examination. There is a three-attempt limit for passing the examination and a three-year limit within which the three attempts must be completed. Individuals requesting reinstatement will not be allowed to report CE requirements completed while under sanction in order to meet the CE requirements for registration. ARRT reserves the right to change its policies and procedures from time to time and without notice to anyone who is under a sanction or is in the process of seeking to remove a sanction.

If the Ethics Committee denies removal of the sanction, the decision is not subject to a hearing or to an appeal, and the Committee will not reconsider removal of the sanction for as long as is directed by the Committee.

From the American Registry of Radiologic Technologists, St. Paul, Minnesota.

APPENDIX B SAMPLE DOCUMENTATION FORMS

PHYSICIAN ORDER FOR
RADIOLOGIC/NUCLEAR MEDICINE
Consultation/Request for Procedure
Department of Radiology

● DO NOT SEND BOTH COPIES OF REQUISITION TO RADIOLOGY. ●
<u>RETAIN</u> WHITE COPY TO FILE IN PATIENT'S MEDICAL RECORD ●

DATE
HOSP. #
NAME
BIRTH DATE
ADDRESS

IF NOT IMPRINTED, PLEASE PRINT DATE, HOSP. #, NAME AND LOCATION

Procedure
Scheduled for Date _____ Time _____

Known Allergies _____

Female of Child-Bearing Age ☐ Yes ☐ No

Patient Transport ☐ Walk ☐ Cart ☐ Chair ☐ Isolette

Oxygen ☐ Yes ☐ No **Diabetic** ☐ Yes ☐ No

Pregnant ☐ Yes ☐ No **Lactating** ☐ Yes ☐ No

Isolation ☐ Airborne ☐ Droplet ☐ Contact
Precautions ☐ Special Organism

☐ **Routine** ☐ **ASAP** ☐ **STAT** ☐ **Portable**

STAT Report ☐ Yes _____
(phone # for report results)

Procedure(s) _____

Clinical Findings/Relevant Diagnosis: _____

Reason for Exam: _____

ICD-9-CM Code _____

Return films with patient
☐ Yes
☐ No

Clinic Code

Physician Name (print) _____ Pager _____

Signature _____ CLP No. _____ Date _____ Clinic/Unit _____ Phone _____

Radiology use only		
14x17	14x36	
11x14	14x51	
10x12	7x17	
8x10		
9x9		
6x12		

Fluoro Time (min) _____ Actual Date of Proc. _____
Room _____ Actual Time of Proc. _____
Procedure _____
Physician _____ Technologist/Sonographer _____
Notes _____
_____
_____
Contrast _____
Date _____

PHARMACEUTICALS AND AGENTS
Radiopharmaceutical Administered _____ Amount _____ Time _____ By _____
Route of Administration ☐ I.V. ☐ Oral Other _____ Lot No. _____

Other Agents Administered _____ Amount _____ Time _____ By _____
Route of Administration ☐ I.V. ☐ Oral Other _____ Lot No. _____

IMAGING INSTRUCTIONS
_____
_____
_____
_____

PHYSICIAN'S RADIOPHARMACEUTICAL/
ADJUNCT DRUG PRESCRIPTIONS
_____
_____
_____

☐ **Outpatient** ☐ **Inpatient**

Technologist's Signature _____

DO NOT FILE IN MEDICAL RECORD

52683/7-05/MH01190/3

UNIVERSITY OF IOWA HOSPITALS AND CLINICS
200 Hawkins Dr., Iowa City, IA 52242

RADIOLOGY COPY

FIGURE B-1 Sample of a diagnostic radiology request form.
From University of Iowa.

ACCIDENT / INCIDENT REPORT FORM
VIRGINIA TECH - OFFICE OF RISK MANAGEMENT
BLACKSBURG, VA. 24061 Mail Code 0310
540-231-7439   FAX-540-231-5064

Name of Responsible Office_____ Date of Report _____

Name of Responsible Virginia Tech Representative _____

Address of Office _____ State _____ Zip _____ Phone _____

Name of Injured Person(s) or Involved Person(s)_____ Age _____ Sex _____

Address _____ State _____ Zip _____ Phone _____

Name of Injured Person(s) or Involved Person(s)_____ Age _____ Sex _____

Address _____ State _____ Zip _____ Phone _____

Name of Parent or Guardian(if minor) _____ Age _____ Sex _____

Address _____ State _____ Zip _____ Phone _____

Name/Addresses of Witnesses (Each Witness Should Attach a Signed Statement of What Happened):

1. _____

2. _____

3. _____

Type of Incident :   ☐   Behavioral   ☐   Accident   ☐   Illness   ☐   Other

_____

Date of Incident/Accident: Hour _____(am or pm) Day _____ Month _____ Year _____

Describe the Incident in Detail

_____
_____
_____
_____
_____
_____
_____
_____
_____
_____
_____
_____
_____
_____
_____
_____
_____
_____
_____
_____
_____
_____
_____
_____

FIGURE B-2 Sample of an accident/incident report form.
From Virginia Tech Office of Risk Management, Blacksburg, Virginia.

Location Of Incident and Diagram Showing Objects and Persons

What Activity was the Injured Participating in at the Time of the Incident_____

Describe any Equipment Involved in the Incident_____

Describe Emergency Procedures Followed as a Result of this Incident:_____

MEDICAL REPORT OF INCIDENT

Were the Parents or Guardian Notified ? ☐ Yes ☐ No
How?_____

By Whom?_____Title_____When_____

Response of Individual Notified_____

Where was Treatment Given ☐ At Accident Site ☐ Doctor's Office ☐ Hospital   Rescue Squad

Describe Treatment Given

Treatment Given by Whom?_____ Date of Treatment _____

Was Injured Retained Overnight in Hospital? ☐ Yes ☐ No   If Yes, Where
_____

Name of Attending Physician _____

Prognosis of Injured at the Time of Report_____

FIGURE B-2, cont'd

Comments_____

_____

Person Completing Report_____Signature_____

Position_____Phone_____Fax_____

THIS ACCIDENT/INCIDENT REPORT IS **NOT** REQUIRED FOR INCIDENTS SUCH AS SCRAPES, BRUISES, SPRAINS, ETC. THIS INCIDENT REPORT IS REQUIRED FOR SERIOUS ILLNESSES, SIGNIFICANT BEHAVIORAL PROBLEMS OR ACCIDENTS INVOLVING INJURIES LIKE FRACTURED BONES, CHIPPED OR BROKEN TEETH, EXTENSIVE LACERATIONS INVOLVING SUTURES, FALLS INVOLVING UNCONCIOUSNESS, DISLOCATIONS, INCIDENTS INVOLVING WATER WHICH REQUIRE RESUSCITATION, OR ANY INJURY REQUIRING HOSPITAL STAY.

THIS ACCIDENT/INCIDENT REPORT IS ALWAYS REQUIRED WHEN THE PROCEDURES OUTLINED ON THE EMERGENCY RESPONSE CARD AND CARRIED BY ALL COOPERATIVE EXTENSION REPRESENTATIVES ARE INITIATED. ONCE COMPLETED THE FORM SHOULD BE FAXED TO 540-231-5064 AND MAILED THE VIRGINIA TECH OFFICE OF RISK MANAGEMENT.

FIGURE B-2, cont'd

C PATIENT SAFETY AND PRIVACY RESOURCES

UNIVERSITY OF IOWA HEALTH CARE PRIVACY NOTICE

OUR LEGAL RESPONSIBILITY

As your health care provider, we are legally required to protect the privacy of your health information, and to provide you with this notice about our legal obligations and privacy practices. This requirement applies to all patients served by University of Iowa Health Care and University of Iowa Student Health Service.

University of Iowa Health Care describes the partnership between University of Iowa Hospitals and Clinics and the UI Roy J. and Lucille A. Carver College of Medicine. Student Health Service provides health services to University of Iowa Students. This notice applies to health information held by both entities.

University of Iowa Health Care and Student Health Service are legally required to follow the privacy described in this notice. If you have any questions or want more information about this notice, please contact our Privacy Officer listed at the end of this notice.

YOUR PROTECTED HEALTH INFORMATION (PHI)

Throughout this notice, we will refer to your protected health information at PHI. Your PHI includes data that identifies you and reports about the care and services you receive at the hospitals, in the clinics, or at Student Health Service.

This notice applies to all of the records, both electronic and paper, about your care. It includes all information created by University of Iowa Health Care or Student Health Service staff. This staff includes physicians, other health care professionals, students, and other departmental staff.

This notice about our privacy practices explains how, when, and why we use and share your PHI. We may not use or disclose any more of your PHI than is necessary, with some exceptions. If state law is more protective of your privacy, we will follow state law.

Changes to This Notice

We reserve the right to change the terms of this notice and our privacy policies. Any changes will apply to your past, current, or future PHI. When we make an important change to our policies, we will change this notice and post a new notice on our Web site, www.uihealthcare.com/hipaa.

You can also request a copy of our current notice at any time from the University of Iowa Hospitals and Clinical registration desks, or the Student Health Service registration desk.

Uses of Protected Health Information

University of Iowa Health Care and Student Health Service collect health information about you and store it in a chart and medical records. The medical record is the property of University of Iowa Hospitals and Clinics or Student Health Service, but the information in the medical records belongs to you.

We use and disclose health information for many reasons. The following examples describe some of the categories of our uses and disclosures. Please note that not every use or disclosure in a category is listed.

Treatment

We may use and disclose medical information about you to physicians, nurses, technicians, physicians in training, or other health care professionals who are involved with your care. For example, if you are being treated for a knee injury, we may disclose your PHI to the Department of Rehabilitation Therapies. Different health care professionals, such as pharmacists and lab technicians, also may share information about you in order to coordinate your care. In addition, we may send information to the physician who referred you to University of Iowa Health Care.

Payment

We may use and disclose your PHI in order to bill and collect payment for the treatment and services we provided to you. For example, we may provide PHI to an insurance company of other third party payor in order to obtain approval for treatment or admission to the hospital.

If you are a University of Iowa student and incur a charge at Student Health Service, and you choose to place that charge on your University bill, the University of Iowa Business Office will receive notice that a visit occurred at Student Health Service and the charge for that visit.

Health Care Operations

We may use and disclose your PHI as part of our routine operations. For example, we may use your PHI to evaluate the quality of health care services you received or to evaluate the performance of health care professionals who cared for you. We may also disclose information to physicians, nurses, technicians, medical students, nursing and other health professional students, and other hospital personnel as part of our educational mission.

If you are a University of Iowa student, Student Health Service is responsible for tracking compliance with University of Iowa immunization requirements. This information is shared with the University of Iowa Office of the Registrar.

Appointment Reminders and Health-Related Benefits or Services

We may use your PHI to provide appointment reminders or give you information about treatment alternatives or other health care services.

Public Health Activities

We report information about births, deaths, and various diseases to government officials in charge of collecting that information. We provide coroners, medical examiners, and funeral directors with information about an individual's death.

Law Enforcement

We may disclose PHI to government agencies and law enforcement personnel when the law requires it. For example, we report about victims of abuse, neglect, domestic violence, and gunshots, or when ordered to do so in judicial or administrative proceedings.

Health Oversight Activities

We may disclose PHI to a health oversight agency for audits, investigations, inspections, and licensure, as authorized by law. For example, we may disclose PHI to the Food and Drug Administration, state Medicaid fraud control, or the Department of Health and Human Services Office for Civil Rights.

Research Studies

We may disclose your PHI to help conduct research. Research may involve finding a cure for an illness or helping determine the effectiveness of a treatment. All research studies are subject to a specific approval process by a Privacy Board or Institutional Review Board. This process evaluates a proposed research study to determine that measures are in place to balance research needs with the need for the privacy of your health information. For some research activities you may be asked to participate in a study, and, if you agree, the researcher will be required to obtain your permission to use your PHI for that study.

Organ Donation

We may use your PHI to notify organ donation organizations, and to assist them in organ, eye, or tissue donation and transplants.

Workers' Compensation Purposes

We may disclose PHI to your employer or your workers' compensation carrier.

National Security and Intelligence Activities

We may release PHI to authorized federal officials when required by law. This information may be used to protect the President; other authorized persons or foreign heads of state; to conduct special investigations; for intelligence and other national security activities authorized by law.

Uses and Disclosures for Which You Have the Opportunity to Object

Hospital Directory

We will use your name, the location at which you are receiving care, your general condition and your religious affiliation for directory purposes. All of this information, except religious affiliation, will be disclosed to people who ask for you by name. If you object to this use, we will not include this information in the directory. You will need to express your objection for each inpatient stay. To object, please notify a member of your nursing staff.

Fundraising

We may use your PHI in efforts to raise money for University of Iowa Health Care. We may provide your PHI to the University of Iowa Foundation for this purpose. We would release contact information only, such as your name, address, phone number, the dates that health care was provided to you, and your insurance status. If you do not want University of Iowa Health Care to contact you for fundraising efforts, you must notify our Privacy Officer in writing at the address listed at the end of this notice.

Disclosures to Family, Friends, or Others

We may provide your PHI to a family member, friend, or other person you tell us is involved in your care, or involved in the payment of your health care, unless you object in whole or in part. If you are unable to agree or object to such a disclosure, we may disclose such information as necessary if we determine that it is in your best interest.

Except as described above, all other uses and disclosures of your PHI will require your authorization.

YOUR RIGHTS REGARDING PHI

You Have the Right to:

Request Restrictions

You have the right to ask that we limit how we use and disclose your PHI. We will consider your request, but we are not legally required to accept it. If we accept your request, we will honor that request except in emergency situations. You may not limit the uses and disclosures that we are legally required or allowed to make. To request a restriction, contact the Privacy Officer listed at the end of this notice.

Request Confidential Communications

You have the right to ask that we send PHI to you at an alternate address. For example, you may wish to have appointment reminders and test results sent to a P.O. Box or an address different from your home address. We will accommodate reasonable requests. To make a request, contact Patient Fiscal and Registration Services listed at the end of this notice.

Inspect and Copy

You have the right to inspect and obtain a copy of medical information that may be used to make decisions about your care. Usually this includes the medical record and billing records. To inspect and obtain a copy of your medical information, you must submit your request in writing to either:

1) Release of Information (for medical information) or
2) Patient Fiscal and Registration Services (for billing)

Both are listed at the end of this notice.

We will make every effort to respond to your request within a reasonable period of time. You may be charged a fee to cover the costs of copying, mailing, or other supplies associated with your request.

Accounting of Disclosures

You have the right to obtain a list of instances in which we have disclosed your PHI. You request must state a time period not longer than six years and your request may not include dates before April 14, 2003. The list will not include uses or disclosures made for treatment, payment, or health care operations. In addition, the list will not include uses or disclosures that you have specifically authorized in writing such as copies of records to your attorney or to your employer. To request an accounting of disclosures, contact the Privacy Officer listed at the end of this notice.

Amend

You have the right to request an amendment of your PHI if you think that information is inaccurate or incomplete in your medical record or in a billing record. You may request an amendment for as long as that record is maintained. You may submit a written request for an amendment to either:

1) Release of Information (for amendment to your medical record) or
2) Patient Fiscal and Registration Services (for amendment to your billing record)

Both as listed at the end of this notice.

UI Health Care may deny your request for an amendment if:

it is not in writing

it relates to information not created or produced by UI Health Care staff

we decide that the information in the record is accurate and complete

Paper Copy of This Notice

You have the right to request a paper copy of this notice. You may pick up a copy at any check-in point throughout the hospitals and clinics; at the registration desk; at Student Health Service; or request that a copy be sent to you. The notice also can be downloaded from www.uihealthcare.com/hipaa.

REVOCATION OF PERMISSION

If you provide us with permission to use or disclose medical information about you, you may revoke that permission at any time. To request revocation of permission, contact Release of Information listed as the end of this notice.

If you revoke your permission, we will no longer use or disclose medical information about you for the reasons covered by your written revocation. We are unable to take back any disclosures previously mad with your permission. Also, we are required to keep all records of the care we provide to you.

COMPLAINTS AND QUESTIONS

If you believe your privacy rights have been violated, you may file a complaint with University of Iowa Health Care or with the Secretary of the U.S. Department of Health and Human Services.

To file a complaint with University of Iowa Health Care, contact the Patient Representative program at UI Hospitals and Clinics. The address and phone number are listed as the end of this notice. You may also contact the University of Iowa Health Care Privacy Officer at the address and phone number listed at the end of this notice. You will not be penalized for filing a complaint and your care will not be compromised.

This notice is in effect April 14, 2003.

Courtesy University of Iowa Health Care, Iowa City, Iowa.

ANSWERS TO CHAPTER REVIEW QUESTIONS

CHAPTER 1

1. A system or code of conduct and morals advocated by a particular individual or group
2. True
3. e
4. d
5. a
6. d
7. personal study and investigations, system of professional conduct
8. contractual
9. priestly
10. covenantal
11. personal, cultural, and professional
12. a. What is the context in which the ethical problem occurred?
    b. What is the significance of the values involved in the problem?
    c. What is the meaning of the problem for all the parties involved?
    d. What should be done to remedy the problem?
13. The Dowd Problem-Solving Model
14. True
15. True
16. d
17. d
18. c
19. d
20. c
21. d
22. b
23. d
24. True
25. True
26. False
27. True
28. False
29. True
30. False
32. False
33. False
34. True
35. False
36. False
37. False
38. False
39. False
40. False

CHAPTER 2

1. d
2. b
3. c
4. nonmaleficence, beneficence
5. a. Action must be good or morally indifferent in itself
    b. Agent must intend only the good effect and not the evil effect
    c. Evil effect cannot be a means to the good effect
    d. Proportionality must exist between good and evil effects
6. True
7. patients
8. beneficence and nonmaleficence
9. Differences should include the active nature of beneficence and the passive nature of avoidance involved in nonmaleficence, as well as the greater importance of nonmaleficence compared with beneficence.
10. acts involving doing good and avoiding harm
11. avoiding harm
12. education; gathering information and their own input and decision making (among other answers)
13. Verbal and written
14. second opinion
15. True
16. b
17. d
18. False
19. d
20. True
21. d
22. d
23. True
24. c

25. d
26. False
27. d
28. d
29. c
30. True
31. False

CHAPTER 3

1. the function in which a person expresses concern for the growth and well-being of another in an integrated application of the mind, body, and spirit designed to maximize positive outcomes
2. characterized by the application of the knowledge of a professional discipline, including its science, theory, practice, and art
3. compassion arising from an awareness of common bonds of humanity and common expressions, fates, and feelings
4. a symbolic interaction
5. a subset of human communication that is concerned with how an individual in a society seeks to maintain health and deal with health-related issues
6. human caring
7. ideal
8. scarcity of time, technical priorities, impact of personal life, lack of training in caring for critically ill and terminal patients, lack of communication, societal pressures, lack of faith in oneself
9. physical noise and environment, inability to see or hear, relationships
10. individual and institutional
11. empathy rotations, communications and critical thinking classes, role modeling
12. objective self-evaluation, desire to change, employing active listening
13. advocacy provides the imaging professional with the opportunity to support the patient in obtaining quality imaging services—this may involve gathering and understanding information concerning an exam, issues concerning helping, nurturing and maintaining autonomy may all be affected by advocacy
14. True
15. False

16. True
17. True
18. False
19. True
20. True
21. True
22. False
23. c
24. d
25. False
26. d
27. False
28. False
29. False
30. True

CHAPTER 4

1. d
2. diagnosis, treatment, prognosis, risks, alternatives, costs, rules, duration of incapacitation, names of persons performing procedure
3. feedback to ensure the patient's understanding of the procedure and opportunity to question
4. The imaging professional may have a limited role in the informed consent process, but it is the physician's duty to provide the information about the procedure for informed consent.
5. a. competence—the ability to make decisions concerning one's life
   b. surrogacy—the appointment of a person to make decisions for another
6. b
7. a prerogative invoked in limited circumstances when health care providers withhold information from a patient because they believe the information would have adverse effects on the patient's condition or health
8. a. The patient must be incapable of giving consent and no lawful surrogate is available.
   b. Danger to life or a risk of serious impairment to health is apparent.
   c. Immediate treatment is necessary to avert these dangers.
9. True
10. True
11. False
12. True

13. False
14. True
15. False
16. False
17. False
18. True
19. False
20. False
21. False
22. False
23. determine patient competency, determine whether patient has given consent, determine if patient needs a surrogate, determine whether patient has advance directive, determine whether patient can cooperate and make choices
24. False
25. True
26. True
27. False

CHAPTER 5

1. conformance with fact or reality
2. a. place of communication
   b. roles of the communicators
   c. nature of the truth involved
3. practical needs
4. right to the truth
5. Confidentiality
6. a. natural secrets
   b. promised secrets
   c. professional secrets
7. professional secret
8. mechanisms for reporting certain types of wounds, communicable diseases, auto accidents, birth defects, drug addition, and industrial accidents
9. when the life or safety of a patient is endangered, when intervention can prevent threatened suicide or self-injury, or when an innocent third party may be harmed as in an abuse situation
10. e
11. False
12. True
13. False
14. False
15. True
16. True

17. True
18. True
19. True
20. True
21. False
22. False
23. True
24. True
25. False
26. c
27. False
28. False
29. False
30. False
31. False
32. d
33. False
34. False
35. False
36. False

CHAPTER 6

1. entire state
2. life cycle
3. a. religious reasons
   b. life is the greatest of goods and should be protected
   c. harm to the community
4. a good death, painless death, mercy killing
5. The advance directive and living will let the health care provider know the desires of the patient.
6. The brainstem continues to function, the body is not dead, the patient seems to be awake but has no awareness of self or environment
7. a. biologic functions
   b. intellect
   c. emotions, also creativity, contact with others, and needs
8. Active suicide is when the person takes his or her own life by inflicting the fatal blow, and active euthanasia takes place when another inflicts the final blow (mercy killing). Each situation may present itself when a person is suffering and believes death will bring relief from that suffering for self or for others involved in the suffering.

9. Patients' rights may be carried out through advance directives, including do not resuscitate orders, living wills, and durable powers of attorney.
10. The imaging professional must always have consent to perform any diagnostic or therapeutic procedure. If a patient refuses, the imaging professional must respect the patient's wishes.
11. when a patient refuses treatment knowing it will lead to death.
12. True
13. False
14. True
15. True
16. True
17. True
18. False
19. True
20. True
21. False
22. False
23. True
24. False
25. False
26. False
27. True
28. True
29. False
30. True
31. False
32. False
33. False
34. False
35. False
36. True
37. False
38. True
39. True
40. True
41. False

CHAPTER 7

1. a. a practice
   b. an approach
   c. a commodity
   d. a collective responsibility
2. a. advertising and marketing practices
   b. managed care and third-party payment practices

3. expensive and scarce
4. a. macro-allocation
   b. meso-allocation
   c. micro-allocation
5. a. egalitarian
   b. entitlement
   c. fairness
   d. utilitarian
6. a. need
   b. equity
   c. contribution
   d. ability to pay
   e. patient effort
   f. merit
7. professional identity.
8. improved efficiency, empowerment of employees, sensible delegation of duties, better scheduling, cross-training, wise application of automation
9. True
10. False
11. False
12. False
13. False
14. False
15. True
16. True
17. False
18. True
19. False
20. True
21. False
22. True
23. True
24. d
25. False
26. True
27. False
28. True
29. True
30. True

CHAPTER 8

1. students and programs
2. Ethical theories
3. contract and covenant
4. d
5. truthfulness and confidentiality

6. justice
7. a worthwhile quality—a value
8. Joint Review Committee on Education in Radiologic Technology (JRCERT) and American Registry of Radiologic Technologists (ARRT)
9. [short essay]
10. a. exchange of information
    b. periodic review and update of information
    c. reading professional literature and participating in professional organizations
11. a. truthfulness
    b. confidentiality
    c. respect and autonomy
    d. justice
12. The Fifth and Fourteenth Amendments to the U.S. Constitution
13. substantive due process, which defines and regulates the rights of citizens and the circumstances when those rights may be restricted; procedural due process, which provides an opportunity to refute attempts to deprive citizens of their substantive rights
14. a. a written statement regarding the reasons for the proposed action
    b. formal notice of a hearing where the student may answer the charges
    c. a hearing at which both sides may present their case and any rebuttal evidence
15. True
16. employment at will, which means that either employer or employee may terminate their relationship at any time for no cause, subject to antidiscrimination or other statute
17. implied contract exception, public policy exception
18. True
19. False
20. True
21. False
22. False
23. True
24. True
25. False
26. True
27. False
28. False
29. False
30. True
31. False
32. False
33. False
34. False
35. False
36. True
37. True
38. False
39. e
40. False
41. False
42. False
43. True

CHAPTER 9

1. the differences that may be rooted in culture, age, experience, health status, gender, sexual orientation, racial identity, mental abilities, and other aspects of sociocultural organization and socioeconomic position
2. adaptation of resources for people of all backgrounds
3. physical and mental health, sexual orientation, age, ethnicity, and gender
4. income marital status, geographic location, education, and religion
5. Interaction patterns
6. at the beginning of the program and through the program
7. Better understanding of patients' differing reactions to the imaging environment, the way patients make choices, and the need to use ethical decision making and provide a variety of ways to help patients understand procedures
8. language courses, visual aids, interpreters, patient advocates, informational sessions, continuing education
9. True
10. True
11. False
12. race, gender, age, national origin, religion, or disability

13. codes of ethics of the American Registry of Radiologic Technologists (ARRT) and American Society of Radiologic Technologists (ASRT) (see Appendix A)
14. employment situations
15. disparate treatment
16. disparate impact
17. a. The complainant belongs to a protected group.
    b. The complainant was qualified for the position.
    c. Despite the qualifications, the complainant was not hired or was discharged.
    d. The employer continued to look for an individual with the complainant's qualifications to fill the position or hired an individual who was less qualified than the complainant and was not a member of that protected class.
18. sexual harassment claims
19. Quid pro quo
20. Hostile work environment
21. a. The employee must be a member of a protected class.
    b. The employee must have been subject to unwelcome sexual harassment in the form of sexual advances, requests for sexual favors, or other verbal or physical conduct of a sexual nature.
    c. The complained-of conduct must have been based on gender.
    d. The conduct must have had the effect of unreasonably interfering with the employee's work performance and creating a working environment a reasonable person would find intimidating, hostile, abusive, or offensive and the employee perceived as abusive.
    e. The employer knew or should have known of the harassment and failed to take appropriate action.
22. If the HIV-infected or AIDS patients are seen as a "direct threat" to the health and safety of others. "Direct threat" is defined as a significant risk that cannot be eliminated by a modification of policies, practices, or procedures or by the provision of auxiliary aids or services.

23. True
24. False
25. True
26. False
27. False
28. False
29. False

CHAPTER 10

1. d
2. organ donor and the recipient
3-6. [short essay]
7. True
8. False
9. False
10. False
11. True
12. True
13. a. PET, detection of Alzheimer's disease
    b. Molecular imaging, monitoring of disease treatment
    c. Virtual colonoscopy, diagnosis
14. Joint Commission on Accreditation of Healthcare Organizations (JCAHO)
15. True
16. Multimodality fusion (PET and SPECT)
17. Real-time magnetic resonance imaging
18. Three-dimensional magnetic resonance imaging
19. radiologist assistant
20. True
21. True
22. a. Patient management and assessment
    b. Performing selected radiographic exams under the supervision of a radiologist
    c. Evaluating image quality and making an initial image evaluation
23. Quality Assurance Guidelines
24. True
25. True
26. False
27. d
28. False
29. False
30. False
31. True

INDEX